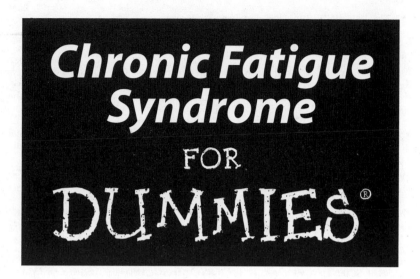

Chronic Fatigue Syndrome FOR DUMMIES®

by Susan R. Lisman, MD,
and Karla Dougherty

BICENTENNIAL
1807
WILEY
2007
BICENTENNIAL

Wiley Publishing, Inc.

Chronic Fatigue Syndrome For Dummies®

Published by
Wiley Publishing, Inc.
111 River St.
Hoboken, NJ 07030-5774
www.wiley.com

Copyright © 2007 by Wiley Publishing, Inc., Indianapolis, Indiana

Published by Wiley Publishing, Inc., Indianapolis, Indiana

Published simultaneously in Canada

For general information on our other products and services, please contact our Customer Care Department within the U.S. at 800-762-2974, outside the U.S. at 317-572-3993, or fax 317-572-4002.

For technical support, please visit www.wiley.com/techsupport.

Wiley also publishes its books in a variety of electronic formats. Some content that appears in print may not be available in electronic books.

Library of Congress Control Number: 2007924221

ISBN: 978-0-470-11772-9

Manufactured in the United States of America

10 9 8 7 6 5 4 3 2 1

WILEY

About the Authors

Susan R. Lisman, MD, received her medical degree at Tufts University School of Medicine in 1978. Her post-doctoral training includes Fellowships in Pediatric Anesthesia, Neuroanesthesia, and Pain Management, all at the New England Medical Center in Boston, MA. She is currently an Associate Clinical Professor at Tufts University School of Medicine and Director, Pediatric Anesthesia, at Newton-Wellesley Hospital in Newton, MA. She is the Chair, Peer Review, Department of Anesthesia, at Newton-Wellesley Hospital. Dr. Lisman was on the OR Management Committee, Director of Quality Assurance, and Risk Management Committees at New England Medical Center. She belongs to several professional societies, including the Massachusetts Medical Society and the American Academy of Pediatrics. She has been the Secretary of the Massachusetts Society of Anesthesiologists for ten years and served as Delegate from Massachusetts to the American Society of Anesthesiologists for many years. She has had numerous articles published in such respected medical journals as *Transplantation*, *Anesthesiology*, *Journal of Clinical Anesthesia, Journal of Oral and Maxillofacial Surgery*, and more. During her twenty plus years as a physician, she has helped patients in all facets of life and of all ages, including those with chronic fatigue syndrome.

Karla Dougherty is a leading writer and editor in the fields of medicine, health, diet, and exercise. She has authored or coauthored forty-one books, including *The Spark: The Revolutionary 3-Week Fitness Plan That Changes Everything You Know About Exercise, Weight Control, and Health* (Simon & Schuster 2001); *Living With Stroke: A Guide for Families;* and *Brain Storms: Living With Traumatic Brain Injury.* She has also ghostwritten a *New York Times* bestselling diet book and has appeared in several publications. She is listed in *Who's Who of American Women* and is a member of The Author's Guild.

Dedication

For Dan, who understands.
— *Susan*

To my uncle, Richard P. Rosenberg
— *Karla*

Authors' Acknowledgments

Acknowledgments from Susan:

I would like to thank my mentors, Dr. Robert N. Reynolds, Dr. Bebe Wunderlich and Dr. Heinrich Wurm, for their professional and personal guidance, encouragement, and never-ending support. I am eternally grateful.

Acknowledgments from Karla:

I would like to thank my husband, D. J. Dougherty, and dear friends, Stefanie Nagorka and Fran Pelzman Liscio, for their support when I needed it most, and to Claudine Wright, for her invaluable help in meeting my deadlines.

Publisher's Acknowledgments

We're proud of this book; please send us your comments through our Dummies online registration form located at www.dummies.com/register/.

Some of the people who helped bring this book to market include the following:

Acquisitions, Editorial, and Media Development

Project Editor: Natalie Faye Harris

Acquisitions Editor: Stacy Kennedy

Copy Editor: Sarah Westfall

Technical Editors: K. Kimberly McCleary, President & CEO, The CFIDS Association of America; Teresa A. Lupton, RN, Coordinator for Educational Opportunities, The CFIDS Association of America

Editorial Manager: Christine Beck

Editorial Assistants: Erin Calligan Mooney, Joe Niesen, David Lutton, Leeann Harney

Cartoons: Rich Tennant (www.the5thwave.com)

Composition Services

Project Coordinator: Jennifer Theriot

Layout and Graphics: Carl Byers, Brooke Graczyk, Joyce Haughey, Stephanie D. Jumper, Laura Pence

Anniversary Logo Design: Richard Pacifico

Proofreaders: Aptara, Jessica Kramer, Todd Lothery, Charles Spencer

Indexer: Aptara

Special Help: Danielle Voirol

Publishing and Editorial for Consumer Dummies

Diane Graves Steele, Vice President and Publisher, Consumer Dummies

Joyce Pepple, Acquisitions Director, Consumer Dummies

Kristin A. Cocks, Product Development Director, Consumer Dummies

Michael Spring, Vice President and Publisher, Travel

Kelly Regan, Editorial Director, Travel

Publishing for Technology Dummies

Andy Cummings, Vice President and Publisher, Dummies Technology/General User

Composition Services

Gerry Fahey, Vice President of Production Services

Debbie Stailey, Director of Composition Services

Contents at a Glance

Table of Contents

Part II: Teaming Up with Treatment Professionals..........79

Chapter 5: Tracking Down the Best Doctor for You 81

Chapter 6: Working with Your Doctor to Sort Out Your Symptoms . . .95

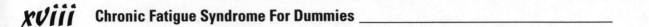

Introduction

. . . .

*C*hronic fatigue syndrome (CFS) is difficult to diagnose because it can look like many other conditions, and for patients with CFS, these conditions, and their associated problems and diagnostic procedures, are often tenfold. On a daily basis, I see patients who have been undiagnosed, misdiagnosed, and overdiagnosed. I see patients who are scared, anxious, and in pain. Unfortunately, a stigma is still attached to CFS; many loved ones and colleagues — even doctors — believe the symptoms many people experience are all in their heads. These patients usually have had a battery of tests, from blood workups to CT scans; they've given a medical history so many times they know every piece of information by heart.

But, despite all this poking and prodding, the patients haven't been properly tested and evaluated. In some cases, their doctors subject them to too many tests, misinterpret the test results, and saddle their patients with medications that not only compromise their quality of life, but can actually increase their symptoms! And, although this illness is rarer in young children, CFS may be at the root of a child's acting-out behavior in school or his introverted depression.

I don't want you or your loved ones to suffer unnecessarily from a bad or nonexistent diagnosis. In *Chronic Fatigue Syndrome For Dummies,* I arm you with the information and insight you need to assess whether or not you may have CFS. I also give you the tools to work with your doctor to identify your symptoms and to rule out other conditions. I give you the information about different treatments, as well as what exciting CFS advances lie ahead in the future. And, most importantly, I give you solid strategies for regaining a better quality of life.

About This Book

Chronic Fatigue Syndrome For Dummies can't and doesn't even attempt to act as a surrogate for skilled and knowledgeable medical care. Your family doctor and specialists play the leading roles in your diagnosis and treatment. This book is designed to play a supporting role, expediting your diagnosis and treatment and enhancing your life by doing the following:

✔ Assisting you in determining whether and when you need to seek professional medical advice for diagnosis and treatment based on your symptoms.

✔ Guiding you in selecting the medical professionals who are best quali-fied to diagnose and treat CFS (and are covered on your health insur-ance policy).

✔ Providing you with the information you need to more efficiently team up with your health care providers to arrive at an accurate diagnosis and obtain the most successful medical treatments, as well as the most effec-tive strategies for a healthier, happier, and more active life.

✔ Empowering you to take control of your illness by presenting practical, plain-English advice, tips, and strategies for living well with CFS at home, work, and school; while having an evening out; and on vacation or busi-ness trips.

✔ Saving your sanity by showing you that you're far from alone, that what you're experiencing is a very real, physical condition.

✔ Giving your loved ones tips and insights on living with someone with CFS — whether it be a spouse, a significant other, a parent, or a child.

Conventions Used in This Book

I don't like to think of my book as *conventional,* but I do have some standard ways of presenting material. For example, whenever I introduce a new, some-what technical term, such as *epidemiology,* I italicize it. Also, when I start a new chapter, I usually only use the full term *chronic fatigue syndrome* upon its first mention; after that, I substitute the acronym, *CFS.* One last convention you also want to be aware of is that when I refer to any medications, I use the generic drug name first, followed by the brand name.

In almost every chapter, I include intriguing stories about people who have suffered from CFS — some of them for years — and who, thanks to what doc-tors now know about CFS and how to treat it, emerged feeling a whole lot better after successful diagnosis and treatment. These stories aren't neces-sarily about specific people; to protect their privacy, I provided composites of real case studies my colleagues and I have diagnosed and treated over our many years as physicians.

In a few chapters, I include fill-in-the-blank forms you can scribble on. Although you can fill out these forms in the book, you may want to make copies to write on, especially if you borrowed the book from your library or plan on reselling it on eBay when you're done with it. These forms are incred-ibly valuable for empowering you to take a more proactive role in your diag-nosis and treatment.

What You're Not to Read

The best way to ingest and digest the information in this book is to read every word of it. I worked hard, along with my coauthor Karla, to provide you with everything you need to know and do to live well with your condition, and I'd hate for you to fast forward through the juicy parts.

You can, however, safely skip anything you see in a gray shaded box. I stuck case studies and technical information you really don't need to know in these boxes, to clue you into the fact that this reading material is optional. However, I doubt that you want to skip the case studies, because they provide real-world examples of people who struggle with the same CFS issues that you and your family now face, and they offer hope for a full life ahead.

Another element you can safely breeze right on by is any text tagged by a Technical Stuff icon. While many aspects of CFS may seem technical by nature, these paragraphs are usually the nitty-gritty details that don't impact your understanding of the illness or treatments. But by all means, if you're pining for additional knowledge, then reading these extra tidbits is a must.

Foolish Assumptions

In some books that cover advanced topics, authors must assume that their readers already understand some basic topics or have acquired beginning-level skills. For example, if this were a book about biochemistry, you'd have to know a little about chemistry first. Reading, understanding, and applying the information in this book to your life requires no prerequisites. This book, along with expert medical care and a moderate amount of cooperation from those around you, is all you need to start feeling better.

I do, however, make a few foolish assumptions about who *you* are. I figure your situation matches one or more of the following scenarios:

- You or someone you know has experienced unexplained fatigue that hasn't gotten better in six months or more, and you think CFS may be the culprit.

- Your doctor has assessed that something is wrong with you, but hasn't yet diagnosed you with CFS or sent you to a CFS specialist.

- Your doctor has diagnosed you as having CFS, and you're determined to know more about the condition and its treatment so that you can live a full life.

- You're a parent or caregiver of someone who has CFS, and you want to know what you can and should be doing to help.

How This Book Is Organized

I wrote this book so you can approach it in either of two ways. You can read the book from cover to cover or pick up the book and flip to any chapter for a quick, stand-alone minicourse on a specific CFS topic. To help you navigate, I divvied up the 21 chapters that make up the book into four parts. Here, I provide a quick overview of what I cover in each part.

Part I: Recognizing and Taking Steps Toward Treating Chronic Fatigue Syndrome

This part begins with a primer that touches on almost every topic covered in the book, so you can accelerate from 0 to 100 in about 18 pages. I proceed to present you with an explanation of CFS, lead you on an exploration of possible causes and common symptoms, point out other illnesses that mimic CFS, and finish up with a prescreening form that can help you in your quest to find real relief.

Part II: Teaming Up with Treatment Professionals

The key to living with CFS is to arrive at an accurate diagnosis and eliminate situations and environments that may be making your condition worse. In this part, I show you how to find and team up with a physician who can assist you in sorting out your symptoms and crafting a comprehensive treatment plan that ministers to both your body and your mind.

Here you can discover the most effective medications and therapies, complementary alternative treatments, and exercise strategies to provide true relief — and help you enjoy a much better quality of life.

Part III: Living and Working Well with Chronic Fatigue Syndrome

After a proper diagnosis, you take a sigh of relief (it's *not* all in your head), but you still need to apply the information your doctor provided you to your workaday and personal world, so you can more safely and fully enjoy your life. In this part, I show you how to gain the knowledge and skills required to cope with your condition at home, at work, on the road, on vacation, and in school or college.

I also offer tips that show you and your loved ones how to play a more active role in managing your illness — sometimes in the daunting face of skepticism and anger. I provide practical advice on what you can do to support a loved one who has CFS and aid children who either have the illness or are living with a family member who does. Finally, I present cutting-edge research that may lay the path to an eventual cure.

Part IV: The Part of Tens

No *For Dummies* book is complete without a Part of Tens. Turn to this part for a list of ten celebrities who also have CFS, ten strategies to make your life with this illness better, ten tips to fight fatigue without drugs, ten things to avoid if you have CFS, and the top ten myths about CFS that perpetuate the you're-just-not-trying-enough syndrome and need to be put to rest.

You can also find a comprehensive list of resources to help you understand, treat, and live with CFS in the appendix. Literally from A to Z, you can find lots of information to help you on your CFS education journey!

Icons Used in This Book

Throughout this book, I've sprinkled icons in the margins to cue you in on different types of information that call out for your attention. Here are the icons you can see and a brief description of each.

If you remember nothing else in a particular chapter, pay attention to anything that's marked with one of these icons.

Tips provide insider insight from behind the scenes. When you're looking for a better, faster, or more effective way to do something, check out these tips.

Whoa! This icon appears when you need to remain extra vigilant, seek professional medical guidance before moving forward, or take certain safety precautions.

You can find material next to this icon that's a little more detailed than the rest. You don't need to read these paragraphs to effectively manage your CFS.

I use this icon when I want to tell a story about someone who also has CFS.

Where to Go from Here

Think of this book as an all-you-can-eat buffet. You can grab a plate, start at the beginning, and read one chapter right after another; you can also dip into any chapter and pile your plate high with the information it contains.

If you're looking for a quick overview of CFS along with its diagnosis and treatment, check out Chapter 1. Chapters 5, 6, and 7 are also key, because they contain everything you need to know to obtain the most effective medical care. So if you're skipping around, don't miss these essential chapters.

If you're already under the care of a doctor and you're satisfied with the results, you can safely skip to any of the chapters in Part III to gather tips and strategies for dealing with CFS in your relationships, your routines, and your everyday life.

When you want some quick pick-me-ups or insights, Part IV is the place to go. Here you can also find a list of CFS myths, CFS strategies, and more.

Finally for some quick tips, tricks, and tools, check out the Cheat Sheet provided at the very beginning of this book, just past the front cover. Better yet, tear it out (preferably not in the bookstore or from a library copy), and carry the Cheat Sheet with you for quick reference.

Of course, after reading the book, you're welcome to dip back into it at any time to pick up something you missed or take a brief refresher course.

Part I

Recognizing and Taking Steps Toward Treating Chronic Fatigue Syndrome

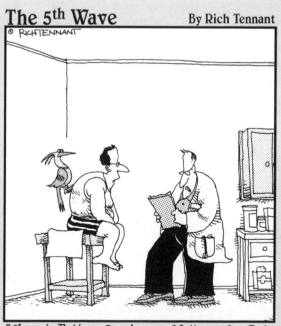

The 5th Wave   By Rich Tennant

"Chronic Fatigue Syndrome? Well, maybe. But like that pain in your shoulder, it could be a lot of things."

In this part . . .

When you first heard about CFS, you probably had more questions than answers. Questions like, what are the symptoms? What causes CFS? How many people have it? Can doctors cure it? When will it go away? How does it go away? Do I have it, or does my friend or loved one have it?

In this part, I answer the most common questions posed by CFS sufferers and their loved ones, and I reveal CFS's common symptoms and treatments. I present you with a prescreening test to help you gauge your own fatigue and determine whether and when you need to see a doctor. I lay out the facts and figures so you know just how prevalent CFS really is. And I fill you in on the possible causes of this often debilitating illness and the hopes for a future cure.

Chapter 1

Dipping into Chronic Fatigue Syndrome: Symptoms, Causes, and Treatments

In This Chapter

▶ Finding out what CFS really is

▶ Understanding how CFS is diagnosed

▶ Discovering a treatment plan that works for you

▶ Helping a loved one who has CFS

Yes, that feeling of tiredness, that low energy, those nonspecific aches and pains — they're all real, and they may be signs of chronic fatigue syndrome (CFS), a condition that affects between 900,000 and 2 million Americans. Worse, approximately 80 percent have never received a diagnosis for their multiple unexplained symptoms.

If you suspect you have CFS, or if you have a loved one who shows signs of CFS, this book can help. In this chapter, I go over the main issues regarding telltale signs and defining symptoms of CFS, the whys and wherefores of the illness, and ways to treat it. I also refer you to the chapters where you can find more information on specific topics.

Taking Your Fatigue Seriously

Wouldn't it be great if you could just pull the covers over your head and not think about your constant fatigue? Being able to just ignore that low energy, the flu-like symptoms that just won't go away, would be wonderful. But unfortunately, pulling the covers over your head is just going to make you hot. If you've been suffering from fatigue in combination with some other symptoms for six months or longer, you may have CFS. In this section, I give you a basic picture of CFS.

What is CFS, anyway?

First and foremost, in order to be classified as having CFS, you need to have fatigue for *at least six months.* This fatigue can't be explained or has been a lifelong condition, and most importantly, plenty of rest doesn't take it away. According to the Centers for Disease Control and Prevention (CDC), you have to have at least four of the following symptoms in addition to the long-term fatigue to be diagnosed with CFS:

- Headache of a different type or length than the headaches you've gotten in the past — a headache like you've never had before
- Aching muscles
- Painful joints
- An increase in symptoms *before* exercise; exercise makes them worse.
- Sore throat that comes and goes
- Swollen lymph nodes in neck, , and underarms
- Short-term memory and concentration problems
- Unrefreshing sleep

In Chapter 2, I go over all these symptoms in depth, including several that aren't listed in the CDC's official definition for the illness but have been reported by people with CFS; these symptoms include chemical or food sensitivity, dizziness, depression, allergies, and irritable bowel syndrome (IBS).

How long does CFS last?

Asking how long CFS will stick around can be a tricky question. Just as CFS can come on quickly (as suddenly as a summertime flu) or slowly, with worsening symptoms over time, the duration of CFS is just as mysterious. Studies show that people who suddenly get CFS tend to have a faster and better outcome, but nothing is written in stone. The best way to improve your chances for recovery is to take care of yourself as outlined in Part III of this book.

Conjecturing about the Possible Causes of CFS

Researchers have been discovering more and more about CFS — what possibly causes it, why certain people and not others get it, and how it takes root — but they don't have any definitive answers. Basically, a variety of causes are being investigated, any one of which may someday be shown to be the illness's raison d'être. These possible causes of CFS include the following:

- **Your family history:** If another family member had CFS (or some of the symptoms of CFS), you may be more vulnerable to getting it; however, the jury's still out as to whether there's a genetic link. Some people with CFS in their family history live their whole lives without getting CFS.

- **Stress, stress, and more stress:** This possible cause can mean day-to-day mental or emotional stress or stressors such as illness or injury. You may have a genetic connection between your symptoms and the way your hormones react to stress. Basically, this hormonal reaction comes down to *allostatic load* (or AL for those in the know). AL measures the wear and tear your body goes through when stress rears its anxious head. Some early studies have reported that people with CFS may have a problem with the physical mechanism that generates a proper stress response, rendering them unable to react effectively to stressors (mental or physical).

- **Body chemistry:** Humans have an amazing messenger system — one that beats FedEx hands down. Your body produces chemicals in response to messages sent to and from the brain — chemicals that don't miss a beat when it comes to getting a good night's sleep or hailing a cab or deciding whether to get that dress in the store window. But as good as your chemical messenger service is, it can get out of whack — whether stress, illness, or emotion is the cause. Think of this chemical imbalance as a blizzard that stops the mail from coming in, one that may or may not bring CFS with it.

- **Viral infections:** You have a powerful immune system in your body, with antibodies and natural killer (NK) cells just salivating for some foreign virus to dare enter your cells. But unfortunately, your immune system isn't always perfect. It can fail to attack with the full force of its fury, not recognize the virus as an enemy, or may even overreact. This whacked-out immune system has also been linked to CFS.

- **Sleep problems:** Yes, it's true: Whether your sleep issues are due to stress, an overtaxed and overworked immune system with no downtime to rest, or just the lack of quality sleep in general, problems with sleep have been linked to CFS.

- **The HPA axis:** Doctors call the hypothalamus in your brain, along with your pituitary and adrenal glands, the *hypothalamus-pituitary-adrenal (HPA) axis.* The hypothalamus sends messages to the pituitary gland via hormonal (chemical) messengers. The pituitary gland, in turn, triggers the production of hormones in your ovaries or testes, adrenals, and thyroid glands. Some people with CFS appear to have abnormally low levels of the hormone cortisol in the blood, which means that a malfunction in the HPA axis may be a possible cause.

✔ **Inflammation:** Think of an inflammation as the way your body fends off viruses and bacteria — the first line of defense in the immune system. However, chronic inflammation can break down the immune system, which may result in CFS.

✔ **Autonomic nervous system dysregulation:** Your autonomic nervous system is responsible for all your critical body functions, from breathing and regulating your heartbeat to keeping your temperature on an even keel. Some people who develop CFS have an autonomic nervous system problem called *orthostatic instability (OI),* which means that staying in an upright position for more than a few minutes results in a feeling of dizziness; this feeling can occur when sitting or standing up. Because OI can be caused by dysfunction in the autonomic nervous system, your autonomic nervous system could somehow be involved in your CFS. However, some physicians believe that OI stands alone, a condition in and of itself; still others consider OI a symptom of CFS, not a cause.

✔ **Physical trauma:** Ouch! The aches and pains of a fall or an accident can hurt your bones, muscles, and even your brain. Not only can physical pain lead to all sorts of not-so-fun things — such as insomnia, depression, brain dysfunction, or even changes on a very basic cellular level in your body — but it has also been explored as a cause, trigger, or perpetuating factor in some cases of CFS.

✔ **Ongoing infection:** Sometimes the flu you caught at the office doesn't go away in the requisite two weeks. Sometimes the infection lingers . . . and lingers. And instead of feeling better, you feel steadily worse. Infection has long been suspected as a cause or trigger of CFS, but researchers haven't identified a specific virus or bacteria as of yet. It could be that by the time a person goes to the doctor after many weeks or months of symptoms, the bug is gone, leaving various forms of damage in its wake.

✔ **Environmental toxins and allergies:** Pollen, dander, mercury, and lead — these damaging substances may be involved in the onset of CFS in the same way infections are.

ANECDOTE

Looking at the onset of CFS

Randall always considered himself one of those regular guys. He worked his 40 hours at a cell-phone chain and stopped at a local bar for a glass of beer before heading home. He had a girlfriend of one year, Cynthia, and they were talking about getting married and having kids. He had good friends, and they never missed a football game or a poker night.

Things started to change gradually. It wasn't like someone waved a magic wand and made him sick. Instead, Randall came down with a bad flu. Cynthia stayed at his apartment and even took off from her receptionist job to take care of him. He got better and thought he'd licked the flu and could go back to work.

But Randall got better only to a point: He didn't have a fever, he was no longer congested and didn't have the chills, but his energy was zilch. Whereas putting in 40 hours on the sales floor was nothing for this 24-year-old before he got sick, it was now a huge effort. He ended up punching out earlier because he didn't feel well. He stopped going to the bar for a drink. He didn't feel like talking to anyone. His throat was scratchy, his body ached all over with the slightest exertion, and he woke every morning feeling as dragged out as he had the night before.

Randall cut back on his social life to hang onto his job and even drew away from Cynthia. He made excuses every weekend until Cynthia came over and confronted him one Saturday afternoon. She found Randall lying on the couch — mail, take-out boxes, dirty plates, and newspapers piled on the counters. The blinds were closed and the television was muted (noise and light just too much for him to handle). The house smelled musty, and the answering machine light blinked, indicating lots of unreturned calls.

It may have looked like Randall was depressed, pure and simple. The lethargy, the isolation, the way he'd let things around him go — all these signs pointed to depression. But there was more to it than that, and it was called life-draining, exhausting, feet-dragging, barely-able-to-tie-his-shoes fatigue, not to mention the other symptoms that pointed to something different.

In addition, whenever Randall tried to get out of his slump, he was even more exhausted for several days afterwards. The day Cynthia came over, he tried to take a shower and get dressed to go out. Before the movie they went to see ended, he was so tired that they had to leave. He didn't get out of bed for days afterwards.

This pattern continued for months, and then gradually Randall began to feel better. But three months later, the fatigue, the aching muscles and joints, the sleep problems, and the sore throat all came back threefold.

Randall went to see his doctor. His job was on the line, and he was worried sick: "When will I feel better? Will it come back?" His family doctor referred him to an internist who had treated other patients with the same symptoms. The doctor put him on a low dose of one of the newer antidepressants that also helps with immune function and pain. He also gave him something to help him sleep through the night. In addition, he recommended making some adjustments to his work schedule and taught him some energy-conservation techniques.

After a lengthy diagnosis procedure in which the doctor excluded other conditions, the doctor gave Randall a name for what ailed him: chronic fatigue syndrome. This diagnosis helped Randall find information about his condition and connected him with others who understood what he was going through. It also gave Cynthia a framework to provide help and improve their communication about what was going on with Randall and their relationship.

Today, Randall is doing better, but he keeps a lighter routine than before. He paces his activities and takes rest periods throughout his day. He sees a therapist every week to help him (and sometimes Cynthia, too) adjust to the changes in his life brought on by illness. He uses coping strategies when faced with stress, and he isn't afraid to reach out and ask for help from people in his CFS support group. And, oh yes, he and Cynthia said "I do."

To find out more about the possible causes of CFS, check out Chapter 3, which gives you all the dirt on the whys of CFS.

Seeing the Right Kind of Doctor

Research from the Centers for Disease Control and Prevention (CDC) shows that the longer a person has CFS without being diagnosed or treated, the less likely he or she is to improve — and the more complicated the symptoms are. So getting an early diagnosis and treatment for symptoms is essential! And that starts with the doctor himself.

Try contacting your local hospital or a local support group for information on doctors who are knowledgeable about CFS. And remember to ask your friends or people in the local CFS support group. You'd be surprised to know that many of them understand what you're going through and may know of an excellent doctor. Of course, before you go to any doctor, check with your health insurance company to make sure the physician is part of the network.

Although you may forget the idea when you see the white coat come into the examination room, the doctor is there for *you*. If you feel your doctor isn't taking you seriously, or if he comes out and says that CFS is all in your head, run (don't walk) to the exit. Remember you're dealing with your health and your life — and you deserve the best. To find out more about finding a good doctor, see Chapter 5.

When you get to the doctor, remember that he may not be fully versed in CFS, but that doesn't mean he's a bad doctor! Work *with* him. Do the research. Bring your questions. CFS is usually the illness of last resort, when everything else has been ruled out, so be patient and make sure you're getting treatment for your symptoms. You can flip to Chapter 6 for more on making sense of your symptoms and Chapter 7 for info on possible treatment options.

Ruling Out the Other Suspects

CFS is more a case of what it *isn't* than what it is. You need to work with your doctor to rule out any other possibilities before coming to a CFS diagnosis. A few conditions that generate symptoms similar to CFS include the following:

- **The plain, old flu:** The flu, an infection with the influenza virus, has many CFS-like symptoms, such as fever, sore throat, and swollen glands; however, unlike CFS, the flu generally doesn't last six months or more.

- **Fibromyalgia:** This condition is also one of the hard-to-diagnose illnesses, with many of the same symptoms as CFS. The main difference between the two is that fibromyalgia's primary symptom *has* to be aching muscles and joints, and the first symptom of CFS *must* be fatigue.

✔ **Lyme disease:** CFS and Lyme disease have a lot of overlapping symptoms, and exploring whether an infection of Lyme may be the cause is worth the effort.

✔ **Hormonal disorders:** From your thyroid to your adrenals, hormonal dysfunction can make you feel tired, foggy, bloated, and just not yourself.

✔ **Sleeping disorders:** Everything from sleep apnea to snoring to insomnia to a bad mattress can interfere with a good night's sleep.

✔ **Depression and other mental disorders:** A clinical depression that makes you feel hopeless and helpless, or generalized anxiety that threatens to overwhelm you can mimic CFS. A thorough evaluation, specialized questionnaires, and some medical tests can help distinguish between common mood disorders and CFS.

✔ **Eating disorders:** If you don't eat, have poor nutrition, or throw up after you eat, you're going to be tired and have numerous unexplained symptoms. Period.

✔ **Autoimmune disease:** The symptoms of certain autoimmune diseases, such as lupus, can mimic those of CFS.

✔ **Obesity:** Lugging around even ten extra pounds can make you sluggish and tired. Being significantly overweight creates significant stress on many body parts, generating multiple and varied symptoms.

✔ **Substance abuse:** Alcohol and other drugs can cause all sorts of side effects — including fatigue.

These conditions and more can all mimic CFS, and you may not have CFS at all. To check out these "fakers," go to Chapter 2. To read about how the doctor rules out other conditions in order to properly diagnose CFS, head to Chapter 6.

Drafting an Effective Treatment Plan

Because CFS is such a complicated illness, with symptoms that can vary from day to day or week to week, having good treatment and a good treatment team are vital to your well-being. See Chapter 7 for a more complete look at different treatments, but in the meantime, here are some treatment success stories in brief:

✔ **Medications:** From painkillers to antidepressants, doctors can prescribe or recommend a host of medications that can help reduce symptoms and improve your ability to do everyday things.

✔ **Individual psychiatric or psychological therapy:** One-on-one mental health therapy can help you sort out your frustrations and your anger about your condition — not to mention how it has changed your life and relationships. Therapy is a vital part of your treatment plan to help with depression or anxiety if these symptoms are present. (You can find more info on therapy in Chapter 8.)

✔ **Family and relationship therapy:** No human is an island, which means that everyone has family or relationships that are important to him or her. In order for you to get the best care — and for those you love to have some respite — therapy for them (or together as a family) is an excellent idea.

✔ **Complementary alternative care:** Although the jury is still out on herbs and supplements, alternative treatments such as massage, yoga, and meditation can help relieve the stress that you may have. (To get the skinny on alternative health care, you can make a beeline for Chapter 9.)

✔ **Restructuring your life and sleep:** Because doctors can't tell when a person with CFS will get better, figuring out how to adapt and cope with the physical, mental, and emotional changes brought on by the illness is vital if you have CFS. Coping mechanisms need to be in place so life doesn't stop.

Many people with CFS have sleep problems, so addressing your sleep is very important, because it may require medications or something as simple as not sleeping for long periods in the daytime. Either way, restful sleep is a big priority. (For more sleep advice, see Chapter 11.)

✔ **Feeding your nutritional needs:** Eating healthy can keep your blood sugar levels balanced — which means more energy, less fatigue, and a better mood for you. Chapter 11 gives you the nitty-gritty details of a well-balanced diet.

✔ **Exercising nice and easy:** Exercise is important to prevent becoming deconditioned, but it must be designed for each individual. The important point is to start very slowly, increase very slowly, and always rest during exercise sessions. Pace yourself to find what works best for you without overexerting. You need to find that happy medium: not too little and not too much. (Chapter 10 has what you need to know about exercise and CFS.)

✔ **Getting rid of stress at work or at school:** You need to take breaks and regulate your schedule. Talking to the guidance counselor or to human resources to see whether you can have a more flexible routine may help. (But make sure your company is supportive before talking.) It may be necessary to involve a doctor, occupational therapist, and the Americans with Disabilities Act (ADA) in this type of workplace disability issue.

Keeping Love Alive in the Midst of CFS

What's love got to do with it? Plenty! Whether you or someone you love has CFS, the illness affects both of you. You need to be conscious of not only how you're feeling and what you're going through but also the needs of your spouse, partner, or other loved one.

Whether you're the caregiver or the person with CFS, there's a give-and-take that must be maintained. The person with CFS has to figure out how to set boundaries, and the caregiver needs to take care of himself or herself, too. In this section, I highlight some of the CFS relationship topics you can find in Chapters 13 and 14.

Appreciating the care others give

If you have CFS, make sure you tell your loved one how much you appreciate him or her. In addition, you may also want to consider doing the following to help out your caregiver:

- ✔ Work out a schedule with a few people to help out with different needs: the kids, the housecleaning, dinners, or even grocery shopping. This way, no one gets the brunt of taking care of you and everyone's happy. It's a win-win situation.

- ✔ Make sure you thank your caregiver — and not just once! A person can't hear thanks enough!

- ✔ Make sure your caregiver takes some time out. If your caregiver can't take care of himself or herself, your loved one won't be able to care for you.

See Chapter 13 for more handy tips on keeping relationships alive when you have CFS.

Supporting a loved one who has CFS

If you happen to be a caregiver, rather than the person with CFS, taking care of yourself is just as important as caring for your loved one. If you don't, you won't have any energy left over to help your loved one and keep up with other responsibilities you may have.

Here are some quick tips for taking care of yourself:

- ✔ Acknowledge your feelings and discuss them calmly and honestly.

- ✔ Don't burden yourself with the responsibility of making decisions alone. Have the person with CFS and other family members help you find solutions to problems.

- ✔ Take a break. Enjoy your hobbies, take a bubble bath, go to the store, or otherwise step back every once in a while. Your friends and family can give the person with CFS a change of company, watch the kids, or take care of chores for you as you recharge.

- ✔ Ask for formal help if you need it. Talk to a financial planner if you're worried about finances, or discuss emotional concerns with a therapist or support group.

By taking care of yourself, you're better prepared to care for your loved one. For an expanded discussion on caring for someone with CFS and attending to your own needs, Chapter 14 is where you want to go.

Guiding a Child through the Trauma of CFS

Children often have a hard time describing exactly how they feel. Not possessed with a huge vocabulary, "It hurts," "I'm tired," "I'm sleepy," and "I feel yucky" may be all they can muster to tell you how they feel. As you and your pediatrician try to figure out what's wrong, your child may have to visit many specialists, be subjected to numerous tests, and be put on a special routine of diet, exercise, and rest. Adding the suspicions of other family members, teachers, and friends that he's only faking can make the process of diagnosis, treatment, and lifestyle adjustments difficult for your child.

How can you help him adjust to the reality of living with a chronic illness? You can't find an easy answer, but the best approach is to be honest with your child. Educate him about CFS in terms he can understand, and involve him in the decisions surrounding his treatment and long-term care. Giving him a sense of control over his treatment can go a long way in giving him a sense of control over his life with CFS.

And kids who have CFS aren't the only ones who can be a concern. If your children see that you're incapacitated or sick, they may get frightened. They need to understand what's going on.

In the following sections, I give you a brief overview about how to help your child fight the battle with CFS, whether he's dealing with it himself or has to adjust to a parent having the illness. For more detailed advice, see Chapter 15.

Educating your child about CFS

The first step in educating your child about CFS is to educate yourself. You can accomplish this by talking to your child's doctor. You can also find numerous publications available free of charge on the Internet from reputable sites such as the Centers for Disease Control and Prevention (CDC), the National Institutes of Health (NIH), and other medical Web sites, such as WebMD. (For a list of these and other CFS resources, turn to the appendix in the back of this book.)

After you feel like you're getting a good grasp on what CFS is and how it will affect your child's life, you need to take the next step of imparting that information to your child. You have many options available to you to help out with this process. Many CFS foundations and organizations offer booklets and brochures for all age groups. The CFIDS Association of America has a useful Q&A section on its Web site with ready answers to many of the questions your child may have about CFS. (You can visit the site at `www.cfids.org/youth/articles.asp`.) But the most important thing to tell your child as you help him understand CFS is that you can do things as a family to help ease his symptoms — and that you love him no matter what.

Attending to your child when you have CFS

The most important element in caring for your child when you have CFS is to keep the lines of communication open. If your child feels secure enough and loved enough to talk to you, you can find out exactly how she feels, how she is coping, and how you can help.

Also, don't forget to allow your spouse or a close friend to help out with some of the daily needs your child may have, such as getting her meals, taking her to school, or doing her laundry. You can focus on helping your child in ways that aren't taxing to you and allow you to spend some quality time with her, such as by helping out with homework, combing her hair, or reading out loud.

Anticipating Future Tests, Treatments, and Possible Cures

The future of CFS has exciting possibilities. From genetic research to studies on the immune system, researchers are finding out more and more about the links to CFS. In the meantime, you can do the following to stay up-to-date with CFS news:

- ✔ **Stay informed with a support group.** Other people with CFS may have heard something you haven't — and vice versa.

- ✔ **Participate in a clinical trial.** If you meet the criteria of the aspect of CFS that's being studied, you can experience new findings firsthand.

- ✔ **Use the Internet.** You aren't alone. Over 900,000 Americans are suffering from CFS, not to mention thousands of others worldwide, and many of them are using the Web to seek out support, answers to questions, and physician referrals (and you can, too!).

See Chapter 16 for more information about exploring future treatments, participating in clinical trials, and finding out the latest information.

Chapter 2

Gauging Your Symptoms: CFS Is More Than Being Tired

*Y*ou've been dragging your body to work every day like a hundred-pound sack of potatoes. You have a flu you can't shake, complete with the fatigue, aches and pains, and a low-grade fever. Maybe you feel like you've been tired, depressed, aching, and in pain forever. Or maybe you just crashed one day after you went on a field trip to a local farm with your son's preschool class. Whatever triggered your malaise and persistent exhaustion and however you arrived at this point, your symptoms began, and you knew something was wrong. Now, you're beginning to suspect that the culprit's initials are C.F.S. — chronic fatigue syndrome.

But do your symptoms really qualify for the official CFS label? Maybe. Maybe not.

Everyone gets tired sometimes and has trouble rolling out of bed and dealing with work and daily chores. But people who suffer from CFS experience specific types of fatigue for extended periods of time, and their symptoms can't be traced back to other causes. In this chapter, I deconstruct the term *chronic fatigue syndrome* and define exactly what each part of that term means. I cover some of the most common and least common CFS symptoms as well as some of the conditions doctors must eliminate before diagnosing CFS.

Evaluating the Onset: When You Recognize Something Is Wrong

One day, you wake up and realize, "Hey, this isn't right." By definition, CFS symptoms must last a long time to qualify as *chronic* (see the section "Recognizing When You've Reached Chronic Status" later in this chapter), but the onset of the illness can strike as suddenly as a bump on the head or over the course of a 24-hour flu; doctors call this fast-paced progression of symptoms *sudden onset CFS.* Or the symptoms can creep up on you slowly like gray hair and wrinkles; the term doctors use for this case is *gradual onset CFS.*

Before I go into more detail about evaluating CFS symptoms later in the chapter, here's what you need to know about the differences between sudden and gradual onset CFS:

- **Sudden onset CFS:** People who are suddenly overtaken with a tiredness so heavy that it feels like a weight dropped out of the sky can often pinpoint the exact day on which CFS entered their lives and the exact circumstances that triggered their symptoms. These people are more likely to have experienced the flu-like symptoms associated with CFS, including a sore throat, chills, swollen lymph nodes, or fever, followed by the sustained, long-term fatigue that's so characteristic of CFS (for more on these symptoms, see the section "Recognizing the Signs and Symptoms of CFS" later in this chapter.). Because of these "infectious" characteristics, sudden onset CFS appears to be the result of problems caused by a virus or bacterial infection — two commonly suspected causes of CFS, which I explore in Chapter 3.

- **Gradual onset CFS:** If your CFS occurred over time, with the fatigue and other symptoms associated with it (such as flu-like symptoms, aches and pains, and terrible headaches) progressively worsening over weeks or months, you've experienced a gradual onset. A study done in Chicago found that 63 percent of the study's participants developed CFS gradually. A different study, this time done in Wichita, Kansas, found that 77 percent of the study's participants developed CFS gradually over time. Because gradual onset CFS is so insidious, creeping up on you while you've been going about your life, it can be more difficult to recognize.

As with any condition, the sooner you discover you have CFS, the better able you are to take care of it — and the better able you are to adapt to a new lifestyle. True, you can't cure CFS, but you may be able to stop it from becoming so debilitating that you become unable to keep up with your daily activities.

Recognizing the Signs and Symptoms of CFS

Although fatigue for six months is the underlying feature in most cases of CFS, other symptoms must be analyzed, because fatigue must be combined with several symptoms to be considered CFS. And doctors must look at the fatigue on an individual-by-individual case.

CFS is difficult to diagnose because of the following reasons (for a more in-depth discussion, check out Chapter 6):

- There isn't a diagnostic laboratory test that can tell you whether you have CFS.

- Elimination is key: Before your doctor can diagnose CFS, she must be able to rule out other "imitators," such as Lyme disease and mono.

- Fatigue can be a red flag for a whole host of other illnesses.

- CFS can look invisible (kind of like concealer for the dark circles), and many people come to the doctor without looking particularly sick.

- The fatigue in CFS can come and go — and you may have a doctor's appointment during the "go."

- Symptoms vary from person to person. CFS is more of an individual illness. Some people can't get up from their beds, and others go about their days, but in a fog, and then collapse later.

- Doctors can't find a pattern to CFS symptoms.

If you aren't getting the help you need, seek out another doctor, preferably one with another specialty or an open-minded primary care professional who sees the whole picture.

Fortunately, or unfortunately for you, CFS - doesn't have just a single symptom, such as muscle pain or headaches. Although a cluster of symptoms adds to your misery, the more you have, the easier it is to paint a more identifiable diagnostic portrait of CFS, simplifying diagnosis and expediting proper treatment as your doctor goes over each symptom in detail, one by one. (For more on reaching a diagnosis, see Chapter 6.)

Based on the latest Centers for Disease Control and Prevention (CDC) guidelines, eight common symptoms shout, "I have CFS!" The following sections name and describe these most common CFS symptoms and list a slew of less common symptoms that are no less distressing (for info on other illnesses or conditions that have similar symptoms as CFS, check out the section "Differentiating CFS from Other Conditions and Illnesses" later in this chapter). According to the CDC guidelines for diagnosing CFS, you must have four or more of the eight primary symptoms to qualify for the CFS diagnosis. See the appendix for more resource information.

Grading the severity of your fatigue

First and foremost, CFS makes you feel overwhelmingly tired, and you don't feel refreshed no matter how much sleep you get. Your body's weak, and you can barely stand up without help. Nothing can pull you out of your free-fall — not sleep, not exercise, and not staying away from sugar. You're eternally exhausted.

Clearly, this overwhelming exhaustion isn't your everyday fatigue, the fatigue most people feel after a busy week, a sleepless night, pulling an all-nighter, or stuffing themselves full of Thanksgiving turkey and mounds of mashed potatoes.

When is fatigue *not* CFS? When it goes away after a good night's sleep, after boarding a plane for a Caribbean vacation, or after you've shaken a bad flu. CFS is a complicated condition — and it doesn't go away that easily. In the following sections, you can see the difference between fatigue and being tired, as well as find out how doctors are trying to narrow the definition of fatigue.

Comparing fatigue to being just plain tired

You know when you're exhausted, and you usually know why. You've been sick. You're burning the candle at both ends. Emotional tensions or financial problems are stealing your mojo. Your boss is overbearing. Maybe you're exercising too much. A good night's sleep, a multivitamin, a day or two off the treadmill, or a couple of weeks on the beach is all you need to recharge your batteries and start feeling like yourself.

However, the most sinister aspect of CFS is that despite how tired you are, nothing you do or don't do makes you feel any better. The tiredness is like some voodoo curse that destines you to an eternity of restless sleep that doesn't leave you feeling at all refreshed, but instead, you may have low energy, a depressed mood, and even short-term memory loss. CFS is more of an erosion of health and spirit than a temporary bout of the blues that you can cure with a little R&R.

In addition, CFS fatigue often deepens with exercise (see Chapter 10 for more details), and you can't even attain some temporary solace with a full night's sleep — you awaken as tired and sometimes more tired than when you went to bed!

If you do have CFS, the fatigue you experience lasts for six months or more. The level of fatigue may ebb and flow slightly, especially if you have gradual onset CFS, but you never feel energized or refreshed.

Narrowing the CFS field with the fatigue scope

Because CFS embraces so many symptoms in addition to plain, old exhaustion, doctors and researchers are working on narrowing the *fatigue scope* — more clearly defining the intensity and duration of fatigue caused by CFS. By narrowing the fatigue scope, they can concentrate on defining the other characteristics of the illness and more easily determining whether a person has CFS or something else.

The best way for a doctor to narrow down the fatigue and make a correct diagnosis is to ask questions. She determines whether the patient's fatigue is indeed as prolonged as he says and performs diagnostic tests to eliminate other illnesses that can cause fatigue to narrow it down. See Figure 2-1 for a visual representation of this narrowing-down process. See Chapter 6 for more information on testing for CFS.

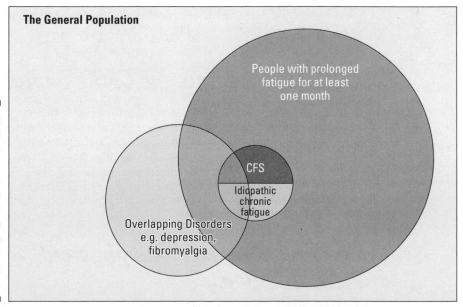

Figure 2-1: A visual look at the narrowing-down process doctors and researchers use to define the fatigue scope.

The General Population

People with prolonged fatigue for at least one month

CFS

Idiopathic chronic fatigue

Overlapping Disorders e.g. depression, fibromyalgia

Feeling the pain of headaches

Suddenly, those tension headaches you used to get have doubled in intensity. Maybe the pounding is a little more intense, or the headaches start in a different part of your head. Instead of a sinus headache, you're feeling it above your ear or in your temples. Sometimes you feel like you've had the same headache forever.

Headaches must be of a different duration and type than the headaches you've gotten in the past. In other words, if you've gotten migraines your whole life, the headaches you're currently experiencing probably have nothing to do with CFS. However, for example, if you start to get sharp, painful aches — like something you've never felt before — then the headache could be a symptom of CFS.

"Ow! My aching muscles!"

Aches and pains can signal a whole host of different conditions, some as benign as the temporary muscle pain that lingers after a tough workout, some as painful and difficult to diagnose as fibromyalgia, rheumatoid arthritis, or lupus. CFS aches can sometimes be localized — around the knees, arms, hands, or legs. They can also be systematic, occurring all over the body in a pervasive "ouch," similar to what you'd feel if you have the flu. Sorting out the pains and the possible causes is crucial to determining whether the aches are indeed a symptom of CFS.

Checking your joints for CFS symptoms

When you bump your elbow or twist a knee, you're likely to feel pain in the injured joint, but that's not the type of pain you typically feel with CFS. With CFS, the joint pain that qualifies as diagnostically significant afflicts multiple joints and isn't accompanied by redness or swelling. The pain may also move from one part of the body to another, unlike common arthritis (another illness of which joint pain is a symptom; see the section "Differentiating CFS from Other Conditions and Illnesses").

Crashing after strenuous physical or mental activity

Forget the fact that exercise is supposed to energize you, or that a crossword puzzle or Sudoku is meant to stimulate your mind. When you have CFS, you can feel out of sorts after walking to the mailbox or going up the stairs in your own home. And forget about the treadmill. If you have CFS, you will be completely exhausted and drained if you try to push yourself and walk two miles — assuming, of course, that you have enough energy to drag yourself to the gym.

As most doctors tell you, physical and mental activity can be quite exhilarating, making you feel more energetic. So, when some people experience persistent fatigue and other unexplained symptoms, their natural impulse is to rest and relax, go walking or jogging, read a book, or go out with their friends. This approach often shakes your average, everyday fatigue, but with CFS, these types of activity have the opposite effect. The harder you work to feel better, the worse you feel.

If you still feel tired to the point where you can barely get off the couch 24 hours after any strenuous physical or mental activity, then chalk up your after-exertion tiredness as a possible symptom of CFS.

Exercise can relieve CFS symptoms to some extent, but the exercise must be carefully monitored and regulated to prevent overexertion. In Chapter 10, I show you how to design a sensible exercise routine and gradually build up to more strenuous activities . . . only when you're ready.

Forgetting stuff: Short-term memory impairment

You're in a fog. The name of someone you met an hour ago is on the tip of your tongue . . . but you can't remember it. You have the attention span of a 3-year-old, minus the energy. What did your boss just ask you to do? Where did your friends say they'll meet you for dinner? Your brain cells feel as though they're covered with Teflon. What's happening to you? Perhaps the short-term memory loss you're experiencing is the result of having CFS.

Having a recurring sore throat

A sore throat isn't necessarily an indication of CFS. A bad cold can often be accompanied by a sore throat that lasts for several days. If you have rhinitis (a sinus infection) with postnasal drip, your sore throat may last for several weeks. A recurring sore throat, one that comes and goes every three or four days, may be a symptom for some people with CFS.

Experiencing tender, swollen lymph nodes

As you can find out in Chapter 3, some doctors and researchers consider CFS to be an autoimmune disorder that's triggered by a viral or bacterial infection. When some people get the flu, they may actually be feeling the effects of their bodies defending them against one of the viruses or bacteria suspected of triggering CFS. When your immune system begins cranking out antibodies to fight infection, your lymph nodes commonly become swollen and tender.

When your lymph nodes are swollen and tender, they usually let you know where they are. Otherwise, you may need to feel around for them. The lymph nodes are located on either side of your neck just below the back of your lower jaw bone, in your armpits, and in your groin. Your doctor can show you precisely where your lymph nodes hang out.

Although a viral or bacterial infection can spark the onset of CFS, CFS isn't known to be contagious. No evidence shows that CFS can spread by casual contact, such as shaking hands or sneezing, or through sexual contact.

Listing the less common symptoms

Although the CDC's list of primary symptoms form the diagnostic criteria doctors use to diagnose CFS, people with CFS report a host of other conditions or symptoms that may accompany the illness:

- Chest pains
- Chills
- Chronic cough
- Depression, anxiety, and panic attacks
- Dizziness, poor balance, and irregular heartbeat
- Dry eyes
- Irritable bowel syndrome (IBS)
- Jaw pain
- Night sweats, low-grade fever
- Sensitivity to light and noise
- Shortness of breath
- Sudden allergies or sensitivities to foods, odors, alcohol, or medications
- Weight changes, either weight loss or gain

Remember, these symptoms must be concurrent with the persistent fatigue of CFS in order to think of them as "clues." They should last for at least a week, or reoccur several times over a month or longer. Otherwise, these symptoms can signal everything from mood disorders to hypothyroidism (without the fatigue, the depression you feel is usually just that).

For more on treating and living well with irritable bowel syndrome, check out *IBS For Dummies,* by Carolyn Dean, MD, ND, and L. Christine Wheeler, MA (published by Wiley).

Recognizing When You've Reached Chronic Status

As I mention in an earlier section of this chapter, feeling fatigued is one thing — but being *fatigued* is a whole new ball game. Even if you feel tired after a full night's sleep, your fatigue still may not signal CFS. You could be depressed or have a sluggish thyroid or have contracted a bug. For your fatigue and other CFS symptoms to qualify as a bona fide case of CFS, they must have lasted for *six months or more.* The definition of six months or more is what puts the *chronic* in chronic fatigue.

In this section, I go over this six-month rule and other CFS qualifiers in more detail to ensure what you're feeling is the real CFS deal.

Examining the six-month rule

According to the CDC's diagnostic criteria for CFS, your fatigue, accompanied by other symptoms, must last for six months before you collectively qualify for the CFS diagnosis. Does that mean you have to tough it out for six long months before seeking medical treatment? Heck no! In fact, the earlier you seek treatment, the better chance you have of preventing symptoms from getting their footing and triggering other conditions, such as depression.

Each CFS sufferer is unique, and according to some experts, close to 50 percent of people who are later diagnosed with CFS didn't initially have its disabling fatigue (but trust me, the severe fatigue of CFS eventually disrupted some aspect of those people's lives). Sometimes the fatigue ebbs and flows; sometimes a month or two can go by before it strikes again. This lack of predictability when it comes to fatigue doesn't mean that a person doesn't have

CFS, especially if your doctor has ruled out other conditions and illnesses (for more on these, see the later section, "Differentiating CFS from Other Conditions and Illnesses"). Genetic research and immunological studies have found that treatment used for CFS has helped both those with clearly defined fatigue symptoms and those who don't fit the criteria.

The take-home message here is that even though your collection of symptoms may not have lasted long enough to qualify for an official CFS diagnosis or you haven't yet reached the six-month mark, don't hesitate to obtain treatment for the symptoms you're experiencing. Proper medical care for any of the conditions that commonly trigger CFS may prevent it from becoming severely disabling and, if you do have CFS, lead to a speedier diagnosis and more effective treatment later down the road.

In fact, by the time a person comes for help, their CFS may have triggered other conditions, such as depression. After all, feeling tired for six months or longer can make anyone depressed.

Qualifying for the eight-hour rule

Some people with CFS can continue to work a full work-week, but other areas of their life are substantially curtailed. When can CFS qualify you for disability benefits? In most cases, insurance companies use the eight-hour rule. Eight hours is the standard working day. If you can work eight hours consistently, for over a week, despite your fatigue, technically the likelihood of CFS is low, and your doctor may lean toward other diagnoses. The ability to work eight hours also means you may not qualify for full disability benefits from your company or the government (see Chapter 12 for more on disability benefits).

Self-screening for CFS

Do you have CFS? Only your doctor can know for sure, and only after she has ruled out other conditions via blood tests, CT scans, failures of other treatment regimens, or time. (See the chapters in Part II about working with health care professionals to treat CFS.) But you can be proactive, especially when you have an illness that's still plagued by the it's-all-in-your-head controversy.

If you think you may have CFS but you aren't sure, a prescreening questionnaire from your doctor may help confirm your suspicions that you may have CFS or convince you to look into other possible reasons for your symptoms. Remember, questionnaires aren't intended to encourage you to play doctor (despite the temptation they may be). See Chapter 6 for more information about working with your doctor to get a diagnosis.

A few facts about fatigue in the United States

A CDC study found that 24 percent of all Americans suffer from some degree of fatigue for two weeks or longer. Around 59–64 percent of those individuals couldn't pinpoint a physical cause. Most people who suffer from fatigue for six months or longer first go to their primary care physician — and 18 percent of them were subsequently diagnosed with an illness other than CFS. In other words, fatigue can sometimes be, well, just fatigue.

If you've experienced unusual exhaustion for an extended period of time, and nothing seems to help, see your doctor immediately, no matter what the results of a prescreening questionnaire may show.

Differentiating CFS from Other Conditions and Illnesses

With some conditions, a diagnosis is in plain sight; a broken arm, measles, sunburn, or the common cold are most likely "what you see is what you got." If only CFS were that simple! The extreme fatigue you feel could very well be something else. In fact, determining CFS as a culprit is more a process of elimination — determining whether your symptoms signal a different illness.

According to the CDC and the Chronic Fatigue and Immune Dysfunction Syndrome (CFIDS) Association of America, over 80 percent of people with CFS haven't been properly diagnosed and aren't getting the treatment that they need. Don't join the ranks of the undiagnosed, untreated masses. Seek your doctor's advice as soon as you notice symptoms are persisting for more than two to three weeks, and certainly for more than four to six weeks.

Because the diagnostic procedure for CFS is often a process of elimination, your doctor is likely to perform a thorough workup, consisting of an interview, a physical examination, a battery of tests, and perhaps even treatment for some other illness or condition before settling on a diagnosis of CFS (for more on the diagnosis process, see Chapter 6).

Common illnesses and conditions that have symptoms mimicking those of CFS include the following:

  ✔ **Addison's disease:** Some CFS specialists suspect that CFS is actually a mild form of Addison's disease — a condition characterized by dizziness, weakness, and fatigue. For full-blown Addison's, the hormonal dysfunction abnormality is more marked than what it would be in CFS, as reflected in blood tests. For more about Addison's disease, see Chapter 3.

✔ **Arthritis:** People suffering from early stages of arthritis may also have aching joints without redness or any observable swelling (a common symptom of CFS), so your doctor must rule out arthritis before you can chalk up your joint pain as a possible symptom of CFS.

✔ **Autoimmune disorder:** An autoimmune disorder means that the very immune system in your body used to ward off infection literally turns on itself. Antibodies get confused and start killing off your healthy cells. Some physicians and researchers consider CFS an autoimmune system disorder, and, indeed, recent evidence points to a possible link. But other autoimmune disorders, including lupus and multiple sclerosis (MS), must be ruled out before your immune system dysfunction is considered CFS.

✔ **Bipolar (BP) affective disorders:** BP is a mood disorder characterized by extreme highs and lows, or mania and depression, with no gray areas in between. If the medications prescribed for bipolar disorder don't improve your fatigue or your flu-like symptoms, chances are that your illness isn't BP. You may find it hard to think of the mania associated with BP to be confused with CFS, but mania can take many forms. In Bipolar II, for example, mania may present itself in anxiety, lack of focus, inability to concentrate, and obsessive thoughts (do these symptoms sound familiar?). (For in-depth coverage of bipolar disorder for both BP sufferers and their family members, check out *Bipolar Disorder For Dummies,* by Candida Fink, MD, and Joe Kraynak [Wiley].)

✔ **Cancer:** Many cancers can make people feel exhausted, as can the chemotherapy used to treat them. With proper tests and treatments, however, your doctor can accurately diagnose cancer and provide effective treatment. If, after treatment, the cancer goes into remission but CFS-like symptoms remain, your doctor may need to run further tests to determine the possible cause.

✔ **Diabetes:** Because diabetes left unchecked can become life threatening, this condition is one of the first ones that needs to be ruled out with a simple blood test. The most common diabetes symptom that is similar to those of CFS is fatigue. Some of the symptoms associated with diabetes that aren't part of CFS include chronic urinary tract infections and a dip in energy after eating foods that contain high levels of sugar or saturated fats.

For information on the latest diagnostic tests and effective treatments for diabetes, check out *Diabetes For Dummies,* 2nd Edition, by Alan L. Rubin, MD (Wiley).

✔ **Eating disorders:** If you mentally can't eat or if you binge and purge, you're sure to feel exhausted and cranky, but an untreated eating disorder doesn't make CFS.

✔ **Fibromyalgia:** This one is tricky. Fibromyalgia is a condition in which you feel pain all over your body, in certain "trigger" spots, particularly in your hips and shoulders (and not your hands and feet). The pain usually starts out gradually, but becomes very intense over time. Because fibromyalgia and CFS have many of the same symptoms (and they can actually occur together), each condition can be mistakenly diagnosed as the other. The key distinguishing factor? In CFS, the more prominent symptom is fatigue (although fatigue can be fairly significant in fibromyalgia, too). In fibromyalgia, the widespread aches and pains are more prevalent than in CFS.

You can find out more about fibromyalgia by checking out *Fibromyalgia For Dummies,* by Roland Staud, MD, and Christine Adamec (Wiley).

✔ **Food allergies or intolerances:** Some researchers have called CFS an allergy (in fact, food allergy is a type of immune system dysfunction), but even minor allergic reactions to food or dust or pollen can make you sleepy. These reactions can even mimic sore throats and swollen glands. In addition, food intolerances (for example, an inability to digest milk) can make you feel tired, achy, and nauseated. Allergies and food intolerances must be ruled out before CFS is ruled in.

For more about diagnosing and treating food allergies and intolerances, check out *Food Allergies For Dummies,* by Robert A. Wood and Joe Kraynak (Wiley).

✔ **Flu:** That scratchy throat and stuffed nose may just need two aspirins, some bed rest, plenty of fluids, and a call to the doctor in the morning. The difference between the flu and CFS is that the flu will eventually go away! Also, the flu's symptoms — sore throat, achy joints, low-grade fever — are more prevalent than fatigue.

✔ **Gulf War syndrome:** Seven percent of soldiers who fought in the Gulf War have come down with symptoms similar to CFS. Fifteen percent of those veterans who weren't on the front lines also have CFS symptoms, characterized by fatigue, muscle and joint pain, brain fog, low-grade fever, weakness, and unsteadiness. Gulf War syndrome is a result of chemical weaponry, post-traumatic shock, and battle wounds. Because its roots are different from CFS, Gulf War syndrome isn't considered CFS in the strict sense — but the stress of war may possibly lead to CFS symptoms.

✔ **Hormonal disorders:** As with autoimmune disorders, hormonal disorders and CFS have been linked. But hormonal imbalance may also signal adrenal problems, depression and other mood disorders, hypothyroidism, and more. Symptoms can include fatigue, swollen glands, anxiety, erratic mood, and weight gain. If you have a hormonal imbalance and symptoms remain even after the imbalance is corrected, CFS may be what's really making you sick. Your physician must make this judgment.

✔ **Hypothyroidism:** Feeling sluggish? Out of sorts? Lacking in energy? Your symptoms could be an underactive thyroid producing insufficient levels of various hormones. Ask your doctor for a blood test to remove all doubt.

In Chapter 3, I discuss the connection between hormones and CFS. (If you or your doctor suspects that your thyroid is playing a role, check out *Thyroid For Dummies,* 2nd Edition, by Alan L. Rubin, MD [Wiley].)

✔ **Lyme disease:** What came first, the chicken or the egg? The bite or the long-term trouble? Because Lyme disease may lead to CFS-like symptoms, you can't rule out CFS just because you have or have had Lyme disease.

The symptoms of the two illnesses are often very similar; both include fatigue, aching joints, foggy memory, and dizziness. The key is whether you've been bitten by a tick that carries Lyme disease. Your doctor can run a blood test to determine whether you have Lyme disease and can often treat it effectively with antibiotics. If your symptoms subside after treatment, you can rule out CFS. If they don't, your doctor may need to do a little more detective work.

✔ **Major depressive disorders:** One of the symptoms of severe depression is extreme fatigue. This level of depression can also make you feel achy and uncomfortable. And like CFS, depression can also affect your short-term memory. And what's worse, because of its debilitating symptoms, CFS can even trigger depression! How do you differentiate between CFS and depression? Antidepressants and counseling often relieve depression, but they will likely have much less effect in relieving the main symptoms of CFS.

✔ **Medication side effects:** When your fatigue or weakness first began, had you recently started any new medications? Your symptoms can very well be a side effect of a medication or combination of medications.

✔ **Mononucleosis:** Although the so-called "kissing disease" is a separate illness in and of itself, mono may actually trigger the onset of CFS. See Chapter 3 for details about the connection between mono and CFS.

The longer mono sticks around, the more likely it is to trigger CFS-like symptoms. Mono can also mimic the illness. If your mono lingers or becomes chronic, make sure you're under a doctor's supervision to keep the symptoms in check until they dissipate.

✔ **Multiple sclerosis (MS):** Both MS and CFS can worsen over time. Both have periods of remission mixed in with the bad times. But MS more often affects the ability to walk (to use muscles and limbs) than CFS. MS can also be diagnosed with A CT scan of the brain and spinal cord, which is one way to see whether your fatigue and pain are the result of two or more lesions in the brain ("multiple" sclerosis), which is a requirement for the diagnosis.

Multiple Sclerosis For Dummies, by Rosalind Kalb, PhD; Nancy Holland, RN, EdD, MSCN; and Barbara Giesser, MD (published by Wiley), offers excellent insight and in-depth coverage of treatment options for this often debilitating illness.

✔ **Normal aches and pains:** An aching back, sore shoulder, or legs that feel like lead may be the result of bending the wrong way or spending a few too many hours at the gym. However, if your aches and pains don't go away after a week or two, you should see your doctor.

✔ **Obesity:** When you're overweight, the slightest exertion can leave you tired and aching. Obesity is one condition that doesn't exactly sneak in under the radar. You know when you're overweight, and, if you start to get your energy back with each lost pound, your chances of having CFS are lessened.

✔ **Subacute infections:** When an infection is subacute, it's "flying below the radar." Recent research points to specific viruses that may cause CFS, even though they remain undetected and hidden from view. Can an infection cause CFS symptoms? Yes. Can an infection mask itself as CFS? Yes. Which is which? If fatigue isn't your number-one symptom, and if your fatigue hasn't hung around for more than a few weeks, then chances are your infection is *not* CFS. Chapter 3 identifies the most common viruses and bacteria suspected of contributing to the onset of CFS.

✔ **Substance abuse:** You know when you're drinking too much or overindulging in pharmaceuticals or illicit drugs (even if you don't want to admit it). Alcohol and drugs are notorious as self-medications for treating depression and chronic pain, but because patients often hide the problem, their doctors may have trouble ruling out substance abuse as a contributing factor. When you see your doctor, come clean about any addictions to ensure an accurate diagnosis and effective treatment.

To read about how doctors can rule out many of the above conditions and illnesses when trying to diagnosis CFS, flip to Chapter 6.

A "tick"ing time bomb

A few weeks after she'd kicked up her heels for a weekend in the country with her boyfriend, Linda's heels started dragging. The weekend getaway had been buggy and humid, and they spotted several deer from the porch of their B & B. They had a great time, but could have done without the itching from insect bites.

Several weeks later, Linda couldn't keep her eyes open, but even after a full night's rest, she woke up weary. What was going on? Did she have Lyme disease? She examined her arms and legs for tick bites, spotting not the slightest sign of a bite.

Over the next two months, Linda grew more and more tired. She'd taken so many sick days at work that she had been forced to go on short-term disability. Her boyfriend did what he could, but between work and caring for his ailing, aging parents, he had little time to spare. Linda's mom had to fly in to help care for her.

Today, Linda still feels overwhelming fatigue, but at least she has a name for it: chronic fatigue syndrome. And proper treatments for her various symptoms have enabled her to return to work. Slowly but surely, Linda is on her way back to a healthier life.

Chapter 3

Looking At the Possible Causes: Where Does CFS Come From?

Chronic fatigue syndrome (CFS) is a mysterious illness with a puzzling past. CFS may develop from something as simple as a bad flu, as tiny as a tick bite, or as traumatic as a loved one's death. Numerous speculative causes for CFS are out there, but the bottom line is that the exact cause is unknown.

To make connecting the cause of CFS to the effect more difficult, CFS doesn't always develop overnight. You may have bumped your head or been bitten by a tick when you were on summer vacation long before symptoms set in — six months later!

In this chapter, I examine CFS from prehistoric times to the present, from when the illness was first diagnosed up to the medical community's current understanding of CFS. I also delve into some of the speculated causes of CFS to reveal the challenges of tracing the onset of symptoms to a specific cause or event, so you can begin to understand when and why your symptoms may have developed.

If at all possible, try to trace back your symptoms from when they first started. Being able to provide a history or pattern to your doctor can help him make a correct diagnosis — and treatment plan — more efficiently.

Examining the History of CFS

You may be thinking, what does CFS in the past have to do with my symptoms today? Simple: The more you know about the background of CFS, the better you can identify the illness. The extra knowledge also gives you a perspective on CFS in general, and on your CFS symptoms.

Chronic fatigue syndrome is a relatively new name for an old condition that has had symptoms on the medical radar screen since the nineteenth century. Centuries prior to that, patients presented similar complaints of the unexplained, debilitating fatigue that's characteristic of CFS, but doctors didn't have a name for it, so they simply chalked it up as some other condition, often a bacterial or viral infection, such as malaria, hepatitis, or influenza (the flu).

The following timeline brings you up to speed on the history of CFS:

- **Prehistoric CFS:** Chronic and profound fatigue, headaches, joint pain, memory loss, and throat and lymph node pain are likely to have affected the earliest Homo sapiens. Unfortunately, the artists who drew on cave walls were more interested in documenting their wooly mammoth hunting trips than describing the history of unexplained illnesses.

- **From ancient Egypt through the European Renaissance:** For centuries, people believed that the body held *four humours* — fluids that needed to be in balance for good health. These humours were blood, phlegm, black bile, and yellow bile. If someone had too much phlegm, the theory went, that person would appear moody, sluggish, and pale (which is where the term *phlegmatic* came from). Too much black bile, and a person would suffer from *melancholia* — a lack of energy and drive. Could these symptoms signal CFS — before the days when CFS existed in the public mind? Quite possibly.

- **1750:** An English physician, Sir Richard Manningham, observed an assortment of symptoms, from fatigue to fever, that were difficult to diagnose. He called this syndrome *febricula* (little fever).

- **1869:** Neurologist George Beard classified the cluster of symptoms characteristic of CFS — the fatigue, fever, and listlessness — as *neurasthenia*.

- **1934:** The first recorded outbreak of this new syndrome in America occurred in Los Angeles, California, when 200 employees of the Los Angeles County General Hospital reported extreme weakness and fatigue.

✔ **1938:** Medical professionals began to use the term *myalgic encephalomyelitis (ME)* in their books and articles. Doctors continue to use this term today, mostly in the United Kingdom.

✔ **1969:** The World Health Organization (WHO) classified ME as a CNS (central nervous system) illness.

✔ **1984 (Outbreaks in America):** A number of people vacationing or living in Incline Village, Nevada, came down with mysterious symptoms. Although they had been perfectly healthy, these people suddenly developed flu-like symptoms, muscle fatigue, and cognitive problems. The same symptoms were also found in people living in upstate New York, in the town of Lyndonville, and in Raleigh, North Carolina. Because subsequent blood tests showed nothing unusual, many physicians become skeptical of the illness. This skepticism still holds true in many doctors' offices today.

✔ **1985:** Studies suggested that people who had higher levels of antibody to the Epstein-Barr virus were more susceptible to CFS symptoms. Although it later turned out that healthy people also had high levels of the antibody, the Epstein-Barr connection stuck. Some members of the medical community referred to the illness as *chronic EBV.* (See the following sidebar, "Probing the Epstein-Barr connection.")

✔ **1988:** A group of researchers at the CDC (Centers for Disease Control and Prevention) developed the first case definition for CFS and introduced the name *chronic fatigue syndrome* (CFS), because fatigue was the main identifying symptom. The term stuck.

✔ **1990s:** To reflect the broader impact of the condition and current science, advocates modified the term to *chronic fatigue and immune dysfunction syndrome* (CFIDS), which is still often used interchangeably with CFS.

✔ **1994:** Researchers at the CDC formed an international group to define the diagnostic criteria for CFS. (See the section "Officially speaking: From the Centers for Disease Control and Prevention [CDC]" for a list of the current diagnostic criteria.)

✔ **Present:** More than 4,000 published research studies have been conducted on CFS, leading to better understanding of the illness. Physicians, psychiatrists, therapists, and others in the medical community are starting to "get it" and accept CFS as a real illness with a defined set of criteria and ways to treat symptoms and advise patients on lifestyle adjustments and coping. You can still find a few holdouts, but the future looks promising.

Probing the Epstein-Barr connection

For a time, many doctors considered the Epstein-Barr virus to be the root cause of CFS, but the evidence suggests that it isn't the complete answer:

✔ The Epstein-Barr virus (EBV) causes infectious mononucleosis, or "the kissing disease," affecting approximately 35–50 percent of people in their teens and early adulthood.

✔ Epstein Barr is one of the most common viruses found in humans — 90 percent of the population has the virus before the age of 30.

✔ Epstein Barr is in the herpes family of viruses. (Yes, the same viruses that can cause herpes in some individuals.)

✔ Most people exposed to EBV are immune to it; they don't get mononucleosis. But, for those who are vulnerable, "sealed with a kiss" can become fatigue, a sore throat, and swollen lymph glands. Yep, that sure sounds a lot like CFS! However, these symptoms don't become chronic in most people who are struck with mononucleosis. After several weeks, most people have few, if any, symptoms remaining.

✔ Because EBV can become chronic, it can lead to long-term fatigue and cognitive problems; many people equate EBV with CFS. EBV is one of several agents that have been shown to lead to CFS. Recent research also shows that Ross River virus and coxiella burnetti (the agent that causes Q Fever) lead to CFS in about 12 percent of documented infections.

People diagnosed with CFS *present with* (show symptoms of) a dysfunctional immune system, which makes CFS somewhat similar to EBV. Patients with EBV have an elevated immunoglobulin G (IgG), one of the antibodies that the body creates to fight illness, that attacks the body it is supposed to defend. The IgG usually coexists with the viral capsid antigen (VCA) — which is associated with EBV.

If you're writing your European pen pal (or another person who isn't an United States citizen), he may not recognize the acronym CFS or the term *chronic fatigue syndrome.* People in other countries know CFS as *epidemic neuromyasthenia, myalgic encephalomyelitis, postviral fatigue syndrome,* or *chronic fatigue and immune dysfunction syndrome.* Of course, they may say it in French, Spanish, or Italian.

Investigating Early Reluctance to Recognize CFS

Doctors and researchers have been more than a little reluctant to label CFS as a bona fide illness. And who can blame them? Would you want to label something you couldn't define (even under a microscope), touch, or test for?

Not until 1988 was CFS recognized as an official illness. Why so long? Because blood tests showed no irregularities, and its symptoms — fatigue, lethargy, muscle aches — are very similar to symptoms of depression and other disorders. Combined with the fact that CFS has multiple and often mysterious causes, the notion that "it's all in your head" is one of the main reasons that the medical community has taken so long to accept CFS as a real illness. Even today, diagnosing CFS is a process of elimination (multiple other illnesses are ruled out as a cause of your symptoms), not a direct hit, which only adds to some doctors' reluctance to diagnose it.

Although your doctor can't see, feel, or test for CFS, you can certainly feel its effects. In your gut (and sometimes in your head, your joints, and your throat), you know something's not right. Because your doctor can't see or test for CFS, your descriptions of your medical history and symptoms are your doctor's only way of *seeing* your CFS. In Chapters 5 and 6, I reveal tips and tests that can help your doctor see more clearly.

When researchers began to bandy about the idea of naming a loose collection of mysterious symptoms that had no single, identifiable cause as an illness, conservative thinkers in the medical establishment protested. Some nonbelievers continue to resist accepting CFS as a real medical condition, but as I reveal in the following sections, well-informed, experienced researchers and doctors have legitimized CFS and continue to work toward identifying the cause and discovering more effective treatments — and possibly a cure.

Officially speaking: From the Centers for Disease Control and Prevention (CDC)

CFS owes much of its current legitimacy to the efforts of research groups under the CDC umbrella. The CDC was the first to define CFS as a medical condition (in 1988) and update the criteria (in 1994).

Following are the official research criteria for CFS direct from the CDC:

✔ Unexplained, unrelenting fatigue that

- Isn't due to strenuous physical or mental activity
- Continues even when you're getting plenty of rest
- Hasn't been a lifelong condition
- Results in a significant decrease in physical or mental activity

✔ This fatigue has to last for at least six months with four or more of the following symptoms

- Decline in memory or ability to concentrate

- Increased exhaustion or –worsening of symptoms, which lasts 24 hours or longer, as a result of physical or mental activity

- Nonrecuperative sleep (you get eight to ten hours of sleep, and you wake up exhausted)

- Muscle pain

- Joint Pain without swelling or redness in

- Headaches that are more painful or of a different type than you've had before

- Frequent or recurring sore throats

- Sensitive cervical (neck) or axillary (arm pit) lymph nodes (groin involvement is not listed in the official case definition.

According to the CDC, one of the most authoritative sources for accurate and timely information about public health and illness, CFS is a real medical condition with a set of clear and identifiable symptoms that point to a reliable diagnosis. Your doctor must still rule out, however, other possible conditions, as I demonstrate in Chapter 6.

Getting the inside scoop: What people now know about CFS

The medical community's acceptance of CFS is growing. Researchers continue to gather new evidence that CFS is a serious medical condition; work to identify treatment options; and progress toward identifying the causes and perhaps even discovering a cure.

Through research studies, census reports, and data collected from patients, the medical community has sketched a statistical portrait that gives CFS a more recognizable face. The following shows you the results culled from this research:

✔ **Prevalence:** Nobody knows exactly how many people are afflicted with CFS, but the CDC estimates that over 1 million people in the United States alone have CFS symptoms.

✔ **Prevalence in women:** CFS generally affects women four times more than it affects men.

- ✓ **Duration:** In studies of a population in Chicago, Illinois, the most common duration of CFS was 2.9 years, but in a CDC study done in Wichita, Kansas, the range varied from 8 months to 44 years, with the average duration of 7.3 years.

- ✓ **Remission rates:** Only 5–10 percent of patients diagnosed with CFS have experienced total remission. (But as they say on your investment portfolio, past results are no indication of future performance.) Following my guidance in this book, you may increase your odds and may feel much better in the meantime

- ✓ **Partial remission rates and relief:** A 2005 study of over 28 clinical trials found that, on average, 39.5 percent of patients diagnosed with CFS improved over time.

Partial remission percentages may be higher than what the official count shows. One of the reasons why pinpointing CFS is so difficult is that follow-up numbers, though critical, are often unavailable. As soon as a person with CFS starts feeling a little better, the last thing they want to do is step into a doctor's office — even if only to report the good news! Also, if 80% go undiagnosed, all of these people may improve without ever having seen a health care professional. Doctors never hear from everyone; as I point out earlier in the section, it's difficult to assess these numbers.

Shaking Your Family Tree

Genes are the building blocks of life — and may play a role in increasing your vulnerability to CFS. According to recent studies, CFS sufferers share more than symptoms: They share a *genetic predisposition* to CFS. A genetic predisposition doesn't mean you're born with CFS, but it would simply increase your susceptibility. Like all the other possible causes of CFS, this theory is still a hypothesis — researchers still don't know why these factors may cause CFS.

A person who's predisposed to CFS, however, could be more likely to experience the onset of the illness whenever the level of physical, psychological, environmental, or emotional stress exceeds a certain threshold. What that threshold is, of course, would likely vary from one person to another. In the following sections, you can further explore the who-done-its of CFS, discovering some of the factors that may prove with more study and research to lead to the condition.

A potential genetic predisposition to acquiring CFS is usually not enough by itself to trigger the onset of CFS. This possible genetic vulnerability would almost always require the addition of a physical or emotional stressor or some other illness to transform the inherent vulnerability into the onset of CFS and the appearance of symptoms.

Investigating the stress-hormone genetic connection

The central component of a groundbreaking CDC study done in Wichita, Kansas (chosen because the population make-up of Wichita is considered to be comparable to the population make-up of United States as a whole) shows the possibility of a genetic connection between people's hormonal reactions and stress (see Chapter 4). The CDC used the Wichita information to conduct a large-scale study of CFS, involving epidemiologists, immunologists, geneticists, physicists, and mathematicians to try to find the causes — genetic and otherwise — of CFS. Dubbed the *CFS Computational Challenge* (or C3), this multidisciplinary study tested blood, genes, and the levels of allostatic load (AL) in a cross section of Wichita residents. (*Allostatic load* measures the overall wear and tear the body experiences as a result of stress — blood pressure, hormone secretions, and other physical signs that remain in the system long after the stressors are removed.)

The C3 found that people with CFS were twice as likely to have a higher AL index than people without CFS. In other words, the researchers hypothesized that the bodies of those with CFS may react differently or ineffectively to stress and, hence, are more vulnerable to physical and emotional stress than those who don't have CFS. Some scientists have categorized this vulnerability as a *fatigue gene*.

The C3 researched more than 20,000 genes, of which 50 genes and 500 *polymorphisms* (the matching markers on a genetic chain) were involved in the hypothalamus-pituitary-adrenal axis (see "Gland-standing with the HPA axis" later in this chapter). These were further broken down into five polymorphisms and three genes that appeared more frequently in peoplewith CFS.

It's a gene thing

Genes are the seeds of life. Although they involve only a few *amino acids* (protein molecules), the way they are paired makes each person unique. (Remember those DNA ladders from science class?) There is an infinite coupling of molecules — which is why the folks on *CSI* are able to make a DNA match during a criminal investigation. You may find it hard to believe that these infinitesimal gene patterns dictate everything from the color of your eyes to the people you like, but they do. In fact, these genes dictate your ability to handle stress, the production of the hormones that make your body work, and the chemicals that respond to signals in the brain.

Digging up the missing genetic link

Just because some people experience different physical reactions to stress doesn't prove a genetic link — but the fact that people without these genetic patterns does make it seem less likely than just a coincidence. It is a powerful link. The C3 (from the preceding section) was able to identify five distinct categories of CFS based on these gene-sequence variations and the way that the symptoms appeared during a battery of tests. These categories of CFS are all related to genetic structure — and the way certain gene lesions make people vulnerable to CFS. The C3 include CFS associated with the following:

- ✔ **A high allostatic load:** A person may be physically unable to generate an appropriate response to stressors (physical or mental).

- ✔ **The brain's chemical dysfunction:** A person may be depressed or moody.

- ✔ **An imbalance in hormonal production:** A person may be moody, nervous, bloated, or sluggish.

- ✔ **Immunologic changes (due to blood cell dysfunction):** A person may get sick more often than others or have other infectious-type symptoms, such as low grade fever or night sweats.

- ✔ **A dysfunction in the central nervous system:** A person may have some memory loss or rapid heartbeat. A study done in Georgetown outside Washington, D.C., found that people with CFS have more of a specific protein in their spinal fluid. As an element in the central nervous system, this protein abnormality may result in neurological impairments, including symptoms of CFS.

Genes may influence the makeup of the chemicals in the brain. A few studies have shown that people with CFS have been found to have imbalanced levels of *serotonin* (one of the chemicals responsible for some depressions and mood disorders). The neuron, or nerve cells, in the brain may get mixed signals and not trigger the production of the right amount of chemicals.

Checking Out Your Body Chemistry

Your body holds an amazing messaging system. The chemicals produced by your body in response to messages sent to and from the brain govern everything from getting a good night's sleep to hailing a cab, from signing your name on a check to protecting you from nasty germs.

A single stressor can throw your body's chemical machinery out of whack and cause a host of minor glitches that can add up to major misery. In the following sections, I reveal a few of the many chemical dysfunctions that may set off CFS.

Examining the virus-CFS connection under a microscope

A *virus* is a molecular particle that enters your bloodstream. As soon as your immune system detects it, specific *leukocytes* (white blood cells) rush to the scene, where they attempt to kill the virus particles before they can penetrate a cell, corrupt it, and make you sick. These white knights consist of phagocytes that literally chew up the invaders and lymphocytes that create the antibodies needed to destroy the virus (B cells produce the antibodies, and a group of T cells, called natural killer cells, do the deed).

Sometimes, however, the immune system doesn't quite do its job. It either fails to attack with the fury needed to evict invaders or it mistakenly identifies the good guys as the enemy and literally attacks itself. When this happens, you develop an autoimmune system disorder, which some researchers believe may be the root of CFS.

Please note, though, that the autoimmune connection to CFS is not yet a significant area of research, and there is still limited evidence to support it.

Triggering Your Immune System . . . or Not

A healthy immune system accurately identifies enemy invaders and mounts a successful attack to purge them from your system. Fever, nasal discharge, diarrhea, vomiting, and most of the other symptoms you suffer from when you're ill are often signs that your immune system is busy killing bad guys and kicking them out of your body.

Your immune system is made up of white blood cells and T cells, some of which are called *natural killers* (NK), which swoop down on invading bacteria and viruses to kill them dead. In the following sections, I discuss your immune system in depth — and how it relates to CFS.

Stressing out your immune system (physically or emotionally)

When you're stressed out with work-related problems, issues at school, or emotional turmoil at home, or you're burning the candle at both ends, you're more susceptible to developing a cold, flu, or other malady. Your immune system, tired of trying to keep up with you, lets down its guard, and the enemy gains ground.

Because CFS may be linked with a dysfunction of the immune system, it is no surprise that an overworked, under-rested body may trigger or worsen CFS symptoms.

For tips on how to minimize stressors in your life or the life of a loved one, flip to Part III.

Looking for sleep in all the wrong places

What's sleep got to do with CFS? Plenty. Researchers have found that that the majority of people with CFS have sleep problems, either too little, poor quality, or too much. When you haven't had a good night's sleep in a long time, an immune-regulating protein called a *cytokine* (a precursor of inflammation) increases, and the number of natural killer cells (one of the generals in the immune system) decreases. Further, a lack of sleep may create stress or exacerbate it. Too much stress combined with a vulnerable immune system may make you susceptible to CFS.

Unfortunately, you can't cure CFS simply by catching up on your sleep, but developing a healthier sleep schedule and working with your doctor to address your sleep problems could possibly help. In Chapter 11, I provide some advice on how to get the optimum amount of sleep.

Looking into the hormone–immune system relationship

Hormones are chemicals produced by your body (anyone who went through puberty is well aware of a hormone's affect on the human body); various organs produce different hormones depending on the messages they receive from the brain. These hormones and certain organs make up what is called the *endocrine system*.

When you have prolonged stress in your life, certain hormones, such as *adrenaline* (produced in the adrenal glands), and *cytokines* (proteins that affect immunity) become imbalanced. The result? A dysfunctional immune system or inflammation.

Hormones are also responsible for stimulating the production of antibodies to fend off germs. Your thymus, located in your chest just behind your breast bone, produces a hormone called *thymosin* that stimulates the production of the white blood cells that create these antibodies. Another hormone produced by white blood cells (and other cells) is *interleukin*. Many hormones have a name and number, and interleukins are no exception. Interleukin-1, commonly referred to as IL-1, produces an interesting side effect on the hypothalamus in the brain, triggering fever and fatigue (for more on the hypothalamus, see the section "Gland-standing with the HPA axis" in this chapter). Some studies have shown that low amounts of Interleukin-6 (IL-6), which is intricately involved in the inflammation process, may be associated with CFS.

Straining your hormones to the point of shifting

When your body or your mind are traumatized by stressors — physical, psychological, or emotional — your body's hormone levels can begin to fluctuate out of their normal ranges. As a result, your immune system may begin to malfunction, either by shutting itself down or by overreacting. In either case, the malfunction may produce symptoms similar to those of CFS, or possibly trigger CFS.

One of the most common causes of hives (swollen areas of the skin that itch intensely) is anxiety. If anxiety alone can trigger your immune system to release enough histamine to make your skin swell and itch, just imagine how tired it can make you feel when your immune system is constantly waging war against known enemies and anything it mistakenly identifies as an enemy.

Gland-standing with the HPA axis

Your hypothalamus, along with your pituitary and adrenal glands, are what doctors like to call the *HPA axis*. When your HPA axis malfunctions, you may be tempted to call it the axis of evil.

Your *hypothalamus* is a structure at the base of your brain that controls appetite and body temperature and sends signals to the pituitary gland via hormonal (chemical) messengers. Your pituitary gland is considered the puppet master of the endocrine (hormone) system, because it releases hormones that control the function of the ovaries, testes, adrenals, and thyroid glands; the pituitary hormones trigger the production of hormones in these glands, which, in turn, fuel their functions.

For example, the hypothalamus tells the pituitary gland to produce *corticotrophin* (a neurotransmitter, or brain messenger), which then stimulates the adrenal glands to produce *cortisol* — a hormone that suppresses inflammation and stress. In some patients with CFS, doctors have observed an abnormally low level of cortisol in the blood (hypocortisolism). Some researchers believe that the low cortisol levels contribute to the onset of CFS symptoms and may indicate a malfunctioning of the immune system somewhere in the HPA axis.

Inflammation is hot

One of today's medical buzzwords is *inflammation,* which research has shown plays a leading role in such conditions as Alzheimer's disease and heart disease. Basically, inflammation is your body's way of fending off viruses and bacteria; it stands guard against new intruders and helps heal injuries.

Sometimes, however, the inflammation doesn't go away. It becomes chronic. The result? An immune system breakdown. Currently, studies are being done to see whether inflammation is at the root of autoimmune illnesses in which antibodies attack healthy cells. Researchers suspect that chronic inflammation may play a significant role in rheumatoid arthritis, lupus, and possibly CFS.

Some CFS specialists consider CFS to be similar to a mild form of Addison's disease — a condition characterized by dizziness when standing, weakness, and fatigue. Patients with Addison's disease usually have lower levels of cortisol in their blood than the levels found in some people with CFS, but various traditional treatments for Addison's disease could be helpful for some CFS patients.

Blaming your period (or lack thereof)

While I've probably already scared any men away from this section by using the word *period* in the heading, hear this: This section is geared toward women. However, if you're a man that's the least bit curious or you want to help a loved one, then by all means, please keep reading.

The fact that CFS affects four times more women than men is an interesting phenomenon. Women wrestle with fluctuating hormone levels every month, some women more than others. Any woman knows what these wild fluctuations do to her body — how they affect her overall health and well-being and what they do to her energy levels. Given the connection between hormones and CFS, most men (who don't have to deal with hormones on a regular basis) may struggle to understand it.

In *perimenopause* (those five or six years leading up to full-blown menopause) and *menopause* (the stage of a woman's life in which her body stops producing estrogen, which stops menstruation and, therefore, makes her incapable of having children), hormone levels can affect women even more than usual. In the following, you can see how the hormonal changes a woman naturally goes through can be quite similar (if not identical) or potentially connected to CFS:

- **Estrogen levels:** Lower estrogen levels can trigger many of the same symptoms observed in CFS patients, including fatigue, headaches, dizziness, lack of concentration, insomnia, depression, and anxiety. A small number of studies have shown that some women with CFS have low estrogen levels. Because of these low levels, and decreased physical activity, women with CFS may be at greater risk for osteoporosis.

- **FSH levels:** Higher FSH (follicle-stimulating hormone) levels can result in hot flashes, night sweats, and flushing, symptoms that have been reported by some women with CFS.

- **Period irregularity:** Women who have CFS or have had CFS in the past - may suffer from irregular periods and even amenorrhea (which means your period stops).

Is it menopause or CFS? As you can see in the preceding list, the symptoms often look alike. One clue is that women in menopause may also have vaginal dryness, a condition that isn't regularly reported by women with CFS.

Other gynecological conditions, which are also common in women without CFS, have been found in women with CFS and may be possible explanation for unexplained symptoms., such as the following:

- *Endometriosis,* a condition in which uterine-lining tissue (the endometrium) is found outside the uterus, has been found in 20 percent of women with CFS.

- Loss of libido was also found in 20 percent of women with CFS.

- Fibroids and ovarian cysts have also been found to be more common in, you guessed it, women with CFS.

- Premenstrual syndrome (PMS) and menopause may trigger or exacerbate CFS symptoms in susceptible women — those who may already have immune system and/or hormonal imbalances. Women who are already vulnerable are standing targets for their imbalances to become worse.

Although CFS may be linked to other gynecological health issues, doctors and patients need to be careful not to confuse the two. One of the best ways to rule out gynecological issues is to visit your gynecologist for an accurate diagnosis and effective treatment.

Troubleshooting your electrical system: Autonomic nervous system dysregulation

Without your autonomic nervous system, you wouldn't last long. Your *autonomic nervous system* (ANS) controls all critical body functions, so you don't even have to think about them. Even when you're fast asleep, your ANS is hard at work keeping you alive.

So, if your ANS does such a great job, why am I mentioning it? Because your ANS, like everything else in your body, can malfunction. And some studies show that CFS patients often have some degree of ANS dysfunction, which typically appears in the form of *orthostatic instability* — a temporary drop in blood pressure when you stand up that may make you dizzy or lightheaded.

How likely that ANS dysregulation is a cause of CFS is still hotly debated, but it may contribute to the onset and perpetuation of symptoms.

Physical Trauma and CFS: Covering the Aftermath

When Sheila slipped on some ice in front of her house, she knew she was in for a long, painful recovery. She'd broken her leg, and the whole right side of her body was covered in bruises. But she assumed that in a few months, when her bones and muscles were fully healed, she'd be fine. She didn't expect the extreme fatigue, the low-grade fever, or the depression.

In the following sections, I explore the potential CFS link to physical trauma — from actual bumps and bruises to serious infections.

Exposing the link to physical trauma

When you fall and hit your head, you expect a headache and possibly some brain injury. When you break a bone, you expect a cast or crutches and a few weeks of pain. But CFS? No way! Of course, you probably know that physical trauma can stress you out emotionally, and that emotional or mental stress can play havoc with your body chemistry and immunity, but that's usually a short-term thing. After you recover, you rarely expect to see any lingering post-trauma symptoms.

Although physical trauma is thought to be more rare than other potential CFS links, a connection appears to exist in some cases. Physical pain can lead to insomnia, depression, cardiovascular problems, diminished brain power, and changes on a cellular level — all red flags for CFS.

Musculoskeletal disorders (MSDs) can be a result of physical stress and are often work related; they don't include slips, falls, or accidents. MSDs affect the muscles, nerves, tendons, joints, and the lower back. Although MSDs such as carpal tunnel syndrome, tendonitis, and sciatica aren't symptoms of CFS, the ensuing pain, repetitive stress, and disability can agitate your emotions, your immune system, and your body chemistry . . . and may possibly indirectly lead to CFS.

Investigating postconcussive syndrome disorder

If you've ever watched a crime show on television, you know what a concussion is — a brain injury resulting from an accident or fight. Postconcussive syndrome can occur days or weeks after a minor head injury. Its symptoms are the same as with major brain injury, including cognitive impairment, fatigue, emotional confusion, and mood swings. Unfortunately, like CFS, post-concussive syndrome disorder doesn't always show up on brain scans. But because it can create neurological impairment in the brain or spinal cord, the syndrome may, in actuality, be CFS. Neurological damage sparks changes in the chemistry and cellular pathways of the central nervous system.

Triggers and susceptibility are only possibilities; no proof exists. People can't know whether they are susceptible anyway, because you can't find any tests to prove susceptibility. It's misleading to point people in the direction of searching whether or not they are susceptible and living in fear that just about anything triggers CFS.

Paining away: Muscle and joint pain

Aching muscles and joints are common signposts of both fibromyalgia and CFS, which frequently leads to misdiagnoses of one or the other condition. But can muscle and joint pain cause CFS? The short answer is maybe. Doctors don't know this for certain. If the pain is a result of physical trauma, the repetitive motions of carpal tunnel syndrome, or the pain of a herniated disc, then the pain may also signal CFS.

Muscle and joint pain alone aren't definitive signs of CFS. They can be signs of another condition, such as fibromyalgia. Only a full medical workup for CFS can deliver an accurate diagnosis. Find out more about proper diagnosis in Chapter 6.

Finding a link in hidden infections

"Oh, it's just a virus." "I have the flu." "After a couple of antibiotics, I'll be fine." Almost everyone has uttered these dismissive statements when they weren't feeling up to par. But sometimes what's supposed to go away in a week or two ends up lingering . . . and lingering. And instead of steadily feeling better, you feel worse — tired, achy, and dizzy. These enduring symptoms may be early symptoms of CFS.

A viral infection can ravage your body — impairing cellular structure and function, throwing your immune system out of kilter, and physically damaging your internal organs. But can a viral infection cause CFS? It appears that this is a possibility.

Riding the train to postconcussive syndrome

The postconcussive syndrome diagnosis got its start in the 1860s, around the time when Freud was examining the symptoms of hysteria. This period also ushered in the early days of railroad travel — when passengers were subjected to frequent collisions and sudden stops.

These mishaps often resulted in frequent headaches, fatigue, depression, and confusion — all symptoms of postconcussive syndrome disorder. Physicians couldn't dismiss every case as "all in the head." Some of the people had to suffer from some sort of brain or spinal cord injury, which was dubbed as postconcussive syndrome.

Known viruses (such as EBV, Ross-River virus, and HHV-6) can undergo adaptations that allow them to hide from the immune system. When they undergo this type of adaptation and behave secretly, they may be referred to as *stealth viruses.* All of these viruses have been implicated as a possible cause of CFS. These stealth-adapted viruses literally sneak up on your body. Usually, when a virus enters your bloodstream and tries to enter a cell, your immune system's antibodies descend on it like a pack of wolves. But stealth-adapted viruses are able to hide themselves from the antibodies. They do their cellular damage on the sly. Think of the Trojan Horse that housed all those soldiers, and you can have a pretty good idea of how these stealth viruses work.

Because stealth-adapted viruses are so skilled at playing the subcellular version of hide-and-go-seek, some of them often remain undetected even after an all-out attack by your immune system. Long after you recover from your more intense illness, just enough of the virus can hang around in your system to make you feel subpar. Some scientists believe that these persistent critters put the *chronic* in CFS.

Although stealth-adapted viruses (and certain bacteria) are experts at hiding from your immune system, researchers have done a pretty thorough job of finding and identifying them:

- **The human herpes virus 6 (HHV-6)**, the cause of roseola in babies, destroys your body's natural killer (NK) cells, the first line of defense against a virus. HHV-6 is different from other herpes viruses because it doesn't lay dormant with periodic or intermittent bouts of activity. Instead, it becomes activated when you have any dysfunction in your immune system.

- **Mycoplasma** is a minute bacteria that has been associated with urinary tract infections and pneumonia and may also be linked to CFS.

- ✔ **Parvovirus B19**, an infection that can cause anemia, nerve damage, and even miscarriage, may be associated with CFS.

- ✔ **Brucella**, found primarily in animals, is an infectious bacteria that can be transmitted to humans via unpasteurized dairy products. Although rare, especially in the United States, people infected with this bacteria may have chronic fatigue, joint pain, and low-grade fevers.

- ✔ **Chlamydia pneumoniae** generally attacks the lining of the arteries and the respiratory system. High amounts of the bacteria have been found in some people with CFS in at least one pilot study.

- ✔ **Bartonella**, the bacteria often associated with cat scratch fever, may also be linked to CFS. Many people with CFS have cats, and studies at the Pasteur Institute in France and the Cleveland Clinic Foundation in Ohio found a connection between cat scratch incidents and CFS symptoms.

- ✔ **Spirochetal** is the bacteria transmitted to people when bitten by the Ixodes (deer) tick. This bacteria causes Lyme disease in susceptible people. Lyme disease is both a separate condition and a possible cause of CFS, and careful diagnosis is critical.

Inspecting Environmental Toxins and Allergens

A study published in the *Journal of Allergy and Clinical Immunology* found that people with CFS are more susceptible to and have more allergies than their healthy counterparts. Allergens in the environment, from pollen to dander, and various toxins, including mercury and lead, may play a role in CFS in the same way that infections do. Your immune system not only launches attacks on enemy invader viruses, but it can also overreact to allergens, which it often mistakenly identifies as invaders, causing you all sorts of misery.

Although people with allergies and asthma typically escape the throes of CFS, these conditions can exacerbate CFS symptoms, especially severe fatigue. In this section, I discuss some of these external cues.

Filling your lungs with polluted air

Pollution can make the least sensitive person gag. For someone who is sensitive to toxic air, it can make life miserable, causing everything from a runny nose and burning eyes to breathing difficulties — all of which may trigger CFS-like symptoms.

Rhinitis, an allergy symptom that may come from airborne allergens, creating a runny nose, has been found to disrupt sleep in 20 to 30 percent of the population. Some CFS specialists think that the disruption in sleep pattern, rather than the allergy itself, may bring about CFS-like symptoms.

Exposing yourself to on-the-job toxins

Dust bunnies. Spray paints. Magic marker pens. Lead. The work environment is filled with potential allergy-inducing triggers. Can the fumes you inhale on a factory line or the recycled office air that engulfs you for eight hours every day trigger CFS? The jury is still out on this question, but doctors do know that on-the-job toxins can cause respiratory illness and allergies with symptoms very similar to CFS — fatigue, achy muscles, and a scratchy throat.

Sucking in the smoke: Cigars and cigarettes

Smoking is a drag, and recent research has revealed a direct link between smoking and the onset of asthma. Whether smoking has a direct influence on other allergies or contributes to the onset of CFS remains unknown, but the fact remains that smoking is a stimulant that can often prevent restful sleep and increase fatigue over time.

If you smoke, stop. Smoking just aggravates your CFS symptoms. Studies have found that second-hand smoke can be just as bad for you as smoking, so steer clear of the smoker hangouts, too. Whether the toxins come from smog, recycled air, or tobacco smoke, they can create conditions conducive to worsening your symptoms.

Experiencing hypersensitivity to chemicals

Your body is a chemical factory, but certain chemicals can throw your system for a loop, especially heavy metals. Some nutritionists suspect that low levels of heavy metals, including lead and mercury, may be responsible for at least some cases of CFS. In fact, one study found that 57–67 percent of patients with CFS have had at least one episode of symptoms after being exposed to certain chemicals, including lead.

Because your body isn't specifically equipped to rid heavy metals from your system, some nutritionists and alternative health care providers recommend a process called *chelation,* designed to leach the toxins from your system. No reliable studies have proven, however, that chelation is an effective treatment for CFS. Treating your condition with chelation can also be quite dangerous to your health to boot, especially if done unnecessarily or improperly .

Coming up short of breath: The asthma link

Asthma is a chronic condition (typically caused by a sensitivity to airborne allergens) that causes tightening of the airway passages and lungs leading to breathing difficulties. Studies show that breathing difficulties are more prevalent in people with CFS than the rest of the population.

Although the anecdotal results provide no clear evidence of a link between asthma and CFS, researchers continue to explore the possibility. Asthma is related to immune system dysfunction, and CFS might be as well. Further research may hold the key to understanding the root cause of various types of immune system dysfunction.

Emotional Stress and CFS: Recognizing the Signs

Many people with CFS can trace the onset of their symptoms to an emotional trauma, such as the following:

- Death of a loved one
- Divorce or relationship issues
- Financial woes
- Problem child
- Loss of job or demotion
- Caring for a needy loved one

Emotionally devastating events or situations can have long-term physical effects. They have the power of rippling through your system and causing long-term health problems. They contribute to chronic stress — which, in turn, may make you vulnerable to CFS.

Emotional distress can make you anxious, depressed, restless, and moody. Can that lead to CFS? The jury is still out, but these symptoms do fuel flames of stress and make your immune system more vulnerable.

Don't dismiss emotionally draining events or situations when searching for the cause of your CFS. Emotional trauma can be as powerful as any physical trauma you may experience.

Emotions can also play a strong role in your successful recovery from CFS or at least in the relief of symptoms. In Chapter 8, I introduce you to various therapies that can assist you in your emotional recovery.

Can You Prevent the Onset of CFS?

After you have CFS, preventing it becomes a moot point. However, if you have a history of CFS in your family, it makes sense to take some precautions, just in case there is a link. Living a healthy lifestyle (see Part III of this book) and reducing the stress in your life — at work, home, school, and in other areas of your life — are ways you can help alleviate symptoms.

As for avoiding physical stressors, including infections, physical trauma, airborne allergens, environmental toxins, and tick bites, you can try your hardest and still experience a shock to your system that's of a sufficient magnitude to potentially trigger the onset of CFS. The best guidance I can provide is to follow the advice of almost every doctor on the planet — eat right, get plenty of rest, exercise, and figure out how to deal with stress. Even if you follow that advice to the letter, however, CFS may still find a way of grabbing hold of you.

You may not be able to avoid all physical, emotional, and mental trauma that appear to play a role in CFS, but you can work toward developing a more low-stress environment. The Chapters in Part III can assist you and your family in developing a low-stress environment that may decrease the possibility of getting CFS.

Chapter 4

Finding Comfort in Numbers: You're Not Alone

• •

In This Chapter

▶ Discovering the vital statistics surrounding CFS

▶ Highlighting at-risk groups

▶ Shining the CFS spotlight on men and children

▶ Peering into future CFS treatments

• •

*J*ust talk to someone who has CFS or has experienced a major depressive episode, and they can give you all the usual lines: "I'm helpless." "I feel hopeless." "I have no energy." People with CFS are often reluctant to say so or seek help because they feel that others may think they're weird. Loved ones may tell them to "snap out of it" or "you're just being lazy."

If you have CFS, these ignorant, insensitive one-liners are exactly what you don't need to hear. What you need to hear is that you're not alone and that CFS is very real. In this chapter, I reveal the statistics and other data to help you prove it. I point out the high-risk groups, shed light on the low-risk groups, and then look ahead to the promising future prospects of CFS treatments and possibly even a cure.

In this chapter and throughout this book, I provide information on the latest research to improve the diagnosis of CFS and its treatment. New discoveries are constantly popping up on the radar, however, so don't stop learning about CFS after reading this book. Check out Chapter 16 to know how to stay up to date with CFS studies.

Examining the Epidemiology and Studying the Statistics

Epidemiological research — studies that examine large groups of people over a period of time — paints a more accurate portrait of CFS. The info gleaned from these studies can be invaluable in estimating the prevalence of CFS, projecting an individual's risk for contracting it, identifying symptoms, guiding diagnosis, and predicting the treatment outcome.

Early on, for example, researchers estimated that about 3,000 to 10,000 people in the United States had CFS. With results from later studies looking at the population, the Centers for Disease Control and Prevention (CDC) now estimates the number at over 1 million. As more studies are performed, researchers anticipate even higher estimates. This is just one example of how research is continuing to change and improve people's understanding and awareness of CFS.

Fukuda's CFS diagnostic criteria

In 1994, the definition for CFS was refined, and the new definition was named after its leading researcher, Keiji Fukuda. CFS specialists still use the new definition as the basis for the majority of CFS studies. The Fukuda definition classifies CFS as the following:

✔ Unexplained, persistent chronic fatigue that isn't the result of ongoing exertion, that isn't lifelong, that isn't alleviated by rest, and that results in a substantial reduction of regular activity: occupational, educational, social, or personal.

✔ Fatigue that has lasted for over six months with four or more of these concurrent symptoms (that didn't start prior to the extreme fatigue):

  • Impairment of short-term memory or concentration

  • Sore throat

  • Tender lymph nodes in the neck or armpits

  • Muscle pain

  • Joint pain — without swelling or redness

  • Headache — that is a different type and has a different pattern or severity

  • Nonrefreshing sleep

  • Energy drain that lasts more than 24 hours after exertion

Sound familiar? If you read Chapter 2, you may notice that Fukuda's definition is the same diagnostic criteria that the CDC uses to identify bona fide cases of CFS. (For more about these diagnostic criteria and other symptoms often associated with CFS, check out Chapter 2.)

There's safety in numbers, or so the saying goes. With an illness that is difficult to diagnose, there's recognition in them there numbers to boot. Since CFS became "legitimate" in 1988, when the CDC gave the illness its name, several landmark studies have hit the streets, pinpointing the who, what, where, and when of the illness.

Epidemiological studies often differ from or seem to contradict one another because population groups studied are difficult to control completely. However, the more results researches gather, the more accurate the estimates become.

The epidemiological studies for CFS are fairly recent and are considered groundbreaking because so little real data was available before the results were published. In this section, I give you the basic findings of the studies, and you discover, in plain black and white, the evidence you need that you're indeed not alone.

Riding the Chicago–Wichita line

Wichita, Kansas, and Chicago, Illinois, have a lot more in common than the fact that they're two major Midwestern cities. These cities have been the sites for two landmark epidemiological studies of CFS in the general population. (See Figure 4-1 and 4-2 for specific details and comparisons of these two studies.)

Lacking CFS diagnoses in Wichita

In 2003, researchers traveled to Wichita to determine how many people had CFS. After studying 100,000 adults over the age of 18 via diagnostic screenings and telephone interviews, they discovered that:

- Out of the 100,000 people, 235 had CFS.
- CFS was four times more common in women than men.
- CFS was most common among Caucasian women ages 50–59.
- Only 16 percent of the individuals with CFS were diagnosed as having the illness.
- CFS lasted, on average, seven years.

If you look at Figure 4-1, you can see some of the results from the Wichita study, revealing that CFS is a significant health issue in the USA.

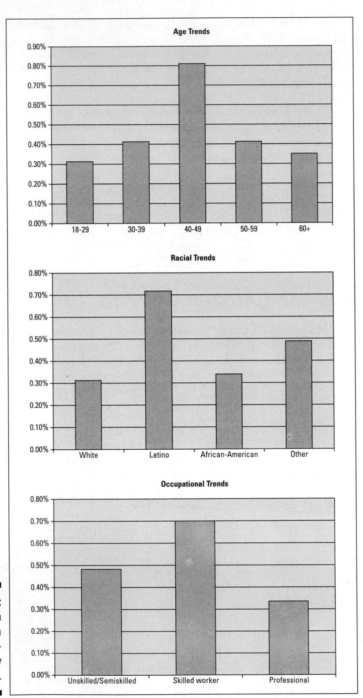

Figure 4-1: Results from the Wichita epidemiology study on CFS.

The conclusion: CFS is a major health problem in the United States. Granted, 235 people out of 100,000 isn't a huge number. That's a little shy of one quarter of 1 percent. The number that's so alarming is the 16 percent of people with CFS actually receiving a diagnosis and treatment. That means 84 percent of people with CFS are suffering in silence. Worse than that, they're suffering unnecessarily. What's even more insidious is the fact that even those people who have been diagnosed with CFS symptoms and are being treated symptomatically are still not provided with much relief!

Growing numbers in Chicago

A Chicago study, published in 1999, in the *Archives of Internal Medicine,* found similar results to those found in Wichita (see preceding section). Approximately 560 per 100,000 individuals had CFS. That's more than double the figure in the Wichita study, representing slightly more than half a percent of the population. Extrapolate that out to the entire population of the United States, and the number translates into about 1 million people.

The study also revealed that the highest levels of CFS were found consistently among women, minority groups, and persons with lower levels of education and low-paying jobs. The conclusion was that CFS is a common chronic health condition, especially for women, that occurs across ethnic groups. It was also contradicted earlier findings suggesting that CFS is a syndrome that primarily affects white, middle-class patients.

Check out Figure 4-2 for some of the findings in the Chicago epidemiology study on CFS.

The bottom line in the Wichita and Chicago studies? Too many people were going undiagnosed or misdiagnosed when it came to CFS.

Taking a global CFS census

Without statistics from other countries around the world, dismissing CFS as an illness that's isolated to a particular country is tempting. Maybe people in the United States simply aren't living right or eating right. Maybe the entire country is populated with hypochondriacs looking for a trendy illness to call their own. Maybe the evil pharmaceutical companies are just trying to sell more drugs.

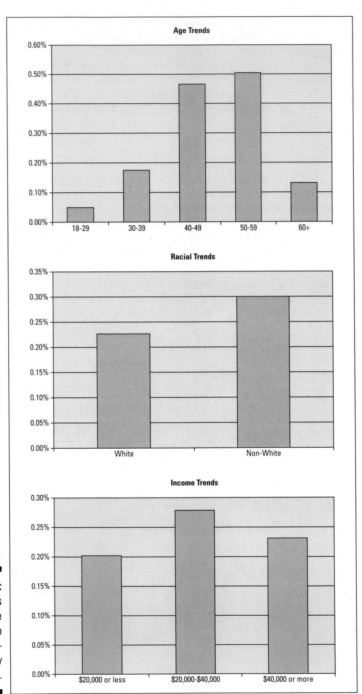

Figure 4-2:
The results
from the
Chicago
epidemi-
ology study
of CFS.

When you factor in the statistics from around the world, however, you find that countries other than the United States have an even bigger problem with undiagnosed cases of CFS. Studies performed in other countries show that CFS crosses the international borders:

- In Iceland, 1,400 of the 100,000 people questioned had symptoms of CFS. Because seasonal affective disorder (SAD) is associated with the chemical imbalances found in depression, as well as hormonal dysfunction, it may signal CFS. And, because Iceland and the other Scandinavian countries have so much darkness during winter, there may be a link between depression and SAD — and CFS. In fact, the typical symptoms of CFS in Iceland even have their own collective name: *Iceland disease!*

- A Hong Kong study in 2001 revealed that 3,000 of the 100,000 people surveyed reported having the symptoms associated with CFS.

- Australia jumped from 37 out of 100,000 cases in 1990 to 1,500 out of 100,000 cases of CFS in 1999.

- In Brazil, 2,000 of the 100,000 people surveyed were reported to have CFS.

- In Great Britain, the numbers have changed over the years, possibly due to different study methods. They jumped from a mere 6 out of 100,000 people with CFS symptoms in 1994 to 2,600 out of 100,000 in 1997. The latest figures, from 2004, show that 800 people out of 100,000 were found to have CFS.

- In the Far East, Japan had only 1 person out of 100,000 report to have CFS in 1996. Only two years later, that number grew to 1,500!

- In some countries, diagnoses of CFS -appear to be less prevalent. These countries include the Netherlands, where only 112 cases have been reported out of 100,000 people studied, and New Zealand, where only 127 people out of 100,000 were reported to have CFS.

CFS isn't some trumped-up illness that's isolated to the shorelines of the United States. Although CFS hasn't been proven to be contagious, this illness is somewhat of a pandemic, affecting people in all countries throughout the world. The less that is known about this often debilitating illness, the more people will suffer unnecessarily.

Profiling groups for CFS

Profiling, or "tagging" a person a certain way because of race or gender, is soooo politically incorrect when it comes to, say, stopping cars on the freeway, often leading to racism and exploited as a tool to enforce injustice. In epidemiology, however, profiling is essential for identifying groups of people who are more prone to contracting a specific illness. Epidemiological profiling assists doctors in providing more accurate diagnoses. Knowing, for instance, that CFS afflicts more women than men or children enables doctors to consider it less probable in some populations and give it more consideration in others.

Although CFS doesn't exclusively attack specific populations, women seem to contract this illness four times more than men, and CFS pretty much restricts itself to people over the age of 18. Women between the ages of 40 and 59 form the group believed to be most at risk. As I discuss later in this chapter, however, this statistic doesn't mean that men and children are immune to CFS.

Early major studies of CFS found that most people with CFS were Caucasian, middle-aged, middle-class women who were well educated. Why? Because most of the data came from clinics and hospitals, the very places where well-educated Caucasian, middle-aged, middle-class women go when they're sick. But they didn't rule out the possibility that CFS is more widespread.

More recent studies, such as the CDC investigation of 13 counties in the state of Georgia, have shown that CFS may be found in all races, all economic levels, and all levels of education. In its Georgia study, for example, the CDC broadened its population scope and found that CFS was even more prevalent in minorities, specifically African Americans, Latinos, and Native Americans. The people in this study were also from a lower socioeconomic bracket — had a yearly income of $40,000 and under. They also found that it isn't just white, middle-class women who are most affected with CFS. Why is that, you ask? It's a hard, cold truth: Minorities have less access to the United States health care system than Caucasians. The predominance of Caucasian women with CFS in prior studies only shows that CFS was being under-diagnosed and under-reported in other populations.

When researchers perform controlled studies of CFS, in which socioeconomic status, ethnicity, gender, age, and marital and parental status are accounted for (to level the playing field), ethnicity seems to have much less influence over which group is at a higher risk. Experts believe that the risk of contracting CFS is more a question of income. The reason why CFS shows up in lower-income minority households is more likely due to economic, environmental, or social factors: poor nutrition, limited medical access, unemployment, discrimination, and the stress brought on by poverty.

Reconciling the results

So is there a CFS profile? As mentioned earlier in this chapter, profiling can be dangerous — and it is here, in studies of CFS. Yes, CFS seems to affect middle-class, white women. On the other hand, as other studies show, it can also affect minority women, women of different economic status, women of different races, men, the elderly, the young, and people all over the world. The result? You can't find one, complete, final answer. The best way to determine whether you have CFS is by reading this book, reading research on the Web, looking at other potential causes of your CFS-like symptoms, and consulting with your doctor. Go to a doctor who will work to get you a good diagnosis so you can get proper treatment. (For more on finding a physician, head to Chapter 5.)

Underestimating the Real Numbers

Like a complex maze, CFS has many characteristics that make it difficult to pin down. When you add in the human factor — the fact that people who have CFS often have trouble identifying their symptoms as CFS or may be reluctant to admit they feel lousy — survey results become more like a murky swamp than a complex maze.

Although a portrait of the CFS patient is becoming clearer, many questions remain unanswered. Who is more "ill" — those with gradual onset or sudden onset CFS? Who may have CFS, but is blaming overtime at the office instead? Who thinks she has CFS, but really has a common condition that mimics CFS, such as Lyme disease or fibromyalgia? In the following sections, I wade through the swamp of misconceptions to reveal some clarity buried in the muck.

Staying in the closet: Under-reporting by patients

The results of every study on CFS have to be taken with a grain of salt, because many individuals with CFS are compelled to hang out in the closet. The fact that's out of the closet is that only 16 percent of the people with CFS have been diagnosed. This means that at least 80 percent of people with CFS are not only undiagnosed, but they're not getting the treatment they need! Why does this happen? Several reasons come to mind, including the following:

✔ **No access to medical help.** In rural areas where the closest hospital is over 100 miles away, people may be unwilling to seek medical treatment, especially for conditions that they think are merely mood related, a bad flu, or overwork. A lack of quality health insurance may also be an obstacle to seeking treatment. If someone has to pay over $50 out of pocket just to step into the doctor's office, costs can quickly add up for the many visits required for an accurate CFS diagnosis. Even if a person does seek treatment, she may give up after the third or fourth visit.

✔ **Type A personalities.** Overachievers tend to think that they can work through anything and therefore put off seeking medical help. A woman executive may think, "Sure, I'm exhausted and my throat hurts. But that's because I'm working too hard . . . burning the candle too brightly at both ends. I have too much stress in my life, in the office, and at home. After life settles down, I'll feel much better."

✔ **Immigrant status.** Maybe you've recently come to America. Maybe your English is limited. For example, researchers are finding that immigrant Latinos in the USA are much more likely to get CFS than other minority groups. They're also much less likely to seek medical care.

✔ **Minority report.** Unfortunately, America still has a fair share of discrimination, which often manifests itself through poor health care, poor living conditions, and poor education. Further, people from some cultural backgrounds are less likely to complain about feeling ill, especially if that illness involves more nebulous symptoms, such as fatigue, weakness, and depression.

✔ **Male machismo.** Not to pick on men, but most guys equate fatigue and muscle aches with weakness. Even when they have another serious illness, they're less likely than women to visit the doctor for advice, if they even have a doctor.

Misdiagnosing the real cause: Under-reporting by doctors

A doctor isn't a mind reader. Yes, doctors are trained to read between the lines, ask the right questions, and be health detectives who put all their knowledge and experience into each patient. But, still, if you don't tell your doctor you've been exhausted for the past three months, or if you have a history of exaggerating your symptoms, she may miss something.

In order for a doctor to do the best she can for you, you have to let her know what's really going on. If necessary, bring a piece of paper with you describing your symptoms and the medications you take. Another tool I suggest to my patients is to keep a medical diary — tracking your symptoms, the times of day that they occur, and your emotional state. Together, you and your doctor can find out what ails you, but only with your help.

Write down a list of your symptoms. Bring the list along to your next doctor's visit and share it with your doctor. In addition, jot down a list of the current medications you're taking. The more information your doctor has about your current condition, the more she can assist you in sorting out your symptoms and offering an accurate diagnosis (for more on diagnosing CFS, see Chapter 6).

CFS has another element to it — what I call the all-in-your-head phenomenon. For years doctors scoffed at CFS, not believing that CFS is a verifiable illness. After all, doctors have no X-ray, no blood test, no physical, and no electrocardiogram that functions as a definitive diagnostic tool. Frustrated by an inability to find a specific physical cause for CFS, doctors were driven to write it off as a psychological malady. Early approaches to CFS were similar to the medical community's early approach to treating many brain disorders, such as depression.

And, because many people suffering from CFS are depressed, unable to get around, their minds in a fog, *all* the signs point to a mental illness, not a physical one. Even worse, CFS is easily misdiagnosed because so many conditions have similar symptoms. When you think about it, you're probably amazed that CFS gets diagnosed at all!

Today, doctors have evidence that shows potential biological indicators that CFS exists — markers in genetic structure, in the immune and central nervous systems, and in the brain chemistry that red flag its existence. The evidence shows dysfunction in multiple body systems — enough to show that something is wrong *somewhere,* but no definitive marker or indicator has been identified. Even armed with the latest research findings, many doctors are still in the dark. Your best bet is to become proactive. Find out what you can about your symptoms and their duration, and then see a specialist. In Chapter 5, I provide strategies and tips for tracking down the best doctor in your area for diagnosing and treating CFS.

Singling Out Women

CFS has a thing for women, particularly women between the ages of 40 and 59. Nobody knows why for sure. Doctors and researchers surmise that the complex hormonal machinery of females may make them more susceptible. Another possibility is that women simply are less likely to put up with discomfort. They recognize when they're not feeling right, and instead of denying it or suffering with it, they do something about it — they head to their doctor. (Of course, I would never imply that a preponderance of men deny or try to suffer through pain, but you can draw whatever inference you choose.)

When the go-to go-getter got CFS

Eileen was a real go-getter. Everyone in the neighborhood knew that if they needed something done, Eileen was the go-to person. She organized parent-teacher nights at school, never missed her kids' soccer games, volunteered to assist students with learning difficulties to learn how to read, and was just one of those people who never said no when a member of the community asked for help.

When she first experienced her fatigue, it was sudden and sharp. She had gotten up out of bed at her usual time, 6:00 a.m., ready to wake her kids, when she felt dizzy. Her whole body felt like lead. She felt as though an invisible force was pushing her back into bed. She was so tired!

Her husband helped get the kids ready for school. He also called her doctor and made an appointment for that afternoon. He worked for the town government, so it was easy for him to drive Eileen to the doctor himself.

The doctor examined Eileen's heart. He listened to her breathe. He checked her ears, eyes, and nose. He took a blood sample. Nothing. The exam and test results showed that Eileen was perfectly healthy. He gently suggested some antidepressants and that Eileen pare back her schedule.

Eileen did more than that — she had no choice. Her symptoms grew worse and worse. She was dizzy whenever she tried to get up, she forgot why she'd walked into a room, and she was exhausted after putting away a single bag of groceries. The antidepressants didn't seem to be doing anything. She felt more depressed than ever.

One of Eileen's friends told her about CFS. Her friend had a cousin who suffered from it and was on disability. Soon Eileen was researching the illness on the Web. At last! She had a name to put to her symptoms. It wasn't in her head.

Eileen found the name of a specialist through that same friend. With the right treatment and lifestyle changes, Eileen was able to resume most of her activities. A year later, like the sun coming out after a storm, her energy slowly returned and she was getting back to being herself.

Whatever the reason, CFS seems to afflict about four times more women than men. In a way, that can be a good thing for women. A doctor is more likely to consider CFS as a possibility in a woman than in a man. In other words, if you're a woman complaining of fatigue, muscle pain, joint pain, and other symptoms characteristic of CFS (see Chapter 2), you're more likely than a man to receive an accurate diagnosis and treatment — if you're visiting a health care professional who isn't skeptical about CFS. Call me sexist, but that's the way it is. In this section, I cover those factors that primarily affect women and can contribute to the reason why women (more than men) are more often diagnosed with CFS.

Factoring in pregnancy

Although I've heard some futuristic discussions on the possibility of male pregnancy, currently only women get pregnant, and when a woman who has CFS gets pregnant, the pregnancy can alter the course of the illness, often worsening it, but sometimes improving it.

The chart shown in Figure 4-3 illustrates the data collected in a study that examined the effects of pregnancy on the dynamics of CFS. This 2003 study, published in the *Archives of Internal Medicine,* points to a hormonal link to CFS.

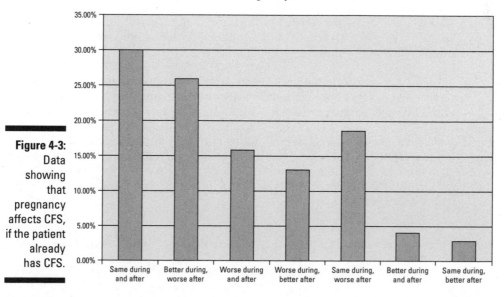

Pregnancy's Effect on CFS

Figure 4-3:
Data showing that pregnancy affects CFS, if the patient already has CFS.

Stimulating the thyroid discussion

Women (more than men) are vulnerable to thyroid problems. Either the thyroid is producing too much of a particular hormone, as in the case of *hyperthyroidism*, or it's producing too little, as in the case of *hypothyroidism*. Hypothyroidism often causes similar symptoms to those of CFS, such as fatigue, irritability, and lack of energy, so women who suspect that they may have CFS should first have their thyroid hormone levels checked in a blood test to rule out a possible thyroid condition.

You can have a thyroid condition *and* CFS. If your doctor diagnoses hypothyroidism and provides treatment, but your systems persist, have your levels checked again. If your thyroid hormones are at normal levels, and you're still feeling miserable, CFS may be the cause.

If your CFS symptoms last more than ten years, you may have other conditions, some that also mimic CFS and can be precursors to it, including shingles, fibromyalgia, IBS, major depression, mono, anemia, cardiac arrhythmia, chronic bladder infection, chronic bronchitis, and asthma. See Chapter 3 for details about these and other conditions that mimic and sometimes interact with CFS.

Putting up with pain

Who puts up with pain more stoically — men or women? Obviously, it has a lot to do with the personality of the person, not the gender. However, women seem to open up about their pain more than men — whatever the intensity.

Scientists, researchers, and physicians have taken great pains (so to speak) to reveal the facts about pain, especially chronic pain. They've grouped the pain that most women or men feel into the following two categories:

- **Paroxysmal pain** occurs randomly and suddenly. This type of pain is intermittent, sharp, and jolting, but temporary, lasting from a few seconds to a few hours. However, periods of paroxysmal pain may be chronic in nature, as when a person has occurrences once a month for twenty years.

✔ **Chronic pain** is duller and lasts longer. This pain is like the fatigue you feel when you have CFS — it doesn't go away after six months.

The key word for women who suspect they have CFS is *chronic*.

Being a middle-aged woman: A double whammy

As a woman, if your thyroid doesn't get you, your menopause may step in and cause other hormonal problems. Menopausal, perimenopausal, and postmenopausal women often experience symptoms similar to those of CFS, such as fatigue, sleep dysfunction, and irritability, but these symptoms may not signal CFS. If a woman is very debilitated by her symptoms, they may be effectively relieved with short-term HRT (hormone replacement therapy).

The hormonal component to CFS in women is often supported by data that shows an increased incidence of the following conditions in women with CFS:

✔ **Endometriosis:** The tissue that lines the uterus travels to areas outside of the uterus.

✔ **Polycystic ovary syndrome:** Ovarian cysts interrupt normal ovulation and menstruation.

✔ **Night sweats:** Both menopause and CFS can cause night sweats. If you're menopausal with CFS, you get a double whammy, which may worsen the night sweats.

Lowering the age limit: Teens and young women

You don't have to be a middle-aged woman to be afflicted with CFS, but if you are a woman, the older you are, the more at risk you become. Young girls are typically less likely to succumb to CFS than older girls and "tweenagers." By the time a child becomes an adolescent, the rates of CFS start to climb. One Chicago study showed that out of 100,000 adolescents between the ages of 13 and 17, 181 experienced symptoms of severity and duration to qualify for a CFS diagnosis.

Although CFS is less common in adolescents than in older segments of the population, the repercussions of CFS can be much more dangerous. Teenagers, who already have a higher incidence of suicide than other age groups, may feel additional pressure from CFS. CFS can inhibit their fun, ruin their social life, expose them to teasing from peers, and negatively affect their classroom performance. An undiagnosed, untreated teenager is at serious risk of suffering a host of other problems.

Counting Heads in the Lower Risk Groups

Although CFS is more attracted to women than men, children, and the elderly, it can afflict anyone at any age. If you experience the symptoms described in Chapter 2, don't rule out CFS or let your doctor rule it out simply because you're not a 50-year-old woman.

In the following sections, I explore some of the groups that see a lower incidence of CFS — but see it nonetheless — and explain exactly why you may be at risk if you're in one of these groups.

No matter what your age or gender, visit your doctor regularly to identify any health conditions as early as possible. Early, effective treatment of other health conditions may be just what the doctor ordered to spare you from adding to your misery with a bad case of CFS.

Singling out seniors: Cranky old fart or CFS sufferer?

Seniors often look forward to the day when their kids move out for good and they can kick back and enjoy their golden years. These golden years, however, are often plagued with minor annoyances or nagging age-related conditions, including fatigue, memory loss, muscle pain, joint pain, and trouble sleeping. Sounds a lot like CFS, right?

While these symptoms may be common in seniors, and most seniors don't have CFS, you shouldn't rule out CFS entirely. Seniors, like any other group, can't be profiled, but it is possible that their fatigue, pain, and lack of energy are due to CFS. Does it matter? Not necessarily. Treatment will most likely be the same: antidepressants for depression, healthier lifestyle for energy, pain killers for aches and pains, and sleep aids for sleep dysfunction.

Hiding his tears: Emotion, men, and CFS

According to the most recent statistics, more than 266,000 men in the United States alone have CFS. As discussed earlier in this chapter, however, the real numbers are likely to be higher, because men are less likely to consult with their doctors about it.

One of the primary symptoms of CFS in men seems to be decreased libido (a lowered sex drive). That's no surprise, because when you feel tired, aching, and exhausted, your mojo is the first thing to roll out of bed. And when that happens, a good number of men seek other ways to solve the problem, including exercise, vitamins, and medications for erectile dysfunction. In some cases, these pursuits of other symptomatic remedies may prevent men from seeking a cure to their real problem — CFS.

Acting out: Children get CFS, too

Can younger kids get CFS? The jury is still out on this question. A study performed by researchers in Chicago found that zero kids from ages 5 to 12 had CFS. In Wichita, a similar study turned up 49 kids (ages 5 to 12) out of 100,000 surveyed who had CFS.

One theory behind the low numbers of children with CFS is that young children often internalize their distress. They feel the same discomfort adults feel — the exhaustion, pain, and general malaise — but because they don't really understand what's happening to them and they can't put a name on it, they express their discomfort in other ways. They may misbehave in school, fail to pay attention, refuse to do homework, and lash out at their classmates. In many cases, kids with CFS exhibit the same behaviors as children with ADHD or depression.

The descriptions of men and kids with CFS tend to be, overall, dismissive. Evidence is limited, but it appears (according to CFS practitioners, kids with CFS, and parents of kids with CFS) that kids with CFS often have symptoms that fluctuate greatly and change with more frequency than adults with CFS. Kids also appear to have more stomachaches, GI distress, and dysautonomia.

Peering into the Future for Potential Cures

Although CFS-like illnesses have probably been around since the dawn of humankind, its discovery is relatively recent. Researchers have only begun to scratch the surface by discovering the differences between people with CFS and those without.

Research results, however, are becoming more and more promising, and research is accelerating very quickly. The following list highlights some of the more promising discoveries and research currently in the works:

- **The length-of-illness connection:** The NIH (National Institutes of Health) and CDC are working together to study the course of the illness and how it changes over the short- and long-term.

- **The neuroendocrine connection:** Some researchers are probing the neuroendocrine system for clues. The neuroendocrine system (the interaction between the nervous system and your hormonal system) goes into high gear whenever you get stressed out, and researchers suspect that overreactions could eventually cause the onset of CFS.

- **The stress test:** Other researchers are busy studying the role that hormones and the immune system play in the body's reaction to stress, hoping to find a link between acute and chronic stressors and CFS.

- **Infections:** Because CFS often shows up after a viral or bacterial infection, microbiologists are constantly searching for bugs that may cause CFS and are examining the immune system's reaction to these enemy invaders.

- **Sleeping habits:** Is lack of sleep a symptom of CFS or its cause? Maybe it's both. Some researchers are currently studying the affect of sleeplessness and pain to determine whether they play a role in CFS onset.

✔ **Gender:** What's so different about men and women? The fact that four times more women than men contract CFS has researchers wondering what it is about women that makes them more vulnerable. Maybe they experience pain differently. Maybe they react differently to certain medications or other substances. Researchers hope to reveal the truth behind this mystery. (For more on CFS and women, see the earlier section "Singling Out Women" in this chapter.)

✔ **Depression:** Like any long-term illness, CFS can certainly cause depression, but researchers wonder if a link between depression and CFS may be even stronger. Can depression cause CFS? Only the results of ongoing research can shed light on the probability.

✔ **Fatigue treatment:** How do you cope with fatigue when rest, exercise, and proper nutrition provide no relief? Researchers are constantly searching for new ways to effectively treat fatigue, no matter what's causing it.

✔ **Cells in the body:** Maybe CFS is the result not so much of what your body's organs and glands are doing or not doing but what the cells in those organs and glands are doing or not doing. Some of the latest research is focusing on the NADH-coenzyme and its effect on degenerative illness (including CFS). The NADH-coenzyme is important for energy production by all the cells in the body. The question is, will increasing levels of NADH increase cellular energy and make you feel perkier? Perhaps.

Part II
Teaming Up with Treatment Professionals

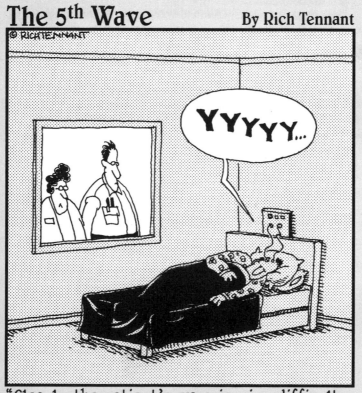

The 5th Wave   By Rich Tennant

"Clearly the patient's experiencing difficulty attaining the deep, final level of restful sleep."

In this part . . .

CFS is a tenacious illness that can sap your energy to the point where you just don't have the spirit to fight back, but you can get help from professionals who are equipped to treat the condition. In this part, I show you how to find and team up with a physician who can assist you in sorting out your symptoms. You also get information on how to form a comprehensive treatment plan that ministers to both your body and your mind.

With the proper medications, therapy, complementary alternative therapies, and a sensible exercise routine, you can begin to silence the symptoms of CFS!

Chapter 5

Tracking Down the Best Doctor for You

....

In This Chapter

▶ Getting ready to meet with your doctor

▶ Playing detective: Is your doctor knowledgeable of CFS?

▶ Discovering what your primary care physician can do

▶ Finding specialists to treat your symptoms

....

Maybe you haven't felt well in a few months. You're not sure if it's due to a serious physical illness or if it's because you're bummed out about something at work or about a relationship. All you know is that your family and friends are getting impatient or worried — you've had to cancel so many social engagements, dinners, parties, and even wedding invites. And at work? Forget about it. Your boss and your colleagues are getting annoyed that you aren't doing your share of work. If things don't change, you just might lose your job!

If any of this sounds even vaguely familiar, consider it time to see your doctor. Whether the problem is in your head or in your body, it doesn't matter. Something is definitely wrong, and trying to sweep it under the proverbial rug is just going to make it worse.

In this chapter, you discover the who, what, and wherefores of getting the right doctor. Keep in mind, though, that even after finding a doctor, it may still take some searching and a variable team approach to help treat your CFS symptoms successfully.

Preparing to Visit Your Primary Physician

You have to start somewhere, and I recommend beginning by setting up an appointment with your primary care physician (PCP). Your primary doctor is your first line of defense. If you need to have any blood tests, CT scans, or MRIs done, he's your man.

If you don't have a PCP, it's high time you got one! Ask your insurance company for the names of doctors, or ask someone you trust for a recommendation.

In this section, I give you tips on making the most of that important first visit: what to expect, what you should ask, and what you should bring to the party.

Although this section is CFS-specific, make sure you also assemble essential documents for your visit to the doctor, such as your insurance information or your method of copayment.

Getting ready for your visit

Going to see your PCP is more than taking a shower and fasting after midnight the night before. Physicians today are busier than ever before; some doctors schedule appointments at eight- to ten-minute intervals! Make the most of your time with the doc by following in the footsteps of the Boy Scouts: Be prepared.

One of the best ways to prepare yourself is by reading this book to get a broad overview of CFS, your treatment options, and some lifestyle changes that may help you feel better. For the most up-to-the-minute information on CFS, also check out the Chronic Fatigue and Immune Dysfunction Syndrome Association of America Web site at www.cfids.org.

Jotting down what you know about yourself

Seeing your PCP for the first time can be heaven for list makers, or drudgery for fly-by-the-seat-of-my-pants folks. Why? Because getting an accurate diagnosis for CFS is no easy task — doctors don't have one definitive diagnostic test for CFS. The more the doctor knows about you and your symptoms, the more likely you are to receive a fast and accurate diagnosis.

ANECDOTE

What's up, Doc? Getting the help you need

Debbie was really nervous. She was 25, single, and, at one time, full of energy. Who needed checkups? No one in her family ever went to a doctor until it was necessary. But her energy was getting more and more zapped as the months went by. She had a pounding headache, something she had never suffered from before, and she had to drag her feet to go anywhere or do anything. Debbie also had achy muscles, joint pain, and swollen lymph nodes that only made her want to do less. She went from party girl to "Debbie Downer."

As a sales rep for a pharmaceutical firm, she needed to have the positive attitude that had made her a consistent top seller month after month — until the last few months. Her job was threatened, her friends were avoiding her, and every time she called her mother, her mom's voice was full of worry.

It was time to see a doctor, so Debbie headed to the local Immedicenter. The doctor checked her blood pressure, listened to her heart, and checked her throat, and she didn't ask any questions. The doctor pronounced: "You have some swollen glands, but that's about it. I'd say you have a low-grade virus. You need to rest." He did a standard blood test that showed an elevated white blood cell count, confirming his "suspicions," and he reiterated: "Rest, rest, rest."

But things went from bad to worse. Debbie couldn't afford to lose her job! And she missed having fun. One night she went on the Internet and searched for "no energy." When CFS came up, she started reading — and reading. The symptoms felt right. The next morning, she called the Chronic Fatigue and Immune Dysfunction Syndrome (CFIDS) Association of America, an organization that had the best information on its Web site. She got contact information for a local support group that provided her with the name of a doctor familiar with CFS in her area, and she made an appointment right away.

Today? Debbie still has periods of fatigue along with some other CFS symptoms, such as swollen glands and muscle aches. But she's figured out how to conserve her energy by pacing her activities and to accept the limitations forced upon her by her illness. The best yet: Because Debbie couldn't go on the road as much as she had before, she got a promotion: a desk job supervising other sales representatives in her territory!

Take some time to jot down a list of your current symptoms, any treatments you've tried so far (and their results), and any new conditions that you think you may have. Also note your medical past, including any previous illnesses you've had and the corresponding treatments; don't forget to add any illnesses that a different health care provider says you currently suffer from (whether you're getting better or not). This way, right there in black and white, you have what's making you sick now and what made you sick in the past. You can then present the list to your doctor — and you can be sure that you haven't forgotten anything.

You should also let your doctor know about your recent sleeping habits, any medications you're currently taking, and your family's health history. The following sections can help you think through and write down all the information you need to take with you to your doctor appointment.

Gauging your current health status

The best place to start when making your doctor list is to determine your current state of health. You can use the following list, adapted from a test provided by the CFIDS Association, to get a good picture of your current state of health:

- Have you not felt like yourself for three months or longer?

- Have you had to curtail your activities, both physical and mental?

- Has your condition had a major impact on work, social activities, and/or school? Is the impact severe enough that you've had to make adjustments in your lifestyle to try to avoid feeling worse?

- Do you have at least four of the following eight symptoms:

    - Weakness and exhaustion that last longer than 24 hours following mental or physical activity

    - Impaired short-term memory or concentration

    - Unrefreshing sleep

    - Muscle pain

    - Pain in the joints without any swelling or redness

    - A new type, pattern, or severity of headache

    - Tender armpits, and/or neck lymph nodes

    - Sore throat

- Did your "unwellness" start suddenly, within a period of hours or days?

Recalling your medical past

The strict definition of CFS requires that other illnesses must be ruled out as possible causes for your new symptoms, so you need to make note of any conditions you've had in the past.

Have you ever been diagnosed with one or more of the following conditions:

- Alcohol or other substance abuse within the last two years

- Anorexia nervosa

- Autoimmune diseases, such as multiple sclerosis or lupus

- ✔ Bipolar disorder

- ✔ Bulimia

- ✔ Cancer

- ✔ Delusional disorders of any kind

- ✔ Dementia

- ✔ Hepatitis

- ✔ HIV and/or AIDS

- ✔ Lyme disease

- ✔ Major depressive disorder (that required hospitalization)

- ✔ Narcolepsy (excess sleepiness)

- ✔ Sleep apnea

- ✔ Thyroid disease

Some conditions can be the result of your CFS or can exist at the same time. Have you ever been diagnosed with one or more of the following conditions:

- ✔ Anxiety disorders

- ✔ Chiari malformation (dizziness caused by a structural brain abnormality)

- ✔ Clinical depression

- ✔ Fibromyalgia

- ✔ Irritable bowel syndrome

- ✔ Multiple chemical sensitivities or environmental illness

- ✔ Orthostatic intolerance (dizziness and/or feeling faint or lightheaded or chest pain when you stand up — as a result of a sudden decrease in blood pressure)

Another list you need to prepare is just as important as the others: What remedies have you tried to alleviate your symptoms, and how did your body respond?

Maybe you've taken an over-the-counter pain killer to ease the pain in your muscles and joints. Maybe you've taken migraine-headache pills. Or maybe you've tried sleep aids, different foods, vitamins and supplements, or more or less exercise. Try to remember everything you've tried and how it affected you.

Logging your sleep habits

Sleep is a problem for many — you only have to look at the medicines now on the market to help people get their eight hours. With CFS, sleep becomes even more of a challenge. You're exhausted, tired, and all you want to do is go to sleep — but you can't. Even after several hours of sleep, you wake up feeling as if you've never slept at all! No amount of sleep leaves you refreshed.

Letting your doctor know about your sleep quality is important, because poor sleep can influence other symptoms. Knowing your sleep habits is equally important, because lack of sleep may be based on something more mundane, like too many lattes from your local java joint, or you could have a sleep disorder, such as sleep apnea or restless legs syndrome.

Also, two weeks before your appointment, be sure to keep a sleep diary in a small notebook, on a pad of paper, or even on your computer (if you're tech savvy). As part of your sleep diary, you want to write down the number of hours your slept each day and the quality of your sleep. You also want to keep a record of the following, as they could also affect how you sleep:

- ✔ How many cups of coffee or caffeinated drinks did I have today? What were the times?

- ✔ Did I exercise today? For how long?

- ✔ When did I eat dinner? Did I have alcohol with it?

- ✔ When did I take my last medication of the day, if any?

- ✔ What did I do before going to sleep?

You can then take your sleep diary with you to your doctor appointment to give your physician a better idea of how to proceed with his diagnosis.

Listing your current medications

Making a list of the medicines you currently take is easier said than done. People can usually remember the medications they take or use on a daily basis — but they frequently forget the dosage. When you make your doctor list, be sure to include any of the following:

- ✔ **Prescriptions:** Whether you take them daily, seasonally, or occasionally, note any prescription medications you take with regularity. Also note the dosage you take.

- ✔ **Over-the-counter medicines:** Include any medicine that you take regularly or that you take as needed, and make sure to include the amount per day. Some examples include pain remedies, sinus or congestion medications, allergy medicine, and so on.

> ✔ **Vitamins, supplements, and herbal remedies:** Don't forget any supplements you take, the dosage, and whether you do so on a daily basis or as needed. Some examples include a daily multivitamin, extra B vitamins when you're feeling low on energy, or an herbal remedy to stave off a cold when you travel by airplane.

Sometimes combining natural medicines with the ones you get at the pharmacy can be downright dangerous to your health. An herbal supplement can sometimes interfere with the work of a hypertension pill or an antidepressant, for example. So be sure to list every pill you pop.

Pulling skeletons out of the family closet

Doctors use the term *family history* so much, it's almost trite. But that family history is vital to your health. The genes passed on from your parents and grandparents often provide clues to why you're sick. (These genes may even skip your brother or your mother but still exist in you.) Perhaps your genetic makeup makes you more sensitive to stress or chemicals, which may put you at higher risk for CFS. Or someone in your immediate family may have had CFS, too, which may also put you at higher risk.

When pulling together your family's medical history, make sure you collect the basics on parents, grandparents, and siblings. You want to be sure to take note of any heart or liver problems, diabetes, eating disorders, mental illnesses, sleeping disorders, and thyroid problems.

Packing a notepad or recorder

Statistics show that people forget a lot more than they remember. A person's brain may have the capacity to store great amounts of memory, but unless there is a trigger, a familiar sight or sound or taste, chances are that memory stays packed away.

When it comes to your health, remembering what to do, how to do it, or when to do it can be a matter, literally, of life and death. What is the best way to remember everything a health care professional says about your condition? A tape recorder. Ask him whether he minds if you record the visit so you can later recall all that was discussed. Most physicians have no problem with this (and, in fact, if he does, that should put a big question mark in your head about his capability!).

If you don't have a tape recorder, don't despair. You can also use an old-fashioned pad and pencil to jot down the important facts. Writing down the important points of your visit with the doctor can trigger even more facts that you thought you'd forgotten. Just make sure you can read your writing later. Another option is to bring along a friend or family member to take notes for you, so you don't have to try to think and write at the same time, freeing you to focus on the discussion with your doctor.

Gauging Your Doctor's CFS Knowledge

An interesting fact about CFS is that any health care professional, from primary care physician to specialist, from family practice physician to internist, from nurse practitioner to physician assistant, can be of some help — *if* he takes you seriously.

Time is precious — and the last thing you need if you're not up to par is to see a primary care physician (PCP) who doesn't take you seriously. But you can't know your PCP's beliefs beforehand, especially about a condition you didn't suspect you had until recently. Before your PCP can help you get the treatment you need, you need to know he's on your side.

Here are the "Mighty Three" CFS questions to bring along on your initial visit:

- ✔ **Do you believe CFS has a physical root?** If he says yes, then you probably won't have to worry about him taking you seriously, because he won't think it's all in your head.

- ✔ **Have you ever treated anyone who has CFS?** If he answers yes, he is most likely sensitive to CFS.

- ✔ **If you've treated someone with CFS, what did you prescribe?** Make sure he notes any medications, relaxation techniques, and diet and exercise changes. You may also want to inquire about the effectiveness of these treatments.

Diagnosing CFS is challenging, no doubt about it. Your PCP, no matter how experienced he is with diagnosing and treating a person with CFS, has many factors to consider before reaching the CFS conclusion (for more on the diagnostic process, see Chapter 6). The following sections help you know what to expect from your PCP.

Don't expect your doctor to be a CFS expert

It's okay if your doctor doesn't know a lot about CFS — as long as he believes it exists. You can help provide education, making your doctor a partner in your condition. You can work together to help you regain your health.

And, speaking of partner, the respect goes both ways. Don't expect to spend the entire afternoon at your doctor's office. He does have other patients! If you bring your CFS lists (see earlier in this chapter), you won't have to spend precious time discussing them.

Above all, remember that doctors are people, too. People forget that they can make mistakes just like us. It just depends on how big that mistake is. If a procedure bothers you, affects your health in negative ways, or you just don't feel comfortable, get thee to another physician anon!

So many physicians want to know more about CFS that the Centers for Disease Control and Prevention (CDC) and the Chronic Fatigue and Immune Dysfunction Syndrome Association of America have teamed up to provide a continuing medical educational (CME) program just for doctors. You can access this course online at www.cfids.org/treatcfs. Another Internet resource is the CFS Toolkit for Health Care Professionals available through the CDC at www.cdc.gov/cfs/toolkit.htm.

Patients often feel intimidated when they're in a doctor's office. They're afraid to speak up or ask a question. But doctors are people, too. And, in order to ensure you're getting the proper care, you need to address your needs — and, even more important, see whether the doctor can address your needs as well.

Knowing what approach your doctor should take

Are you unsure what to expect from your PCP when it comes to treating your symptoms and diagnosing your CFS? Well, you can know you're in good hands with your PCP if he does the following:

- ✔ Performs tests to exclude any other diagnoses before concluding you have CFS. This diagnostic process means a battery of tests — from blood tests and perhaps CT scans and more. (See the Chapter 6 for the skinny on the diagnostic process.)

- ✔ Knows the official definition of CFS and understands that symptoms are different from person to person and can come and go. For the definition of CFS and its symptoms, see Chapter 2.

- ✔ Realizes that CFS can affect many different faces, from African American to Caucasian, from rich to poor.

- ✔ Takes into account medication sensitivities that are common in people with CFS and starts with the lowest effective dosages.

✓ Offers patients the choice of lying down on the examination table, because standing up during exams may cause dizziness.

✓ Makes your sleep a priority. Poor sleeping habits can make other symptoms worse.

✓ Allows more time for office visits.

✓ Provides you with the opportunity to tape visits or take notes.

✓ Takes an interest in your diet and exercise regimens. Healthier diets and energy conservation may help alleviate symptoms.

✓ Treats the symptoms *and* offers support and a sympathetic ear.

✓ Believes you and treats you with respect, which is a *must* for a good CFS doctor.

To make things just a little more complicated, your PCP needs to understand that CFS symptoms can also be similar to or overlap with symptoms of other illnesses. (For more info, see Chapter 2.)

If your PCP has a specialty, like endocrinology, neurology, rheumatology, or immunology, he may believe CFS is a physical illness; but some of the most adamant naysayers belong to these specialties. Researchers in these areas have been more focused on finding a physical cause, but it hasn't always translated into the clinical realm; clinical practitioners are still often unaware of research literature.

Finding a CFS Specialist for a Thorough Workup

Your PCP may suggest you see a CFS specialist after your initial visit to avoid delays if he suspects CFS could be an eventual diagnosis or if he thinks a specialist can provide more expertise in treating you. Or you may have come to this conclusion on your own. At any rate, you need someone who speaks the CFS language and who understands what the illness is, what its symptoms are, and, most importantly, how to treat it. A CFS specialist may be just what you need.

In this section, I discuss some of the best strategies for finding the right CFS specialist to fit your needs.

Gathering recommendations

In today's world, with the Internet and e-mail, making a list of CFS specialists to contact is easier than ever. Here are some suggestions, though, to get you started on your search for the right CFS specialist:

✔ Check with your insurance company (always a must!). Your insurance company has resources to help you find a physician in your area who is covered under your policy.

Be sure to get all the details of your coverage before proceeding with a CFS specialist. Not doing so may end up costing you a lot of money.

✔ Contact the Chronic Fatigue and Immune Dysfunction Syndrome (CFIDS) Association of America at www.cfids.org or by calling them at 704-365-2343. CFS can give you a list of local support groups that can be useful in recommending a CFS specialist.

✔ Contact the International Association of Chronic Fatigue Syndrome (IACFS) at www.iacfs.net or by calling them at 847-258-7248 for a list of physicians it recommends. This group also has annual conferences where you can find out a lot about CFS as well as meet specialists in person.

✔ Ask your PCP for a referral.

✔ Ask your friends, family, and co-workers whether they know anyone with CFS, and if so, ask who that person sees.

✔ Check with your local hospital. Some doctors specializing in CFS may be affiliated with the hospital — or the hospital may point you in the right direction of another hospital or physician that would know.

✔ Check with a local CFS support group. The support group should have the names of some good doctors.

✔ Research online. Try investigating doctors who have authored journal articles on CFS. By finding the location of where the study took place, you can usually bet that the main doctor who authored the article (his name comes first) is also located in that area. You can also check out Web sites, message boards, and chat rooms. (For more online resources, check out the appendix of this book.)

But beware: Gathering research on the Internet should only be an information-gathering process. You don't know who is who and what is what online. If the Web site ends in .gov, you can almost bet your right leg that it's accurate and trustworthy. Organizations with a Web address that ends in .org or .edu are usually accurate as well, but proceed with caution. You should always make sure an organization or Web site is credible by searching for information on it. If you aren't convinced that a Web site or organization is legit, I suggest you steer clear of it.

ANECDOTE

More than just a little teenage trauma

Ginger was your typical 16-year-old girl. She loved going to the mall, putting on makeup, and spending half the night instant messaging her friends. She was a pretty girl, with a fresh, open face, and she got good grades. And then something happened.

It was the night after the PSATs. Ginger remembers it vividly. She'd studied and studied for weeks and had gone to special classes to be more prepared. She was dying to get into Harvard and knew she needed a high score to even be considered. But she was also enough of a teenager to want to hang out with her friends. She had a crush on a boy at her school, and they had had a soda together at the food court! She was pushed and pulled on all sides. To add to the frustration, her mom got sick with a bad flu, and Ginger had to pick up the slack, helping with more chores than she usually did.

But she was fine. Fine. She knew she'd aced the tests when she left the room. She was confident she had done well. Ginger and her parents went out to dinner to celebrate, and it was on the ride home that it happened. The sky suddenly started pouring, the rain beating on the window of her dad's Toyota. It was loud and her father had to go very slowly; it was a sheer veil of water in front of them. Ginger held her ears and started to cry.

Her parents immediately wanted to comfort her. While her dad drove, her mother turned around and took Ginger's hand. "We're almost home, baby," she said. When they finally drove into the garage, and the rain stopped pounding, Ginger crawled out of the car. She told her parents she was okay, just really tired. She went right to bed.

The next day, Ginger couldn't get up. She had no energy. She also had a sore throat and swollen lymph nodes. Her mother was sure it was mononucleosis; a lot of kids at school were coming down with the infamous kissing disease. But things got worse. Ginger couldn't concentrate; she couldn't even sit up in class. Her whole body felt like one giant pain.

Worried sick, Ginger's parents took her to the family doctor, who, after talking to Ginger a bit, said she was just depressed. Maybe she also had a bout of mono, too. But he took some blood just in case.

It turned out Ginger didn't have mono — and the antidepressants he gave her weren't doing any good. But Ginger was lucky. Her doctor had had a patient a year ago who had CFS. He remembered it distinctly because he thought at first she'd had Lyme disease. But blood tests showed no indication that she had been bitten by a tick. The patient had found a specialist from an online CFS support group, and, a year later, she'd come to see Ginger's doctor again for a regular physical. She told him she had CFS and with treatment and lifestyle changes, she'd been able to go back to a relatively normal life although she still had some ups and downs. Ginger's doctor no longer believed that CFS was all in your head. He'd even gone to a one-day conference for family physicians on diagnosing CFS.

As soon as the blood tests came back reporting that mono was out of the question, the doctor referred Ginger to a CFS specialist. No more waiting! With time, good medical care, and learning to work within the limits set by her illness, Ginger has slowly improved. Although Ginger isn't about to try out for cheerleading any time soon, she has been able to go back to school. She's been able to keep up with her homework with extended deadlines for bigger projects, so that she can pace herself. And the best news? She got into Harvard.

Verifying the doctor's credentials

Your doctor may be doing the physical checkup, but you can do a checkup, too. Besides using the Internet and checking physician referral services, specific organizations can provide information about the doctor or other health care providers you see. These organizations include the following:

- The American Medical Association (AMA), Department of Physician Data Services, 515 N Street, Chicago, IL 60616; phone 800-621-8335; Web site www.ama-assn.org.

- The American Board of Medical Specialties, 1007 Church Street, Suite 404, Evanston, IL 60201; phone 866-ASK-ABMS (275-2267) or 847-491-9091; Web site www.abms.org.

- The National Commission of Physicians Assistants, 12000 Findley Road, Suite 200, Duluth, GA 30097; phone 678-417-8100; Web site www.nccpa.net.

Calling for an appointment

Now comes the easy part: Calling the doctor's office for an appointment. Have a few days and times for an appointment in mind when you call so you aren't going, "um . . . ah . . ." or, worse, making an appointment and hanging up only to realize that that was the day your sister was coming to visit.

You also want to make sure that the appointment time is good, because the last thing you need is more stress. Don't push yourself for time or cram too much into one day.

It also doesn't hurt to check with the doctor's office about how they deal with insurance companies. Some offices have policies where they send bills for charges directly to an insurance firm, but others expect payment up front. Getting reimbursed then becomes your responsibility.

Consulting Additional Specialists for Specific Symptoms

No human is an island. And no doctor does everything you need. Your doctor, for example, may be an excellent endocrinologist and may have been able to prescribe medications to keep your hormones in balance. But he isn't a therapist — and you may need to consult a trained specialist to deal with your emotional issues related to changes in your life brought about by CFS.

Similarly, you may need to see a pain or sleep specialist if your symptoms are seriously interfering with your life — and if the medical treatment you're getting from your current doctor isn't working.

Don't be afraid of hurting your regular doctor's feelings. First of all, he may be the one to suggest that you see a specialist. And, secondly, his goal should be your good health. If he balks, that's a sign that you may want to go elsewhere for all your medical needs.

Chapter 6

Working with Your Doctor to Sort Out Your Symptoms

. . . .

In This Chapter

▶ Understanding the difficulty of diagnosing CFS

▶ Measuring your fatigue: How tired are you?

▶ Figuring out what diagnostic tests you need

▶ Knowing what to do if you're not happy with your doctor

. . . .

*N*o matter how knowledgeable and experienced your doctor is about chronic fatigue syndrome (CFS), she can't simply draw a vial of blood, send it to a lab, and call to let you know whether the test came back positive or negative for CFS. The diagnostic procedures are much more complicated than that. Your physician is likely to take a detailed history followed by a physical examination, identify one or more medical conditions that may be causing your symptoms, and perform tests to rule out those other potential causes before arriving at a probable (often not definitive) diagnosis.

This chapter points out the many challenges your doctor faces, so you won't be too disappointed if your doctor seems a little unsure of her diagnosis. I also step you through the diagnostic process so you can know what to expect.

Preparing Yourself for a Case of Chronic Confusion

You may not have considered CFS at first. You thought you were just tired, sick with a bad flu that wasn't getting better, or stressed out. But after some time has passed and you still don't feel better, you realize you may need to begin to explore other reasons for your condition.

If determining what's wrong is difficult for you, you have to expect that it's probably difficult for your doctor, too. She's not going to say, "Aha! You have CFS," as soon as you enter the examination room. This section helps you understand why CFS is challenging to diagnose and how to prepare yourself for those first few doctor visits.

Acknowledging the challenges of diagnosing CFS

CFS had no detailed classification before 1988. It was called everything from a bad flu to "it's all in your head." As a result, many people who struggled daily with specific symptoms were left undiagnosed — and frustrated.

It's now known that specific characteristics must be met in order for your illness to be called CFS, which I describe in the following list (for more details, check out Chapter 2):

✔ Fatigue that affects your daily activities must be the number one symptom and must have been present at least six months.

✔ The fatigue must be combined with at least four of these eight symptoms:

- Memory loss and/or inability to concentrate

- Sleep difficulties, or sleep that doesn't leave you feeling rested

- Sore throat that comes and goes

- Muscle pain

- Joint pain without redness or swelling

- Headache that's different from ones you've had in the past

- Swollen, tender lymph nodes in armpits, or neck

- Increased fatigue and worsening of other symptoms after physical or mental activity

Even though the symptoms of CFS are more defined, actually diagnosing the illness is still difficult for the following reasons:

✔ Doctors don't have one diagnostic test to pinpoint the illness. Unlike cancer or a bladder infection or a good old stomachache, CFS is a diagnosis made as a result of *many* tests. And, even then, some doubt may still exist. Some of these tests may include lab studies or X-rays and such, while others may be written questionnaires. (For more on the testing process, see the section "Painting Your Diagnostic Portrait.")

✔ The doctor can't make a diagnosis of CFS until she's been able to rule out any other condition that has symptoms, such as swollen lymph nodes, muscle pain, and restless sleep, that are similar to those of CFS.

✔ Sometimes the medications you're currently taking can also mimic the symptoms of CFS. For example, certain antidepressants may make you fatigued and may also cause sleep problems. Allergy medications may make you feel brain-fogged and de-energized. Steroids may lower potassium level, which, in turn, lowers your blood pressure — and can make you feel dizzy and unhinged when you stand up.

✔ To make it even more complicated, your CFS symptoms can beget other CFS symptoms. For example, your restless sleep may cause more severe fatigue. The severe fatigue can cause depression, interfere with thinking, cause greater pain, and so on. The confusion comes from the fact that depression can make you feel very tired. It can create restless sleep. It can even make you feel achy — all symptoms of, you guessed it, CFS.

✔ Only a few studies have looked at treating CFS. Believe it or not, although you can find over 4,000 case studies of CFS, the majority of them focus on its possible causes and how many cases of it are in the population.

✔ Your doctor may be just as ignorant as you are about your CFS. The illness can be confusing because it mimics so many other conditions. However, this lack of understanding doesn't mean she's a bad doctor. It just means she needs to keep an open mind. If you think you have CFS, she shouldn't dispute it. Instead, she should give you diagnostic tests to rule out other conditions and research the condition herself.

Despite the quality care your doctor may have been able to provide in the past, you may find yourself wanting a physician who is more familiar with CFS. If so, check out the section "Seeking a Second Opinion When Your Doctor Doesn't Work Out" later in this chapter.

Improving your odds of an accurate diagnosis

Because less than 20 percent of Americans who have CFS have actually had an accurate diagnosis, becoming a proactive patient is very important. The odds of getting an accurate diagnosis can only be as good as the information you give your doctor. "To thine own self be true," as Shakespeare said.

To help you improve your odds of receiving an accurate diagnosis, you can do the following:

✔ You, the patient, need to be clear on what you're feeling. You can find a few quiet minutes and write down your symptoms. You can jot down your feelings at different times of the day. Bring your notes to the doctor.

✔ You need to have done your homework and prescreened your illness to make sure you communicate successfully with your doctor.

Rating Your Fatigue

Because the severity of your fatigue and the significant impact it has on your life is the number-one symptom separating CFS from a whole host of other conditions, you can't just tell your doctor, "I'm tired all the time," or "Yeah, I'm really, really tired." These statements are just too general. Fatigue is a very common complaint heard by clinicians, but it frequently doesn't disrupt a person's life to the same degree that CFS does. How bad is your fatigue? What is its "personality"?

One of the written questionnaires that your doctor might use to rate your fatigue is the *Multidimensional Fatigue Inventory*, or, as we doctors like to call it, the *MFI-20*. This questionnaire consists of 20 questions in five fatigue categories:

- ✔ General fatigue
- ✔ Physical fatigue
- ✔ Reduced activity
- ✔ Reduced motivation
- ✔ Mental fatigue

Each question has a rating scale of 5, from not true, sometimes true, and true. (See Figure 6-1 for a sampling of this test.)

I feel tired

yes, that is true ☐☐☐☐ no, that is not true

I think I do a lot in a day

yes, that is true ☐☐☐☐ no, that is not true

Figure 6-1: Sample Multi-dimensional Fatigue Inventory (MFI-20).

When I am doing something, I can keep my thoughts on it

yes, that is true ☐☐☐☐ no, that is not true

Physically I can take on a lot

yes, that is true ☐☐☐☐ no, that is not true

ANECDOTE

Here today . . . still here tomorrow

Jon was in college when he came down with CFS. He had been infected with a flu that had been spreading around the campus. Most of his fraternity brothers recovered after two weeks, tops. But Jon continued to have a sore throat and low energy beyond those 14 days. In fact, Jon's symptoms got *worse*. He was depressed, his muscles ached, and he was so tired that he had to take two incompletes. By the time Christmas break came along, he couldn't wait to go home and go to bed. Joining his friends on a skiing trip they'd planned wasn't even an option for him.

Jon went to his family's doctor, toting along the records from the college infirmary, which stated he had Epstein-Barr. But blood tests didn't indicate that he had the virus, although the doctor couldn't rule out the possibility that he'd had Epstein-Barr at one time. At first, the doctor diagnosed Jon as being overworked and stressed — a common-enough malady in college kids. He recommended bed rest for the whole time Jon was home. He also referred Jon to a psychotherapist who could help him cope better with school.

But Jon tossed and turned; he couldn't sleep. But he couldn't stand up, either. When he tried to get up to go to the bathroom, he'd feel shaky and dizzy. Therapy wasn't doing any good either. Jon couldn't focus enough to talk — or to listen.

His parents were worried sick and brought their son to the hospital. Fortunately, a young resident there recognized the symptoms of CFS. She suggested that Jon immediately make an appointment with a specialist she knew.

However, it took several visits for even the specialist to determine whether he had CFS — it's that hard to diagnose! After a battery of different tests, Jon's new doctor decided to treat his symptoms: pain killers for muscle and joint aches, an antidepressant for his depression, and a gentle exercise and structured sleep program that provided relief without overexertion. Within another two months, Jon started to see improvement: His sleep was better, and he no longer felt as sore all over.

By the time Jon graduated from college, two years later, he felt so good that it was hard to believe he'd ever been sick. Maybe it was his age, maybe his constitution, his genetic make-up, or the fact that he got help early in his illness, but Jon never experienced that same degree of illness again.

Painting Your Diagnostic Portrait

You may have heard the saying, "It's not the quantity that counts, but the quality." Unfortunately, when it comes to testing for CFS, what counts is usually a combination of both.

CFS has many layers and can't be diagnosed with a single test. So when you visit your doctor, be prepared to spend time taking a battery of tests, from interviews, question and answers, blood tests, and more — all of which may take several preliminary visits, or trips to a laboratory or radiologist. When it comes to diagnosis, the tests and questionnaires have three goals:

✔ Ruling out other causes for your symptoms (such as thyroid disease, Lyme disease, and so on)

✔ Determining how severe your symptoms are and how they're affecting your life

✔ Determining appropriate treatment

This section details exactly what those tests are and which ones are the most important for your doctor to administer.

Because CFS can mimic many other conditions, resisting the urge to self-diagnose your symptoms is important. Many people have thought they had CFS when in actuality they had another illness that needed different treatment. Self-diagnosis not only doesn't help, but it can also make you sicker. However, you can share your knowledge about CFS and speculations that it could be CFS.

You have to keep your perspective when it comes to CFS testing. The process itself can be very lengthy, and getting a diagnosis takes patience on your part. If one test is inconclusive, another test may be ordered. Your doctor may also want to retest you to see whether you get the same results. In other words, the testing process can take months — and, in some cases, years — to be diagnosed. The important thing is that you're getting treatment for your symptoms while the doctor is determining a diagnosis. Unfortunately, even with the best of efforts, a diagnosis can remain elusive no matter how many tests you take.

Your medical and family history

When you have your initial doctor visit, the first thing you should be asked to do is fill out a medical and family history questionnaire. In fact, the receptionist will likely give you the form to fill out when you check in with her.

Your doctor then meets with you first in her office, where she goes over your history and asks specific questions to fill in any blanks. (Some offices have a physician's assistant who does the interview and then gives it to the doctor during your exam.) Some of the things you can expect in taking a history include questions about the following:

✔ **Your past health.** Most people are familiar with those lists of diseases, everything from asthma to urinary tract infections, that have Yes and No boxes for you to check off.

✔ **Your mental health.** Although depression and other mental disorders are on your Yes or No list of conditions, you may be asked for more details, especially because your doctor wants to rule out any psychological causes for your symptoms.

✔ **Recent illnesses.** Because so many different conditions may result in CFS, informing your doctor about anything — from minor ailments such as a "bug" to more serious conditions like fibromyalgia — is important.

✔ **Armed service.** If you served in the United States armed services, your symptoms may possibly be a result of Gulf War Syndrome, or other battles where chemicals may have been used.

✔ **Your lifestyle.** The way you live affects your health. Are you the outdoors type? Are you a person who is more at risk of getting bitten by a tick? Do you live near woods? Do you work in a hospital? Do you sleep a lot as part of your routine? Do you work every day? Do you party too much?

✔ **Your travel history.** Did you visit a foreign country in the weeks before your illness began? Were the sanitary conditions in the country adequate? Do you recall being bitten by an insect or having a rash while you were there?

✔ **Your sexual history.** Have you or your partner had unprotected sex with other people in the weeks or months before your illness began?

✔ **Allergies and chemical sensitivities.** To eliminate chemical sensitivity as a diagnosis, your doctor may ask you about any detergents, soaps, or perfumes that make you break out in a rash or cause a sore throat, or any chemicals you're exposed to at work.

✔ **Your family.** No, your doctor doesn't want to pry, but the fact is that, for better or worse, you inherit more from your family than their blue eyes and ability to throw a ball. If your mother or father had been diagnosed with CFS, you, too, may be more vulnerable. On the other hand, if someone in your family had, say, Epstein-Barr, your doctor may be more inclined to see whether that was the cause of your fatigue leading to CFS.

Your family history doesn't involve your third cousin Alice or your great Uncle Morris on your father's side. Your immediate family means your parents, your grandparents, and your siblings, although your doctor may want to know about your first aunts and uncles as well.

When you meet with your doctor for the first time, your doctor also ask you some more unusual questions. The purpose of these questions is to make an accurate diagnosis. These questions may include:

✔ Since you've fallen ill, how would you describe a typical day?

✔ What are your usual activities and routines, at home and on the job?

✔ Do you exercise? How do you feel afterwards?

✔ What are your three greatest problems or fears about your symptoms?

✔ What kind of specific goals are you looking for in treatment?

When does another illness *not* exclude CFS?

Sometimes a cigar, as they say, is still a cigar. You may have a diagnosis of an *imitator disease* (such as fibromyalgia), but still have CFS at the same time. You may find yourself in this type of situation when:

✔ None of your other conditions can be confirmed via any diagnostic test.

✔ You're currently being treated successfully for the other condition — but still have CFS symptoms.

✔ A different condition was diagnosed and treated *before* the onset of your CFS.

✔ Physical examinations, blood tests, or imaging tests (such as x-rays or CT scans) are inconclusive.

Your doctor may also call you the next day to follow up and see how you are.

A basic physical

After your family and medical history has been taken, you are given a basic physical examination, which includes checking the glands around your neck, taking your blood pressure, and looking at your eyes, nose, and throat. Blood may also be drawn for routine testing, ruling out other conditions, and determining any viral connection. These elements of an initial exam are all normal and necessary.

Key medical tests for CFS

Here's a list of the most common tests given to a person who is suspected of having CFS:

✔ **Complete blood count (CBC) and blood chemistry:** These all-inclusive blood tests confirm that your kidneys and liver are functioning well, that your blood sugar is normal, and that protein levels are good, among other things. They can help rule out anemia, leukemia, and other blood disorders, as well as collagen vascular diseases.

What's a *collagen vascular disease?* Basically, this term is medical-ese for autoimmune diseases that work away at the collagen (which, in addition to making your skin smooth, is responsible for the structure and strength of your tendons, cartilage, and other connective tissues) in your body. These disorders include lupus and rheumatoid arthritis.

✔ **Thyroid function study:** This test checks whether your thyroid function is normal. An abnormal result can be the reason for your fatigue and muscle pain.

✔ **Sedimentation rate:** This test can determine whether you have any inflammation, infection, or lupus in your body via a urine test.

✔ **Urinalysis:** This test can also exclude some infections, kidney disease, and lupus (and other collagen vascular disorders).

✔ **CT scan and/or MRI:** These examinations are both imaging tests. A *CT (computerized tomography) scan* is a sophisticated X-ray. A CT scan gives high-quality detail of specific areas of the body and can help your doctor rule out some brain disorders, back problems, or issues with your joints.

An *MRI* (or *magnetic resonance imaging*) is even more sophisticated. It can come up close and personal and is particularly helpful in determining whether your fatigue is caused by multiple sclerosis (MS) by highlighting the lesions in your brain. Two or more of a certain kind of lesion in your brain means MS (hence, the word *multiple*).

People have complained that an MRI makes them feel claustrophobic, but listening to music in earphones or taking an anti-anxiety medication beforehand can help ease the feeling. Open MRIs are also available, which make claustrophobia obsolete. If tight spaces concern you, be sure to talk to your doctor about your options before committing to an MRI.

✔ **Ultrasound:** An ultrasound (or sonogram) uses sound waves to show an organ on a nearby screen. In CFS, an ultrasound can be useful to determine whether you have any inflammation (which may signal an autoimmune disease — or another reason for your symptoms), or any problems with your colon, gall bladder, or stomach, all of which can cause pain (and all of which could rule out CFS).

Some doctors also suggest the *tilt table test.* This lengthy test is used exclusively to see whether you have *orthostatic intolerance* (a fancy name for problems standing or sitting upright for more than a few minutes at a time, particularly a dizzy, faint feeling). In this test, you're first wired up to an electrocardiogram (ECG) machine and a blood pressure cuff and intravenous line. (In case you have a reaction, the doctor administering the test needs to be able to give you medicine quickly via the line.) After all is in place, a baseline in the supine position is measured. The table you're on then tilts head-up 30 degrees for five minutes. Another measurement and ECG is taken during this time. The table then moves you up to a 60-degree angle (you're strapped in place) for 45 minutes while your blood pressure, heart rate, and ECG are monitored.

In her shoes

Orthostatic intolerance (OI) has nothing to do with fallen arches and those supports people put in shoes. It may be a symptom of CFS, as well as being a condition in its own right. In fact, studies show that up to 97 percent of people diagnosed with CFS have OI, especially if they're young. Two types of OI are associated with CFS, both of which can be diagnosed with a simple test: taking your blood pressure while lying down, then while standing up. In people with CFS, the OI is delayed. It takes a few minutes before you feel faint or your heart begins

to race. OI also results in poor blood circulation if you have CFS. The two OIs of CFS are

- **Neurally mediated hypotension (NMH)** is a sudden drop in blood pressure when you stand up. The drop usually causes an increase in CFS symptoms.

- **Postural orthostatic tachycardia syndrome (POTS)** is a sudden rapid heart rate (read: pulse) within ten minutes of standing up. You may also hear POTS called *chronic orthostatic intolerance,* or *COI.*

Filling out questionnaires

Part of the testing process requires you to fill out a variety of questionnaires. Pretty painless, if you ask me. Check out the following list of questionnaires your doctor may recommend:

- **Short Form McGill Pain Questionnaire:** You use a pen and a preprinted form for this test. See Figure 6-2 for an example.

- **A sleep quality questionnaire:** Although a variety of sleep tests are out there, your doctor can cut to the chase with the *CDC Brief Sleep Questionnaire,* which easily helps your doctor discover your sleep patterns and quality.

    The Pittsburgh Sleep Quality Index is a comprehensive self-rated questionnaire that offers a picture of your sleep patterns, your sleep quality, and your sleep habits. This questionnaire is used primarily for older adults in whom sleep may be a problem in and of itself.

Because restless sleep can be a symptom of CFS as well as a cause of fatigue, being able to determine whether your fatigue was brought on by lack of sleep, increased because of lack of sleep, or caused by your lack of sleep is important for your doctor's diagnosis. Therefore, a dialogue with your doctor, where she asks direct, often very specific questions and you answer honestly, is crucial.

- **The SF-36 Health Assessment Tool:** Because CFS is so difficult to pinpoint, this general health questionnaire can be a valuable tool not only to help your doctor diagnose your condition, but also to help you clarify and organize your physical, emotional, and mental symptoms, as well as your state of well-being. And, when charted over time, it can also help show a pattern of symptoms that do — or don't — respond to treatment.

✔ **The Patient Health Questionnaire (PHQ-9):** Developed by Pfizer Inc., this simple, useful questionnaire asks nine questions that can help a doctor determine whether you may be clinically depressed — and if that depression is directly related to your CFS.

✔ **Beck Depression Inventory:** Although this test can be important to determine the scope and depth of your depression, administering it initially isn't important. You know if you're depressed — and the other tests your doctor administers are enough to validate that claim. It is primarily given if your depression gets worse or doesn't improve with treatment, only then should you take this test.

Questioning the tests being performed on you

Every doctor has her own protocol — what is unnecessary to one physician may be considered extremely necessary to another. One doctor's "normal" can be another doctor's "Are you crazy??" The types of tests your doctor wants you to take all comes down to your doctor's experience, preference, and results she's witnessed.

Scrutinize all tests with a certain degree of common sense in mind. True, diagnosing CFS takes a battery of tests, but at a certain point, you may suspect that more is being done than absolutely necessary. The best way to see whether you're being overtested, undertested, or used as a guinea pig without your prior knowledge is by speaking up. Ask your doctor what she's doing. Ask why she thinks the test is necessary.

A diagnostic test doesn't have a set price. The cost of each test can vary from state to state, laboratory to laboratory, and doctor to doctor. In order for you to determine how much out-of-pocket money you have to pay (if any), I advise that you call your insurance company *before* having any tests done to see what the insurance company covers and what it doesn't.

Some insurance companies still don't recognize CFS as a bona fide illness. If your coverage doesn't pay for certain tests or you don't have any insurance coverage, you may have to work out a payment schedule with your doctor. Sometimes you can negotiate costs to decrease your out-of-pocket expenses — it's worth asking. The important thing to remember here is to go in with your eyes open. In other words, don't let the bill that comes in the mail be a shock.

I. Pain Rating Index (PRI):
   The words below describe average pain. Place a check mark (✓) in the column that represents the degree to which you feel that type of pain.

		None		Mild		Moderate		Severe
Throbbing	0		1		2		3	
Shooting	0		1		2		3	
Stabbing	0		1		2		3	
Sharp	0		1		2		3	
Cramping	0		1		2		3	
Gnawing	0		1		2		3	
Hot-Burning	0		1		2		3	
Aching	0		1		2		3	
Heavy	0		1		2		3	
Tender	0		1		2		3	
Splitting	0		1		2		3	
Tiring-Exhausting	0		1		2		3	
Sickening	0		1		2		3	
Fearful	0		1		2		3	
Punishing-Cruel	0		1		2		3	

II. Present Pain Intensity (PPI)–Visual Analog Scale (VAS).

No pain |————————————————————————————————| Worst possible pain

III. Evaluate over all intensity of total pain experience.
    Place a check mark (✓) in the appropriate column:

Evaluate		
0	No pain	
1	Mild	
2	Discomforting	
3	Distressing	
4	Horrible	
5	Excruciating	

Figure 6-2:
Sample
Short Form
McGill Pain
Question-
naire.

Seeking a Second Opinion When Your Doctor Doesn't Work Out

The fact is that doctors are there to help *you*. Seeing a doctor isn't like wanting to join a sorority or a bridge club. You don't have to worry whether she likes you. Sure, you want a good rapport with your doctor, but you don't have to (and shouldn't want to!) be best friends with her. What all this leads up to is this: If your doctor isn't giving you the help you need, if you aren't getting better, then you need to find someone else. Be honest.

A good doctor will wholeheartedly agree and, many times, refer you to a CFS specialist if one is in your area. Sometimes, working with an open-minded doctor who is willing to take the time to partner with you on a diagnosis and treatment plan can help lead to an outcome as successful as a "specialty" professional. Friends, colleagues, support groups, and hospitals are all good resources for finding a doctor that fits your needs. (See Chapter 5 for more in-depth information on finding a physician.)

Chapter 7

Crafting Your Medical Treatment Plan

In This Chapter

▶ Looking at the different medicines used to treat CFS symptoms

▶ Considering alternative therapies in combination with your medical treatment

*E*verybody is different. Some people have no problem swallowing a half dozen pills each day, while other people cringe at the thought of it. Some people have a higher pain threshold while others feel the "ouch" every time they bump into a wall. Some people have hormonal problems along with their CFS — and still others don't. Many possible routes lead to a variety of CFS symptoms, and you can find an equal number of medical treatments.

A successful treatment plan usually focuses on the following four areas:

✔ **Medications** for symptomatic relief

✔ **Psychological therapies** for possible emotional and psychological factors and to treat emotional and psychological issues that arise from CFS

✔ **Lifestyle adjustments** to accommodate for fatigue and other incapacitating symptoms

✔ **Light exercise and other activities** to prevent deconditioning and increase muscle strength and tone and promote energy conservation

This chapter shows you how to proceed with putting these approaches to work and setting up your own treatment plan.

 Instead of asking yourself, "What's right for me?", ask yourself (and your doctor), "How do I relieve my fatigue/pain/nausea/depression?" or whatever symptom for which you want to find relief. The more specific you are about your symptoms, the more effective your treatment can be.

Soothing Your Symptoms with Effective Medications

Today, physicians usually treat the symptoms of CFS along with symptoms from other conditions you may have, which can mean several different types of medication. For example, if you developed CFS symptoms following Lyme disease, your doctor may treat both concurrently. The same goes for a bad flu or depression.

In addition to what ails you, your doctor needs to know how serious your symptoms are — and if they can be treated with lifestyle changes rather than with medication.

To make some order out of your symptom chaos, doctors tend to look at *primary symptoms,* which are incapacitating ills such as restless sleep, pain, fatigue, headaches, and confusion. Some of the facts doctors must take into account when deciding on medicinal treatment for you are the following:

- ✔ Your sensitivity to medications, especially those that make you sleepy.

- ✔ Your allergies, if any, to certain medicines, such as penicillin.

- ✔ Avoiding overmedication: Some antidepressant medicines, for example, not only treat your moods, but can also alleviate your pain and help with sleep, so additional pain medicine may not be necessary.

- ✔ Any herbs, supplements, or vitamins you may be taking that, combined with your prescribed medicine, can either cause harm or enhance the prescribed medicine.

Starting out slowly is often best — and that includes medication. Because patients with CFS have a lot of symptoms similar to known side effects of some medications, your doctor may have you start out small and increase doses slowly — and only until the problem is treated. An even better option, your doctor may decide to use medicines that combine treatments for more than one problem. That way, you can kill two birds with one stone and save some money, too.

In this section, I go over the primary symptoms of CFS and what your doctor can prescribe to ease your discomfort.

Cranking up your energy level with stimulants

Fatigue can cause more than restless sleep. It can also have a lot to do with the lack of energy you have throughout the day. If you find yourself staggering from room to room, unable to get dressed and get to work, and so exhausted that your daily routines are compromised, your doctor may suggest a stimulant to get you through the day. Table 7-1, courtesy of www.cfids.org, shows stimulants that some clinicians reportedly have prescribed to treat CFS.

Persons with CFIDS generally don't tolerate standard, "usual" doses of many medications. It is advisable to start at lower than usual dosages and gradually increase to therapeutic range, not to exceed FDA-recommended amounts.

Table 7-1	Commonly Prescribed Stimulants		
Medication Chemical Name	*Medication Brand Name*	*Common Side Effects*	*Additional Information*
Phentermine HCl	Fastin; Adipex-P; Ionamin; Oby-Cap	Overstimulation; constipation; diarrhea; sleep problems; high blood pressure	Potential psychological addiction; multiple potential drug interactions
Methylphenidate HCl	Ritalin; Ritalin-SR	Sleep problems; nervousness; abdominal pain; abnormal heart beat; blood pressure changes; drowsiness	Caution in patients with anxiety disorders; potentially addictive; several potential drug interactions
Dextroamphetamine sulfate	Dexedrine	Excessive restlessness; overstimulation; sleeplessness; rapid heart rate	Potential drug dependence; multiple drug interactions possible
Modafinal	Provigil	Headache; dizziness; blurred vision; insomnia; changes in thinking; nervousness; difficulty controlling body movements	May interfere with birth control medicines; potentially habit-forming; persons with mitral valve prolapse and other cardiovascular diseases should avoid use of this drug

Stimulants aren't appropriate for just feeling tired – and they aren't for everyone. They can significantly interfere with sleep and rest and should be prescribed only after your sleep patterns have been studied and treatment addresses any existing sleep disorders like sleep apnea. As with many medications used to treat CFS, they appear to help some people, yet make other people feel worse.

Narcolepsy is an illness in its own right, a chronic neurological disorder in which your brain is unable to regulate your sleep-wake cycles. In addition to swift urges to sleep during the day (including actually falling asleep for several seconds, minutes, or even hours), people with narcolepsy may even have rare symptoms such as sudden loss of voluntary muscle control *(cataplexy)*, vivid hallucinations, and even short-term paralysis. Your physician will determine, based on symptoms, if you need tests to determine if you have this condition.

Muting your aches and pains

You may want to sing, "Pain, pain, go away, come again some other day," but without the right treatment, your little song is just a play on words. The following are the five types of CFS pain:

- ✔ **Deep pain** occurs in the muscles.

- ✔ **Arthralgias pain** describes pain in the joints.

- ✔ **Headache pain** in CFS is often described as "pressure-like."

- ✔ **Allodynia pain** indicates that the skin feels sore when touched.

- ✔ **Neuropathic** or **nerve pain** is experienced as a constant burning or "pins-and-needles" sensation.

In this section, you get the real scoop for keeping these pains in the neck (and other places) away. A list of different pain medications doctors prescribe, courtesy of `www.cfids.org`, is shown in Table 7-2. Read on for more details.

The medications in Table 7-2 have not been studied and approved for use specifically in people with CFS. This list is comprised of FDA-approved standard drugs used for pain management and may have been prescribed by physicians treating people with CFS.

Table 7-2	**Pain-Relief Medications**		
Medication Chemical Name	*Medication Brand Name*	*Common Side Effects*	*Additional Information*
Aspirin	Bayer; Ecotrin; various others	Nausea; heartburn	Buy over-the-counter
Ibuprofen	Advil; Motrin	Abdominal pain or discomfort	Buy over-the-counter
Acetaminophen	Tylenol; Panadol; Aspirin-Free Anacin	Allergy-like rash, itching, etc.	Possible food and drug interactions
Propoxyphene napsylate plus acetaminophen	Darvocet-N; Darvon Compound 65	Drowsiness; nausea	Mild narcotic: dependence possible
Naproxen	Naprosyn	Abdominal pain; indigestion	Food and drug interactions
Morphine sulfate	MS Contin; Oxycontin; Oramorph	Anxiety; depression; constipation	*Narcotic:* dependence possible
Hydrocodone bitartrate plus acetaminophen	Vicodin; Anexia; Co-Gesic; Hydrocet; Lorcet; Lortab; Zydone	Dizziness; nausea; sedation	*Narcotic:* dependence possible
Pentazocine HCL plus aspirin	Talwin	Confusion; dizziness; disorientation	Drug dependence possible
Oxycodone HCl plus acetaminophen	Percocet; Roxicet; Tylox	Sedation; dizziness; nausea	*Narcotic:* dependence possible
Ketoprofen	Orudis; Actron; Orudis KT; Oruvail (extended release)	Abdominal pain; stomach ulcers; changes in kidney function	Drug and food interactions
Hydromorphone HCL	Dilaudid	Drowsiness; anxiety; fear; constipation	*Narcotic:* dependence possible

Table 7-2 (continued)

Medication Chemical Name	Medication Brand Name	Common Side Effects	Additional Information
Meperidine HCL	Demerol	Dizziness; light headedness; nausea	*Narcotic:* dependence possible
Piroxicam	Feldene	Stomach ulcers and bleeding; abdominal pain	Drug and food interactions

Treating aches and pains with NSAIDs

The first line of defense in treating CFS-related pain is the NSAIDS, *nonsteroidal anti-inflammatory drugs* — those over-the-counter (OTC) medications, such as ibuprofen (Advil and Motrin), naproxen (Aleve), and plain, old aspirin. Prescription NSAIDS may also be recommended. They work by attacking *prostaglandins,* chemicals in your body that cause inflammation and create pain. Unfortunately, these same prostaglandins may also cause indigestion, which means stomachaches, heartburn, and possible ulcers.

Many OTC NSAIDs contain more than just their anti-inflammatory ingredients. Some combine cough, migraine, or allergy-reducing agents as well. So don't take two different NSAIDs at the same time! Combining the different pills can cause more gastric upsets. You want to keep your NSAIDs pure.

In order for you to have pain relief, many doctors recommend taking your NSAID with an antacid, like Tums or Rolaid. Some people have found the side effects lessen when they take their pill with food.

You may have heard talk about *COX-2 inhibitors* — a newer prescription-strength NSAID that doesn't cause stomach upsets — such as celecoxib (Celebrex). While these newer prescription-strength NSAIDS are very effective in reducing pain and inflammation, studies have found that they may also increase the risk of heart attack and stroke. These studies have also concluded that the same severe side effects can occur with large doses of the nonselective over-the-counter brands as well. Always check with your doctor before taking any NSAID and make sure he supervises your intake.

Suppressing depressing pain with amitriptyline

Believe it or not, antidepressants can treat more than emotional pain. Studies have shown that a particular antidepressant, *amitriptyline,* can ease physical pain — and even help you sleep. Amitriptyline (brand name: Elavil) is one of the earliest types of antidepressants, created way back in the 1950s, and is a tricyclic antidepressant. Lower doses of amitriptyline are given for CFS pain.

Tricyclic isn't the three-wheeled bicycle you got on your third birthday. It's a scientific term for a particular classification of antidepressants that have three connecting atoms in their molecular structure — which works on the chemical *norepinephrine* in the brain that has been known to cause depression.

Other tricyclic antidepressants that also work like amitriptyline are doxepin (Adapin), desipramine (Norpramin), and nortriptyline (Pamelor). So if amitriptyline doesn't work for you, others may.

A word of caution: These other types of tricyclic antidepressants may also make orthostatic intolerance worse, so people with CFS who have orthostatic instability should take them with care.

Going old-school with opiates

When you hear the word *opiate,* do you picture a dark, smoky room, oriental rugs, and hookahs? Although opium dens really did exist in London, China, and other places, the opiates you take for your CFS pain have nothing smoky about them.

Opiates duplicate your body's own pain-blocking properties — those chemicals in the brain and spinal cord, such as endorphins, that block pain signals in the nervous system. The opiates used in clinical settings are quite effective, but may also be addictive. Morphine, codeine, and oxycodone are all opiates often used in hospitals and as short-term painkillers after surgery.

Some opiates, such as morphine, can release *histamines* — those same culprits that are released during allergic reactions and why antihistamine medicines are effective. The result of taking opiates can be a rash or hives. Taking an antihistamines such as Benadryl may reduce symptoms due to histamines. Other side effects of opiates can include dry mouth, stomachaches, and constipation.

You can relieve constipation caused by opiates by eating a diet rich in fiber, drinking prune juice, taking a fiber supplement (such as Metamucil) or a stool softener, and drinking at least eight glasses of water a day.

After several days of use, opiates can cause physical dependence. This dependence isn't technically an addiction because you aren't craving the stuff — but you must taper off the medication to avoid withdrawal symptoms, such as a stomachache, chills, rapid heart rate, diarrhea, goose bumps, sweats, runny nose, and even more body aches and pains. If you're concerned that you're becoming dependent on any type of opiate, be sure to talk to your doctor right away. (For more on opiates and addiction, see the nearby sidebar.)

Treating your pain with over-the-counter pills

Looking for the right pain medication on a pharmacy shelf is like looking at the many different brands of yogurt in the dairy section of the supermarket. You see extra-strength, migraine-strength, decongestants, and sleep aids, not to mention plain, old, tried-and-true aspirin — both generic and popular brands.

Over-the-counter NSAIDs, such as Motrin and Aleve, are one choice that can relieve pain symptoms. But they can also cause stomach upset. (See the previous section on NSAIDs for more info.) Another choice is the *analgesic* (pain relief) medicine called *acetaminophen* (such as Tylenol and aspirin-free Anacin). These analgesics can help relieve your pain, but they won't do much for your inflammation. But if you have an ulcer or can't tolerate NSAIDs, they may do the job. They won't cause stomach problems, but you can have too much of a good thing. Taken in excess, acetaminophen can cause liver problems. Be sure to talk to your doctor about the right dosage for you.

An over-the-counter drug may help alleviate your symptoms, but it won't cure your illness. But making life even a little easier is, well, priceless.

Myth: All (opiate) roads lead to addiction

Yes, opiates can become addictive. You only have to watch one of the cop shows on television to see how people will kill for oxycodone (such as Percocet, Tylox, or Oxycontin). But, believe it or not, most people *don't* become dependent on the opiates when taking them to treat pain. In fact, less than 1 out of every 100 people become addicted when taking opiates for pain. How do you know if you're in danger of abusing your medication? Here are some warning signs:

✔ Constant use and compulsive need — even if it harms you

✔ Avoiding doctor visits

✔ Cravings that don't stop until you take the drug

✔ Stealing, wheedling, and forging prescriptions

✔ Behaving as if the only thing in the world is that drug

Patching up your pain with a pain patch

Patches are in. Medications from birth control to smoking cessation aids or motion sickness remedies to wrinkle smoothers have a patch. Why are they so effective? Patches don't have to go through your whole digestive system to get to work. The medicine in the patches is absorbed into the skin, and then quickly spread to where the body needs it via the bloodstream.

One of the strongest pain patches is fentanyl transdermal system (Duragesic), which provides relief from chronic pain for up to 72 hours. However, it has been known to cause complications (including coma!) if overdosed, so your doctor may choose a less potent medication first — and only under his strict supervision. Another pain patch used to treat pain in CFS is lidocaine transdermal patch (Lidoderm), which is also prescription-only.

You can find over-the-counter pain patches as well, including Bengay and Tiger Balm, which provide analgesic relief.

Patches are different than capsules. Because the medicines in them are absorbed by your body over time, your pain symptoms may wax and wane. Leave the patch on for about an hour or so before removing it to determine whether the patch is working.

Medicating your clinical depression

Another symptom that many people with CFS experience is depression, which can be a condition in and of itself or a result of your *having* CFS — and the impact the illness has had on your life. (This type of depression is called *secondary depression* because it isn't the main illness or condition.) In either case, doctors have several ways to treat depression, and I go over some of them. See Table 7-3, courtesy of www.cfids.org, for a quick list of depression medications, and then keep reading for more information.

Note that the medications in Table 7-3 haven't been studied and approved for use specifically in people with CFS. This list is comprised of FDA-approved standard drugs in the antidepressant class and may have been prescribed by physicians treating people with CFS. Also, these medications must never be taken in combination with an MAO inhibitor.

Table 7-3	Medications Commonly Used to Treat Depression		
Medication Chemical Name	**Medication Brand Name**	**Common Side Effects**	**Additional Information**
Amitriptylene (tricyclic)	Elavil	Dizziness; anxiety; dry mouth; weight gain	Multiple potential food and drug interactions
Bupropion HCl	Wellbutrin; Wellbutrin SR; Zyban*	Abdominal pain; anxiety; agitation; may interfere with sleep; seizures	Don't take if you have a history of an eating disorder
Doxepin HCl (tricyclic)	Sinequan	Dizziness; drowsiness; confusion; weight gain	Potential drug and food interactions
Fluoxetine HCl	Prozac	Drowsiness; anxiety;	Multiple potential drug and food interactions
Nefazodone HCl	Serzone	Blurred vision; confusion; dizziness; drowsiness	Multiple potential drug and food interactions
Paroxetine HCl	Paxil	Nausea; dry mouth; drowsiness	Multiple potential drug and food interactions
Sertraline HCl	Zoloft	Nausea; dry mouth; anxiety; drowsiness	Multiple potential drug and food interactions
Trazadone HCl	Desyrel	Dry mouth; abdominal or stomach problems	Potential drug and food interactions
Nortriptyline HCl (tricyclic)	Pamelor; Aventyl	Abdominal discomforts; drowsiness	Potential drug and food interactions
Citalopram hydrobromide	Celexa	Abdominal discomforts; agitation; anxiety; dry mouth	Potential drug and food interactions

Medication Chemical Name	Medication Brand Name	Common Side Effects	Additional Information
Venlafaxine HCl	Effexor; Effexor XR (XR = extended release)	Abnormal dreams; anxiety; dizziness; drowsiness; dry mouth; nausea	*Caution:* If you have high blood pressure, heart, liver, or kidney disease is present; take with food.
Amitriptyline HCl *plus* Perphenazine	Triavil	Drowsiness; sedation; nervous system abnormalities	Multiple potential drug and food interactions
Imipramine HCl (tricyclic)	Tofranil	Drowsiness; abdominal discomforts; sun sensitivity	Special warnings; multiple potential drug and food interactions
Phenelzine sulfate (MAO inhibitor)	Nardil	Stomach, intestinal discomforts; dizziness; drowsiness	Multiple potential food and drug interactions
Mirtazapine	Remeron	Dizziness; drowsiness; abnormal dreams and thinking	Special warnings; potential drug interactions
Desipramine HCl (tricyclic)	Norpramin	Abdominal discomforts; drowsiness; sun sensitivity	Special warnings; potential food and drug interactions

Although antidepressants can help reduce secondary depression, they aren't a cure for CFS. In fact, they should be prescribed judiciously. Some antidepressants may increase other CFS symptoms and cause other unwanted side effects.

When it comes strictly to treating depression, most physicians use the newer antidepressants, those *selective serotonin reuptake inhibitors* (SSRIs) that have had so much success ever since Prozac came on the market. These medications improve the imbalance of the chemical *serotonin* in the brain, which can cause depression.

But having CFS presents other issues. In order to cut down on the number of medicines you need to take, some physicians use one tricyclic antidepressant to treat both depression and pain (see the section "Suppressing depressing pain with amitriptyline" earlier in this chapter). Tricyclics work on restoring the imbalance of norepinephrine, another chemical associated with depression. They may also help improve sleep for some people.

Some studies and anecdotal reports of SSRI and NSRI use in CFS show that they don't appear to help; in fact, some symptoms get worse, particularly sleep problems and fatigue.

Tricyclic antidepressants block your body's use of *norepinephrine,* the chemical that can constrict blood vessels in your extremities and increase blood pressure. When the norepinephrine is blocked via an antidepressant, blood pressure may become lower — resulting in lightheadedness and fainting. If you have problems with dizziness (orthostatic intolerance) already, tricyclics may not be right for you at the typical dosages used to treat depression.

Another type of antidepressant that has had some success with CFS patients is MAO inhibitors, such as Nardil and Parnate. (These pills have nothing to do with a former Chinese leader). MAO stands for *monoamine oxidase,* an enzyme in the brain that has been associated with depression when imbalanced. MAO inhibitors block the production of this enzyme. Because the chemicals serotonin and norepinephrine are both monoamines, MAO inhibitors essentially work the same way as the SSRIs and the tricyclics do — but they carry additional risks. People taking MAO inhibitors have to very carefully watch their diet. In combination with certain foods, medicines, or alcoholic beverages, these drugs can be life threatening. The upside is that they work faster than tricyclics. One study of depressed patients with CFS found that 50 percent improved with MAO inhibitors.

MAO inhibitors can cause a dramatic rise in blood pressure and possibly result in death if taken with food or drink high in the chemical *tyramine.* These foods and drinks include smoked or pickled meat or fish, sauerkraut, cheese, liver, sausages, and red wine. MAO inhibitors also shouldn't be taken with certain medications. *Always* check with your doctor before taking an MAO inhibitor and before discontinuing it; and when it comes to food and drink, use the axiom, "When in doubt, throw it out."

Still other antidepressants your doctor may prescribe work on the imbalance of dopamine (another brain chemical) or a combination of serotonin and nor-epinephrine (called SNRIs, which stands for serotonin norepinephrine reup-take inhibitors). Some brand names of SNRIs are Effexor and Wellbutrin (which has also been found to work on nicotine withdrawal).

Some studies and anecdotal reports of SSRI and NSRI use in CFS show that they don't appear to help; in fact, some symptoms get worse, particularly sleep problems and fatigue.

Antidepressants do have side effects, however, but each one can have differ-ent side effects in each person. For example, Effexor has been found to increase blood pressure in some individuals, but not in others. Zoloft has been found to add on the pounds in some people, but not in others. See Table 7-3 for a complete low-down on antidepressants commonly used in CFS patients.

Knocking yourself out for a restful night's sleep

Fatigue is the number-one symptom of CFS, but, as you know too well, feeling tired doesn't translate into being able to sleep. In fact, every bone and muscle in your body may be screaming, "Sleep!", but you're still going to toss and turn and be, well, plain miserable to boot. Worse, the less sleep you get, the more depressed, anxious, and uncomfortable you will be. Your symptoms will get worse, and you'll do anything for a good night's sleep.

Short of having someone konk you over the head, you can get the sleep you need via sleep aids. Over-the-counter medications such as Tylenol PM and Benadryl have been effective as sleep aids for some people with CFS.

Prescription drugs are a different story. Yes, prescription sleep aids may become habit forming, but what's more important — the need for a pill or the need for a full eight hours? See your doctor for more information.

Table 7-4, courtesy of www.cfids.org, is a list of common sleep aids along with their side effects and risks.

The medications in Table 7-4 haven't been studied and approved for use specifically in people with CFS. This list is comprised of FDA-approved standard drugs for the treatment of sleep problems and may have been prescribed by physicians treating people with CFS.

Figure 7-4		Common Sleep Aids	
Medication Chemical Name	*Medication Brand Name*	*Common Side Effects*	*Additional Information*
Alprazolam	Xanax	Drowsiness; abdominal discomforts; abnormal muscle movement	Drug dependence possible; many drug and food interactions.
Clonazepam	Klonopin	Drowsiness; coordination problems	Multiple, severe potential drug interactions.
Temazepam	Restoril	Drowsiness; dizziness; fatigue; headache	Drug dependence possible.
Diphenhydramine	Benadryl (antihistamine)	Sleepiness; dry mouth; nausea; coordination problems	Potential drug interactions.
Zolpidem tartrate	Ambien	Daytime drowsiness; dizziness; headache; indigestion; may cause amnesia or confusion	Works rapidly; potential drug interactions; potentially habit forming.
Flurazepam HCl	Dalmane	Dizziness; drowsiness; falling; may increase depression	Drug dependence possible; use caution if patient is depressed.
Quazepam	Doral	Drowsiness; headache	Potentially addictive; use caution if patient is depressed.
Estazolam	ProSom	Drowsiness; coordination problems; headache	Potentially addictive; potential drug interactions.

Suppressing your allergy symptoms

Some people who develop CFS have a history of allergies. So how do you deal with your allergies when you have CFS? In this section, I go over some of the remedies used for CFS patients with allergies.

Lubricating your eyes

Because even eye drops can affect other parts of your body, use your Visine Plus discriminately. If you suffer from dry, itchy eyes, artificial tear eye drops may do the trick. Be sure to use the preservative-free ones, because any preservative may create a reaction in your CFS-sensitive body. (But make sure you check the expiration date periodically, and don't touch the dropper tip to your eye!)

If artificial tears don't do the trick, speak to your doctor before trying any other over-the-counter brand. He can also prescribe a prescription-only eye drop that is less likely to make your CFS worse.

Checking out some useful over-the-counter antihistamines

Why not? If an antihistamine can help your symptoms, I'm all for it! I would suggest one of the current "top three" nonsedating pills for daytime:

- ✔ Desloratadine (Clarinex)
- ✔ Fexofenadine (Allegra)
- ✔ Cetirizine (Zyrtec)

Because some antihistamines can make you drowsy and even up your symptoms, I suggest taking them in the evening. Benadryl, which has sedating elements, may help you sleep. But, again, and I can't say this enough, check with your doctor before taking any medication or supplement — and that includes over-the-counter allergy meds.

Banishing nausea from your system

Being extremely tired is bad enough. But on top of that, you're nauseated, you have diarrhea or constipation, and you're bloated. Yikes! What can you do? In this section, I go over some gastrointestinal (GI) remedies to keep your nausea and other stomach problems at bay.

Although gastrointestinal symptoms aren't officially part of the CFS case definition, many people with CFS do complain of GI issues, so your GI tract deserves its day in the CFS sun.

Stimulating your immune system with gamma globulin

No, this isn't a science-fiction story. *Gamma globulin* is a drug that mimics human immune proteins called, you guessed it, globulins. This drug is rich in antibody molecules that can fight a whole host of infections and is used primarily to rev up an immune system that's not working right. It has had limited success with CFS patients, but the jury is still out on its usefulness.

Calming your gut with antinausea pills

Physicians usually prescribe antispasmodics for cramps and stomachaches; antidiarrheal medications for . . . well, you know; and even anti-anxiety medications to keep stress at bay and soothe the mind. (Stress can make your GI symptoms even worse.) You can find a list of these GI medications in Table 7-5, courtesy of www.cfids.org.

The medications listed in Table 7-5 haven't been studied and approved for use specifically in people with CFS. This list is comprised of FDA-approved standard drugs used to treat gastrointestinal symptoms and may have been prescribed by physicians treating people with CFS.

Table 7-5	Gastrointestinal Medicines		
Medication Chemical Name	*Medication Brand Name*	*Common Side Effects*	*Additional Information*
Phenobarbital *plus* hyoscyamine sulfate *plus* atropine sulfate, *plus* scopolamine hydrobromide	Donnatal; Bellatal	Drowsiness; agitation; bloating; decreased sweating; constipation	Potentially addicting; multiple drug interactions possible
Dicyclomine HCl	Bentyl	Blurred vision; dizziness; drowsiness; nausea; nervousness	Multiple warnings and potential drug interactions
Hyoscyamine sulfate	Levsin; Levbid; Anaspaz; Levsinex	Decreased sweating; dry mouth; drowsiness; bloating; blurred vision	Several warnings and potential drug interactions

Medication Chemical Name	Medication Brand Name	Common Side Effects	Additional Information
Chlordiazepoxide HCl *plus* clidinium bromide	Librax	Sedating; dry mouth; blurred vision; coordination problems; constipation	Potentially addictive; many potential drug interactions and warnings
Nizatidine	Axid	Abdominal pain; diarrhea; constipation; dimmed vision; sleep problems	Caution when taking with aspirin; drug interactions possible

Although GI medicines may help with your nausea and cramps, they may also increase your GI distress. Work with your doctor to find the right solution.

Knowing when to avoid over-the-counter antinausea medication

Avoiding certain medicines isn't as important as knowing what OTC medicines can help your symptoms and which ones can put you at unnecessary risk. Certainly, OTC pain medications may be preferable before going on to the pre-scription-strength stuff. After checking with your doctor, you can also help yourself with OTC medications for upset stomachs, such as Tums or Gas-X.

Be warned that Dramamine can help your nausea, but it can also make you tired (which is great at night, but not so great during the day).

Lashing out at suspected triggers: Lyme disease, autoimmune conditions, and viral infections

What came first, the chicken or the egg? The Lyme disease virus or the CFS? Let's face it — who cares? The important thing is you feel sick and need help. In this section, I go over some of the treatments that are being used to help you fight back.

My, how you've grown!

Human growth hormone is currently being tested as a drug to suppress a malfunctioning immune system in people with CFS. It's only in the investigation stages, but be on the lookout for this possibly successful new treatment.

Getting your flu shot: Yes or no?

The benefits of an annual flu shot must be weighed against the possibility of making your CFS symptoms worse.

The pros:

✔ A flu shot can protect you from getting an infection — and feeling even worse.

✔ A flu shot can prevent you from spreading an infection to others.

✔ A flu shot is recommended if you're in a high-risk flu group, such as the elderly and the very young.

The cons:

✔ A flu shot itself has the potential worsen your CFS symptoms or cause a relapse.

✔ A flu shot isn't recommended if your CFS symptoms include swollen glands, sore throat, and fever.

✔ A flu shot is never recommended if you have had severe adverse reactions to a flu shot before you came down with CFS.

The bottom line? Work with your doctor and see whether the advantages outweigh the disadvantages. Ultimately, the decision is yours.

Hitting on the right antibiotic

If you have an infection, the right antibiotic can help knock it out of your system. But your CFS means that you're extra sensitive to medications — so a blood or saliva culture is important for matching the bacteria with the correct antibiotic. As a rule, doctors give antibiotics only if a person with CFS has a clear sign of infection.

Regulating your immune system with interferon drugs

Ampligen is a synthetic nucleic acid (the real nucleic acid helps form your DNA and RNA) that stimulates the production of interferon. Why is interferon good? It helps modify immune systems so that your body is more able to fight off the bad infection.

As an added plus, interferon also works like an antiviral drug. Studies have shown that some people with CFS have improved when taking Ampligen; they are less confused and more able to perform daily activities. But the drug is still in the clinical trial stages in the United States and isn't yet approved for widespread use by the FDA,. Ampligen also has a risk of liver damage.

Alpha-interferon is the real deal, produced by the immune system when attacked by a viral infection. But treatment with Interferon-A2 (its official drug name) was found to be successful only if a CFS patient's immune system had an imbalance of natural killer antibodies.

Some studies say that alpha-interferon may also make CFS symptoms worse! So be sure to consult with your doctor.

Combining Medicine with Other Treatments

Medical regimens are only a part of the CFS picture. Yes, certain drugs can alleviate your pain, flu-like symptoms, depression, and fatigue. But studies have found that you can have much more success if you combine your medicine with other therapies: one-on-one talk therapy, stress counseling, sleep management, and more. I give you a brief introduction to these treatments here, so you can begin to determine whether they may be right for you. However, you can read more about these alternative treatments in Chapters 8, 9, and 10.

Seeking psychological and emotional counseling

Put two people on antidepressants side by side. One of them combines their medicine with psychological counseling; the other just pops the pills and sees a doctor only when a prescription needs refilling. Which person do you think will have more success in battling depression?

Easy. Medicine can only go so far. Like diet and exercise, medicine and therapy go together for success. CFS is a burden — you have no getting around that, and depression, whether the cause or a result, can only make all your symptoms worse. Although most types of counseling may be beneficial, some talk therapies have had more success with CFS than others. Look for all the details in Chapter 8.

Combining traditional medicine with alternative therapies

Although medical doctors and alternative therapists (homeopaths, nutritionists, and more) don't always get along, even the most scientific physician today believes that certain alternatives are a good thing. Healthy eating, meditating, journaling, taking multivitamins — these have all become mainstream. You can find the details on alternative therapies in Chapter 9.

Team discipline counts!

An ideal medical treatment for CFS consists of an *interdisciplinary team:* a group of health care professionals in different fields who work towards a common goal — your health. This team may include a primary care physician, a mental health specialist, a physical therapist, an exercise trainer, a sleep expert, and a neurologist or other specialty physician. This team works in concert with each other; each health care professional has a record of what the others are doing, their diagnoses, and their progress. The team isn't constant — you may need only one or two training sessions with a personal exercise trainer or a sleep expert. But no matter how many times you see a health care professional, his records become a part of your treatment plan.

Popping a multivitamin once a day

Good health is the primary goal of any CFS doctor worth his salt. Maybe a multivitamin isn't considered to be medication by some physicians, but vitamins are still pills that you gotta swallow, and doctors may recommend taking a multivitamin along with other medications being used to treat CFS. Taking a multivitamin can't hurt, and it may help your immune system and your general health. Sometimes additional B12 and essential fatty-acid (EFA) supplements are suggested.

Work with your doctor to see what vitamins you should and shouldn't take in relation to your other treatments. (See Chapter 9 for more details on supplements.)

Developing a realistic exercise routine

Unfortunately for CFS sufferers, exercise, that mainstay for cardiovascular health and coping with stress, may do more harm than good. Too much and you can feel even more exhausted and more fatigued than before. But *too much* doesn't mean *never.* Working with a physical therapist, occupational therapist or personal trainer, you can develop an exercise routine that works for you — giving you the benefits without the repercussions. See Chapter 10 for more information.

Restructuring your life to accommodate your treatment

CFS brings a lifestyle change — there's no denying it. The fatigue, the depression, the flu-like symptoms — these and other symptoms may seriously curtail your daily routines, especially if those daily routines can exacerbate your condition. Some of the hard life lessons CFS patients may face — or feel they may face — include the following:

✔ The unpredictable course of CFS makes it almost impossible to schedule things.

✔ Memory loss and lack of concentration can affect the way you work or study.

✔ Less energy translates into less activities. You can't do everything you did before.

✔ Uncertainty about the future course of your CFS makes it hard to plan for your own future.

✔ Debilitating symptoms makes it hard to work and get around — giving you a loss of independence and financial security.

✔ Worries about your ability to raise your children may or may not be unfounded.

✔ You have a rocky road ahead for your relationships. Intimacy may not be possible.

✔ A lack of understanding about CFS can affect your daily life. People may think you're faking it. You may even begin to wonder about that yourself.

But despite some of the life adjustments you may have to make, have hope. Combining several approaches to treatment can help find a new balance of rest and activity that allows some predictable pattern and structure for redefining a meaningful life. See Chapters 11, 12, and 13 for the full scoop.

Chapter 8

Handling Your Emotional and Psychological Issues

• •

In This Chapter

▶ Discovering how much you're being affected on an emotional level

▶ Tracking down a quality therapist

▶ Finding out how one-on-one therapy helps

▶ Getting friends and family involved in your recovery

• •

If you think having chronic fatigue syndrome is hard enough, CFS can also cause emotional and psychological distress. Some people who have CFS show signs of depression, irritability, antisocial behavior, agoraphobia, or additional psychological and psychiatric conditions that often intensify other symptoms of CFS.

Whether or not your depression and anxiety *became* one of your symptoms or was the *result* of your symptoms doesn't matter. What does matter is the emotional, mental, and psychological toll it is exacting from your already overtaxed mind, body, and soul. In this chapter, you see how CFS can affect you emotionally and how to deal with the changes. You can also discover how to recognize the signs of depression and figure out when and how to seek out the help you need.

Your brain can get sick just like any other part of your body. Many people struggling with emotional and psychological issues are ashamed of what they're experiencing or try to handle the illness on their own, but this move is a faulty one. You need to get treatment for any symptoms associated with your mind and your emotions just like you would a physical symptom, such as a cough or a swollen kneecap. Hey, you'd go to the doctor if your kidneys were acting up — and you need to treat your brain the same way.

Recognizing the Vicious Emotional Cycle in Action

Have you ever noticed how a snowball gets bigger and bigger as it rolls downhill? This snowball effect can apply to your condition — and your emotions, and you don't even need the snow. Picture this scenario:

> You come down with CFS symptoms. You try to minimize the symptoms, but you can't. You become depressed in addition to your fatigue, aches and pains, and sore throat.
>
> Scared, you go to your doctor. She tries to treat your condition, but ends up sending you to a specialist. Soon, you're on a full regimen of medical treatment, from painkillers to sleep aids, from antibiotics to antidepressants.
>
> At the same time, your life changes. You can't focus as well at work or in school. Some days, you can't even get out of bed! Depression, anxiety, and fear become your companions. The more you try to hide your emotions away, the stronger they come back.
>
> Your feelings mix with your symptoms, and your anxiety homes in on your depression. Your pain becomes both physical *and* mental. In turn, your symptoms get worse and your feelings more intense. Your depression worsens, which only makes you more anxious. Your physical pain becomes even more intense with its dose of mental torture.

Here, the CFS snowball is ready to become an avalanche — unless you get help for the emotions you're feeling. In this section, I help you understand this vicious cycle in more detail, so you can stop it in its tracks.

Tipping the scales: The beginning of the cycle

When does the snowball effect start to form? Where does your emotional cycle begin? As you probably suspect, it all starts with CFS. Living with CFS is difficult, no doubt about it. The frustration of not being able to do what you usually do or feel healthy or energized can cause havoc to your emotions and psyche. The fatigue, a difficulty in concentrating, the swollen glands, the inability to do things like before — these symptoms of CFS can create an emotional disorder, even if you had no hint of a problem before.

CFS has an impact on every facet of your life, and on every person you know, love, and work with. Not only do you deal with your illness, which looms large over your every waking moment, but you may feel the need, to a larger or lesser extent, to hide your condition from view. Then you also have to deal with the fact that, when you do tell people, they may not believe you. These factors alone, especially when combined, can play nasty games with your mind and your emotions.

In addition to the emotional stress, you must constantly battle with the physical stress — the very real pain you feel every day. Trying to push through your inability to get out of the chair (for example) can add a tremendous amount of stress to an already overwhelmed mind.

As if that weren't enough, you must also face the financial stress. A million questions about how you will make ends meet may be running through your mind: What if you can't keep your job due to your CFS? How will you earn money? How will you support yourself and your family? How will you get or keep your health insurance? How will you survive?

These emotional and psychological stressors can create a vicious cycle — like a snowball, it builds and builds, making everything worse. Getting the psychological help you need sooner rather than later aids progress. If you find that your mind and body are stretched thin, consider it time to say, "Stop! I can't take this anymore!" It's time to get some help.

Knowing when you need to break the cycle

So how do you know when you may be dealing with more than just a down day? When is the right time to see a mental health care professional so you can stop the cycle? Ask yourself the questions in the following list. If you say *yes* to any one of them, you may very well have emotional or psychological issues for which you need to seek professional help to reclaim your life:

- Has your circle of friends begun to shrink?
- Have you used up all your sick days and vacation time because you were too ill or lacked motivation or desire to go to work?
- Have your loved ones become less patient with you?
- Have you stopped going to the gym because the subsequent fatigue you feel isn't worth it?
- Have you found you can barely tolerate the sound of the TV? Or, on the flip side, are you watching TV more and more?

✔ Have people been asking you what's wrong, perhaps due to changes in your behavior?

✔ Have you started to say something, but then forgot what you were going to say midstream?

✔ Are you getting less and less to do at work, even though you've asked for a new project?

✔ Has making dinner — even a frozen one — become more than you can handle physically, emotionally, or both?

✔ Have you stopped your personal grooming, such as avoiding the shower for over a week?

✔ Do you find yourself crying at things that haven't impacted you in the past, such as a stupid TV commercial?

If you find that you need to seek out the help of a professional, turn to the section "Finding a Good Therapist" to get you started. Don't wait.

Avoiding the slippery slope

I can't say it enough: Recognizing that you may need to seek a mental health professional and then doing it is vital to your well-being. Otherwise, the snowball effect (that sounds a little fluffier than it is) can soon take a drastic turn down a slippery slope.

If you don't seek out help to deal with any emotional or psychological issues you may be facing regularly, you're putting yourself in harm's way. The longer you wait, you're at more risk of spiraling down, your feelings of helplessness or lack of hope getting the best of you. You may even begin to have self-harming or suicidal thoughts. If you're having or have had such thoughts, talk to your doctor or a close friend or family member that you trust. Keeping these thoughts to yourself only puts you at more risk.

Self-Screening Yourself for Depression

Everyone gets down now and then. And sometimes feeling down is appropriate! Something would be wrong with you if you didn't feel bad if you were fired or your significant other broke up with you. But although unhappiness feels like an albatross you may wear around your neck forever, it passes. Within a month, you'll be more like yourself. In clinical depression, however, the albatross just gets heavier and heavier. You don't snap out of it.

At least half of the people suffering from CFS also suffer from depression at some point, which makes sense. Adjusting your life to a chronic and debilitating illness such as CFS is difficult. Don't wait until you are so down that all your other CFS symptoms flare up. Your unhappiness over having CFS can turn into full-fledged clinical depression.

Here are the signs that may signal depression. Notice how close some of them are to CFS symptoms (for more info on CFS symptoms, check out Chapter 2):

- Apathy and lack of enthusiasm
- Excessive crying
- Excessive irritability
- Extreme fatigue
- Feelings of helplessness and hopelessness
- High anxiety
- Inability to concentrate and focus on the task at hand
- Insomnia (or too much sleep)
- Irrational guilt
- Lack of joy in all things
- Lack of self-esteem
- Loss of appetite (or eating too much)
- Loss of sexual feelings
- Physical pain with no apparent reason
- Suicidal thoughts

  If you're having suicidal thoughts, make sure you see your health care professional right away! (And bring a family member or close friend if you feel like you need the support.)

- Withdrawal from others
- Worried, ruminating, or obsessive thoughts

Because CFS can make you depressed, and because so many CFS symptoms are similar to depression, you should talk to your doctor to help make sense of what you're feeling. Most likely your doctor will suggest therapy and possible medication that can help with both your CFS symptoms and your depression. Although these medicines and talk therapy won't cure your CFS, they can make your life more bearable and your outlook much better. (See the section "Finding a Good Therapist" later in the chapter for more information.)

The five stages of grief

Over 40 years ago, the renowned psychiatrist Elisabeth Kubler-Ross outlined five stages people with terminal illness go through before they die. Her five stages have been interpreted through the years to apply to all things traumatic: losing a job, getting a divorce, or even having a chronic condition. In the wake of any traumatic experience, you need to go through the following five steps in order to be emotionally healthy (the order and length of time people experience these steps vary from person to person):

Stage 1: Denial ("This is just the flu. I'll be fine before you know it!"): When you first find out you have a chronic illness, or when your symptoms begin to take over, you can't believe it. Of course, you can get up. You just need iron, or you're depressed, whatever. But one thing is for sure: If someone said you have CFS, you'd turn away.

Stage 2: Anger ("I can't believe this happened to me! It's not fair."): As the shock of your diagnosis wears off, anger sets in. Being furious that you came down with a debilitating illness is only natural.

Stage 3: Bargaining ("Dear God, if I can only get my energy back, I promise I'll be a better person."): Whether you believe in God, Allah, Buddha, or the Universe, it makes no difference. You can even be a devout atheist, and yet you will try to make a bargain with the powers that be, that somehow, someway, a miracle will occur and you will immediately be yourself again.

Stage 4: Depression ("My life is ruined. I'll never be happy again."): Half of the people with CFS get stuck at this stage for quite a while. They may even revisit it in the future. The fact is that your life isn't what it once was. You can't do the things you used to do. You're a different person. And, boy, does that suck.

Stage 5: Acceptance ("Okay. This is it, at least for now. I have to make the best of it and learn how to live again."): Dr. Kubler-Ross's last stage means that you have literally tried everything not to have CFS, but you do. You know it, your family knows it, your friends know it, and your doctors know it. Yes, things will be different, but they can still work. Realizing what's what is called a healthy reality.

I always like to add a sixth stage: Hope — because from the depths of despair comes hope. Not a false hope, like you will wake up perfectly fine tomorrow, but a realistic, valid hope that with support, love, and knowledge, you can get through the worst of your illness.

One difference between clinical depression and CFS is in relation to post-exertional malaise, or relapse after mental or physical exertion. In depression, exercise usually helps the symptoms you're facing, but exercise only exacerbates CFS symptoms. Another difference is that people who are depressed rarely have a sore throat or swollen lymph nodes, which are common symptoms of CFS.

The biggest red flag, the one that you have to pay attention to above all else, is suicidal thoughts or attempts. What's worrisome here is that if you're depressed, you may not push yourself to go to the doctor to get help. Telling *someone* about what you're feeling and thinking is vitally important, because he can make sure you see a health care professional immediately. Share the previous list of depression signals as well as the following list with your loved ones, and they can be on guard for any behavior that may spell danger. Some warning signs that you may be having suicidal thoughts include the following:

- Giving away personal objects that mean a lot to you.

- Social isolation so extreme you don't go out of your house, and no one's heard from you in weeks.

- Throwing away the soap and toothbrush and laundry detergent. When you're depressed, you don't care about your looks, but if giving up on grooming keeps up for weeks, your condition could be more serious.

- Calling people you haven't spoken to in years just to say hello (or goodbye).

- Thinking about the different ways you can kill yourself.

- Stopping your medications or stockpiling them.

- Writing a goodbye letter to friends or family members.

Finding a Good Therapist

Therapy can be very effective and is often essential in stabilizing your emotions and psychological ups and downs. You have such a wide variety of therapies and therapeutic treatments to choose from that separating the "wheat from the chaff" is sometimes hard. Yes, charlatans are out there. Yes, some doctors aren't as good as others. But with a little legwork, you can find a good therapist — one that understands what you're going through and helps you through it.

The most important thing to remember in getting a therapist is that she *must* understand that CFS is real, that it is a physical disorder, and that the emotional pain and mental confusion you're suffering are a result of your symptoms. She *must* believe that CFS isn't all in your head.

If you can find a therapist who has experience treating CFS, so much the better. But it isn't imperative. As long as she has an open mind and is willing to work with you — and you have a good rapport — then you're in good hands. In this section, I go over exactly that: how to find the right therapist for you.

Therapy, like medicine, isn't a perfect science. A good therapist can help you create a strategy to cope with the stress in your life, as well as how to live with debilitating symptoms. She is there to listen and lend a sympathetic, an objective, ear. But you have to do some work. Therapy isn't as easy as remembering to pop a pill, but if you're willing to meet your therapist halfway, try out her suggestions, and be honest with her, your emotional pain can ease.

Gathering recommendations

First things first: Before picking up the phone to make an appointment, you need to make sure as best you can that you're going to the right therapist. Sure, you can do a consultation, and in fact, most therapists prefer a session where they talk to a potential patient to see whether she can help and whether the two of you have a rapport. But consultations cost, and feeling that you're going to the right therapist right off the bat is always better.

So how do you do this? Recommendations, recommendations, recommendations. Consider the following sources:

- ✔ **Your physician:** Your primary care physician should be able to give you the names of a few therapists. He may also be aware of therapists who either specialize in CFS or also think that CFS is physical.

- ✔ **Your loved ones:** You may feel like you're the only person who needs to see a shrink, but you may be surprised when you start to ask around. More people than not have gone to therapists at various traumatic times in their lives — and are better for it. A trusted friend or family member can suggest a good therapist for you and even ask his therapist whether she knows a therapist who specializes in CFS.

- ✔ **Your support group:** If anyone should know the name of a good therapist for your problems, you can count on the members of a CFS support group. If you aren't a member of one, find out more about them later in this chapter.

✔ **A CFS-specific organization:** Several excellent nationwide organizations may be able to help you with information. Two good ones that you should check out are the Chronic Fatigue and Immune Dysfunction Syndrome (CFIDS) Association of America via its Web site, www.cfids.org, and the International Association of Chronic Fatigue Syndrome (IACFS) at www.iacfs.net. Please note that neither organization gives referrals, but both can give you good advice on finding a therapist. (You can find more resources in the appendix.)

✔ **Someone in your church or community center:** Church members and other community leaders may be able to recommend a therapist to you or know someone who can.

Checking your insurance coverage

Okay . . . so you have your list of therapists in hand and you've narrowed it down, say, to the top three. The next step is to check your insurance company for their policies on mental health visits.

Be sure to find out the answers to the following questions:

✔ **Are any of the therapists on your list in its network?** Most insurance companies give you the option of going in-network or out-of-network, but the latter costs more. If you're in an HMO, you must go to one of its affiliated professionals.

✔ **How many visits to the therapist are allowed?** The number of allowable visits vary from plan to plan. Some companies allow for CFS having an "organic base" and cover your therapist as any other doctor. Others have set limits for the number of allowable visits for which they'll pay.

Many plans require that you go to one of the company's providers for an initial assessment phase (one to three appointments), and then the insurance company tries to match you with the right therapist. If you go to a therapist directly, some companies won't pay for the costs or will pay only a small percentage of benefits.

Verifying your doctor's credentials

After you've decided on a doctor, you need to make sure she's not on any "Wanted" list. You can check on your doctor via the American Psychiatric

Association (if she is a psychiatrist) at www.psych.org or the American Psychological Association at www.apa.org, if she is a psychologist. (See other resources in the appendix at the back of this book.)

A mental health professional can have several different types of degrees — and all are acceptable. The degrees are as follows:

- ✔ **Psychiatrist:** Like the character Lorraine Bracco plays on *The Sopranos,* a psychiatrist has a medical degree. She went to med school and did an internship and residency just like other doctors. She is able to prescribe medications.

- ✔ **Psychologist:** Instead of a medical-school degree, a psychologist may have a Ph.D. in psychology. He can do individual therapy, but has to refer you to a psychiatrist (or your primary care physician) for medications. Some psychologists don't have a Ph.D., but as long as they are board-certified, it doesn't matter. (You just can't call him "doc.")

- ✔ **MSW:** This acronym stands for *master in social work.* She has exactly that: a master's degree in social work. The downside is that someone who has an MSW can't prescribe medication, if necessary.

- ✔ **PN:** The *P* is for Psychiatric and the *N* is for Nurse. A PN spent time practicing in a mental health facility and may have a master's degree.

When you go for your first visit, the mental health professional's college degree, master's and/or Ph.D., and board-certified certificates are likely prominently displayed in her office. If they aren't, don't be afraid to ask to see them. And don't be afraid to ask her why she doesn't have them on her wall. You may be suspicious of the doctor if her credentials aren't readily visible.

Board certified doesn't mean a medical doctor is qualified to be a carpenter. Each specialty of medicine has an official accrediting board and members must meet exacting standards to be board certified. They must first pass a test. Although doctors don't officially have to be board certified to practice, certification is one of those things that can affect your confidence in that practitioner.

Getting Individual Therapy

The majority of people who have CFS as well as another emotional or psychological issue do individual therapy, either once or twice a week. The therapy session is usually informal, with both the therapist and the patient sitting in comfortable chairs or sofas. Sometimes the therapist sits behind a desk.

You should be able to feel comfortable while at your therapy session. The office itself should be peaceful, calming, and quiet — like a haven from the rest of the world.

In individual therapy, you do most of the talking. Your therapist may interrupt you to ask you a question, to guide you in a specific direction, and to help you see something in a whole new (and more objective) light. She may also suggest coping strategies to work on at home.

Individual therapy doesn't happen overnight. In order to be effective, you need to have several visits. You can't find a quick miracle cure for your emotional or psychological issues you're facing. But over, say, two months, you should feel that you're getting better, as if the cloud has lifted. It won't be a "Eureka!" moment, but more of a gentle smile. If combined with prescription drugs (which is generally recommended for the clinical depression in CFS), the therapy may be able to progress a little quicker.

Here, in this section, is everything you need to know about one-on-one therapy for someone with CFS.

Improving your understanding of CFS with psycheducation

Knowing the psychological underpinnings of the emotional side of your CFS is invaluable. For psycheducation 101, understanding the different therapy techniques that are out there can give you a jumpstart on help, so take a look at the following technique descriptions:

- ✒ **Free Association:** This technique focuses on connecting a perception, a smell, or a taste with an experience in the past. A connection can also be linked to different air temperatures, times of the year, or day and night. For example, Ellen hates spring — it's when her symptoms first started. She begins to get even more depressed every March. A therapist can help her see the link between the two and help her learn to understand her illness and, in term, accept it.

- ✒ **Dream interpretation:** Old-fashioned Freudian analysts aren't the only ones who ask you about your dreams. Many therapists encourage their patients to keep a dream notebook on their night tables to jot down details about dreams that woke them up so they won't forget them in the morning. These dreams can help you and your therapist determine what's bothering you, what you're afraid of, and what's stopping you from being able to cope with your CFS.

✔ **Behavioral and social-skill training:** Here your actions speak louder than words. Instead of talking about how your illness is making you feel, your therapist asks you to be aware of how these feelings are affecting your day-to-day routines. You have homework in which you keep a diary of when you feel really depressed — as well as what triggered it and what you did. This technique is also part of cognitive-behavioral therapy (CBT). See the details about CBT in a following section.

Keeping a journal isn't just for writers. Studies have found that putting down your thoughts in a notebook, a blank book, or even a legal pad can have a calming effect. Writing about your feelings can help you cope with them. As you write, ideas and coping strategies may come to you. The pages not only help you become more aware of your symptoms, but they also become a barometer of how you're progressing. Another reason to journal: If you find your memory impaired, the journal can provide clues to what you may have forgotten.

Journaling isn't for everyone. Sometimes, it can have the opposite effect, and some people begin to focus even more on the issues they're dealing with. If you find that journaling doesn't help you or even aggravates what you're feeling, talk to your mental health professional about finding other coping methods.

Establishing healthy thinking through cognitive-behavioral therapy (CBT)

You're probably asking yourself what exactly this CBT is (besides sounding like something a little too technical for your taste). Basically, *CBT* is a *biopsychosocial treatment* (even more off-putting), which means that the therapy concentrates on how the mind and body interact to trigger or exacerbate CFS symptoms. Studies have shown success with CBT in helping people with CFS better handle the emotional trauma of their condition.

Although your doctor, specialist, or physical therapist can help administer CBT techniques, seeing a CBT therapist who has had special training in it is always the best option. (It's like seeing your eye doctor for plastic surgery: It can work, but you're usually better off going to a plastic surgeon to get rid of your wrinkles.) To find a licensed CBT therapist in your area, contact the National Association of Cognitive-Behavioral Therapists at www.nacbt.org or by calling 800-853-1135 or 304-723-3982 (for callers outside the United States). You can also contact the Association for Behavioral and Cognitive Therapies at www.aabt.org or 212-647-1890.

Here's what you need to know about CBT:

✔ You have biochemical signals that "spark" in your brain and travel to and from your body, providing the fuel for bodily function and conscious and unconscious thought. Your conscious thoughts — the ones your brain allows you to hear — can be either harmful or positive. You can either feel hopeful about your CFS treatment plan — or horribly depressed.

CBT works on these conscious thoughts, turning the bad to the good, to improve function, behavior, and symptom management. And, because these conscious thoughts spark different biochemical signals, your unconscious thoughts will be biochemically changed as well.

✔ *Stress* is the key word in CBT: awareness of how stress is affecting your CFS symptoms and how to better cope with the stress stemming from your illness. Through the CBT process, you discover how to recognize and more successfully manage your particular brands of stress.

✔ CBT also involves relaxation exercises that alleviate stress. Deep breathing, meditation, and visualization are all used to help you have a better life, despite your CFS.

✔ Your CBT therapist may introduce light physical exercise into your program, designed on your present activity levels. Even if you can barely lift your head, some exercise can be gradually introduced into your life to help reduce stress and help you relax. By supervising your exercise, you can help stop the destructive everything-or-nothing way of exercise, where you push too hard when you're feeling better — resulting in even more fatigue and exhaustion. CBT helps you figure out how to pace your physical activity.

✔ In comparison to traditional therapies, CBT is usually more short-term. You and your therapist together may make, say, an eight-week goal to find relief from your emotional trauma with every-other-week visits to ensure you're still on track.

✔ The most important rule of all: You must do the work, too. You have to form a partnership with your therapist in which you work together to recognize your negative reactions to stressors, those thoughts that keep you down, and, ultimately, change them to enhance your quality of life. You have to be an active participant for CBT to work. In other words, if you are given "homework assignments" (in reality, tools to help you recognize your negative thinking), you can't say your dog ate them.

✔ You have to stick with the program. If your symptoms get worse, one of your first thoughts can be to get rid of the once or twice weekly gab sessions with your therapist. Who wants to visit a therapist when your glands are swollen, you have a terrific headache, and you can barely get out of bed? Quitting midstream is the most common reason for CBT not to work. Stay with it. If necessary, you and your therapist can work out a way for the therapy to continue when you can't leave your home.

CBT can work — but it's not a cure-all. Yes, it can help with your coping abilities, help soothe your emotions, and help you move forward with your life. But you still need treatment to deal with your other CFS symptoms — CBT doesn't get rid of fatigue. It may improve fatigue somewhat, but appears to help less with pain and other physical symptoms. You may also need to continue on your medications.

Not all insurance companies recognize CBT. Always check with your health insurance company to find out its policies before proceeding with the therapy. If your insurance company doesn't cover CBT, you may want to stick with a therapist it recommends first. But if you have the money and want to try CBT, go for it. Costs of CBT vary from therapist to therapist and region to region.

Just because your doctor suggests you try CBT doesn't mean he thinks your CFS is all in your head and you need to see a shrink. By discussing CBT, he is acknowledging that you have this physical illness that CBT therapy has been found to help in a short amount of time.

Participating in Relationship, Family, and Group Therapy

No one lives in a vacuum, and if you have CFS, your loved ones are affected as well. Therapists often recommend that other family members join in on therapy sessions to assist those members in gaining better insight into CFS and to help the patient maintain a lifestyle and relationships that are more conducive to improving the patient's health and well-being. Families who unite against CFS often report improvements in their relationships and a strengthening of family ties.

Whether it's a significant other, a spouse, siblings, or children — your family plays a crucial role in helping you cope with your CFS. In this section, I go over the role of your loved ones in detail. I also introduce the idea of group therapy, where you can get the professional counseling you need and be connected with other people who have CFS at the same time.

Repairing relationships on the rocks

Staying together is hard enough for couples who don't have the added stress of a chronic illness — so imagine how difficult it is if you have CFS and can no longer go out to dinner, go to a movie, or even havefewer conversations or laughs. Couples therapy can help you iron out your differences and better communicate what's troubling both you and your significant other — including your complaints and disappointments.

Couples therapy involves a therapist and the two of you. The therapist's role is to encourage you both to speak up honestly. And when, say, you get angry that your other half dare complain when you're lying in bed, in horrific pain and unable to move because of exhaustion, the therapist can interject, stopping the flow of anger before it gets ugly and getting both of you to understand each other's point of view.

Sometimes your individual therapist is licensed to also do couples therapy, but it may be better if she recommends someone different, so you're both new patients at the same time (you may say that you're leveling out the playing field).

Making CFS a family affair

Family bonds run deep. Most people are tied to their families in one way or another — even if they've had problems. However you define it, the structure of your particular family gives it order. Each member has a role to play — on both a conscious and unconscious level. For example, your family may have two breadwinners, one nurturing caregiver, a teased sibling, or even a scapegoat. As long as everyone knows his or her role (usually unconsciously), order is in place and peace is maintained.

But a debilitating, chronic illness like CFS changes all that. The balance gets off-kilter and order turns into discord. Why? Because change — both good and bad — threatens the continuation of the way the family has always operated, it is fought both consciously and unconsciously. The consequences of CFS can be highly disruptive and fraught with tension — especially if your symptoms are severe or if you are, say, the breadwinner, nurturer, or leader of the pack.

The result? Stress with a capital *S*. Until a new hierarchy shifts into place or until balance is restored, your family may feel anger, betrayal, confusion, and, yes, depression.

Family therapy can help bring balance to the family system faster, easier, and more efficiently. Instead of one-on-one talk, you and your family meet with a therapist and air your problems and worries out loud in a safe environment — where no one can walk out without explanation, throw a lamp, or break a wall.

Your family and significant others may also consider seeing their *own* individual therapist, to help them sort out their feelings without you being present (a good idea, in my mind).

Developing effective problem-solving skills

Solutions — not delusions — are the order of the day. Problem-solving within your family involves both the practical and the emotional. Your therapist can help guide you to those solutions, especially when it comes to stress and coping with your CFS. But here are some basic skills that you and your loved ones can start working on right now:

- ✔ **Taking care of someone else means taking care of *you* first.** Encourage your caregiver to get in his exercise, a massage, or alone time in order to be strong enough to help you.

- ✔ **Find yourself a quiet room.** Whether the abode is a corner of a studio apartment or a room on the top floor, you can create a peaceful sanctuary where anyone can go to ease stress. The room should be sparse, painted in soothing colors, and should have a pillow, a sofa, or a comfortable chair to sit on where you can easily meditate, write in your journal, or just lie still.

- ✔ **Create a support list.** When someone has a chronic illness like CFS, having more than one person helping out is a great idea. This way no one person gets so tired and stressed out that the problems are doubled. You should have a list of names and phone numbers of your doctors, therapists, relatives, and good friends in an accessible place.

- ✔ **Treat each problem as unemotional as possible.** Sure, if your symptoms are in full gear, not getting emotional about your inability to do the things you used to is difficult. But if you take a step back and look at the problem as if you were back in math class, you may find a better solution than crying into your pillow. Check out the following scenarios:

  - Can't make your sandwich? Get someone, like a friend, family member, or co-worker, to make several meals to keep in the refrigerator. Or have someone buy you some frozen dinners.

  - Can't finish your report? Ask your boss or your professor for an extension. You can't hide your CFS under your bed, and eventually colleagues and peers will have to know. You also may want to consider taking a semester off, using short-term disability benefits, or finding a different job, one that isn't as taxing. (See Chapter 12 for more details on having a job and CFS at the same time.)

Viewing your problems as logically as possible, with problem-solving in mind, is always a better option than becoming upset and overwhelmed.

Swapping insight and support in group therapy

You may have heard that old adage, "There's safety in numbers." I'd go further and say, "There's recognition in numbers." Group therapy offers both that safety and recognition via other people who have CFS and who have had similar experiences. Group therapy works when someone feels particularly isolated from the outside world.

This type of therapy is different than a support group, because a licensed therapist is in charge. She sets up specific guidelines and rules and ensures that each member of the group gets a chance to speak, and that no one gangs up on another person. Anonymity is a must, and no one uses surnames.

Group therapy offers you the opportunity to see you aren't alone, and that other people not only have CFS, but also have trouble getting out of bed or talking to their co-workers, or are feeling the stress in their relationships. You get a double benefit: therapy plus support.

Your individual therapist either runs the sessions himself, or he can recommend you to someone who does.

Chapter 9

Checking Out Some Alternative (Therapy) Routes

. . . .

. . . .

*Y*ou may have heard the saying that "two heads are better than one." Well, the same goes for medicine. Herbs and supplements, for example, can't take the place of proven antibiotics or traditional medical treatment, but they can supplement it. Herbs, supplements, aromatherapy oils, massage — all of these alternative therapies may help ease your pain and increase your energy in conjunction with traditional medicine. If you think that alternative therapy is also called *complementary medicine* just for fun, think again. Side by side, traditional medicine and alternative therapy can increase your odds of beating CFS.

Unfortunately, the alternative therapy community has a fair share of quacks and charlatans who are willing to take your money without providing any additional relief. In this chapter, I give you tips on how to spot the fakes and find truly good alternative therapists, and I steer you in the direction of alternative therapies that promise the greatest potential benefits.

Studies have found that many people with CFS are very likely to try alternative therapies, including massage therapy, nutritional supplements, megavitamins, and meditation. Although most of them found alternative routes helpful, only 42 percent discussed these treatments with their doctors! What's wrong with this picture? Although these treatments have helped others, communicating with your doctor about alternative routes you're interested in is important. Using alternative medicines alone can be a dangerous game — causing life-threatening illness or doing nothing to help. You may also be unaware of a complication or a symptom that makes the therapy harmful to your health.

Looking for the Best Alternative Caregivers

Almost everyone has heard the hype, those promises that sound too good to be true — "Loose ten pounds in ten minutes!"; "Get your energy back after one dose!"; or "Fatigued? I guarantee it will disappear after one session." Sadly, these promises are almost always empty. Just like there aren't any free lunches, you can't find any overnight cures for weight loss, lack of energy, or CFS.

But because CFS doesn't have one set treatment, you may be more inclined to look outside the traditional realm of medicine for relief and seek alternative therapies. But you have to be careful: Alternative health care professionals don't have the same stringent certifications and regulations as their traditional counterparts.

However, certain signs can steer you in the right direction. In this section, I detail how to differentiate the real deal from the fakes, so that after you decide upon an alternative therapy (detailed later in the chapter), you can know how to look for the right professional.

Checking for health insurance referrals

Alternative therapies are becoming more and more accepted in today's world, so much that many health insurance companies have a referral list of alternative health care professionals who not only pass the insurance seal of approval, but also are discounted for members. Check with your health insurance company to see what it covers. Your coverage may include the following:

- ✔ Nutritionists
- ✔ Massage therapists
- ✔ Acupuncturists
- ✔ Chiropractors
- ✔ Hypnotists
- ✔ Yoga instructors
- ✔ Exercise experts and gyms

Look before you leap

Ask yourself these questions before beginning any alternative therapy:

✔ What does my doctor or specialist say about this treatment?

✔ Did I research the therapy on the Internet?

✔ What is this treatment supposed to do?

✔ Do any scientific studies show that this treatment is safe and effective?

✔ Are there any ways the treatment can harm me instead of help?

✔ Did I ask the alternative health care professional what the risks are?

✔ Am I satisfied with what he's saying? Does it sound okay?

✔ Is this person licensed by the specific alternative therapy association?

If the alternative therapy and the alternative health care professional checks out, you can feel good about proceeding with the therapy.

However, you need to continue to ask yourself one important question: Am I feeling better with this treatment? If you aren't feeling better or are feeling worse, you should discontinue the therapy.

If your insurance doesn't cover a particular type of alternative therapy like yoga, but you'd still like to try it, you can see whether the therapy offers a free trial or session. For example, yoga classes often advertise that the first class is free, or maybe you can go to a class as a guest of a friend who is enrolled. Then if you think that the alternative therapy is worth the money, you can decide whether or not to pay for it out of your own pocket.

Using licensing associations

Even though many alternative therapy fields don't have the backing of the prominent American Medical Association, they have their own ways of regulating their practitioners. Before you book an appointment, check to see whether the person you're going to see is accredited with his specific organization.

Just because someone doesn't have credentials from a specialty organization doesn't necessarily mean he's mediocre. (Only a few states actually license these alternative therapy practitioners, but more and more are doing so.) But always ask the three-letter question: "Why?" If you're satisfied with his explanation as to why he doesn't have a license, you can try out the therapy — but only after you've spoken with your medical doctor about your plans.

You can find some of the professional associations of alternative therapies by checking out the following resources:

- ✔ **HolisticBenefits.com Resource Directory:** At this Web site, www.holisticbenefits.com, you can find listings of organizations literally from *A* (for the Aquatic Bodywork Association) to *Y* (The International Yoga Association).

- ✔ **National Certification Commission for Acupuncture and Oriental Medicine:** This organization can help you find an acupuncturist in your area. You can contact them via the following: NCCAOM, 11 Canal Center Plaza, Suite 300, Alexandria, VA 22314; phone 703-548-9004; Web site www.nccaom.org.

- ✔ **Massage therapist organizations:** The following are the three main organizations that massage therapists join:

  - **International Massage Association (IMA):** 25 South 4th Street, Warrenton, VA 20188; phone 540-351-0800; Web site www.imagroup.com.

  - **American Massage Therapy Association (AMTA):** 500 Davis Street, Suite 900, Evanston, IL 60201-4695; phone 877-905-2700 or 847-864-0123; Web site www.amtamassage.org.

  - **Associated Bodywork & Massage Professionals (ABMP):** 1271 Sugarbush Drive, Evergreen, CO 80439; phone 800-458-2267 or 303-674-8478; Web site www.abmp.com.

- ✔ **Chiropractic organizations:** The following are the leading national and international associations for doctors of chiropractics:

  - **American Chiropractic Association (ACA):** 1701 Clarendon Boulevard, Arlington, VA 22209; phone 703-276-8800; Web site www.amerchiro.org.

  - **International Chiropractors Association (ICA):** 1110 N. Glebe Road, Suite 650, Arlington, VA 22201; phone 800-423-4690 or 703-528-5000; Web site www.chiropractic.org.

- ✔ **American Dietetic Association:** As the largest group for food and nutrition professionals, you can not only find professional, certified dietitians on its Web site, but also a lot of healthy eating tips. To contact the ADA about finding a dietician, you can use the following info: American Dietetic Association, 120 South Riverside Plaza, Suite 2000, Chicago, IL 60606-6995; phone 800-877-1600 ext. 4844; e-mail findnrd@eatright.org, Web site www.eatright.org.

If you're considering a different type of alternative therapy that isn't covered on this list and want to check the professional's credentials, you can most likely find phone numbers and member information through an Internet search engine. Just type in "alternative therapies for CFS" or the specific therapy, such as yoga or massage therapy for CFS.

Getting referrals from your friends

Does someone you know look particularly relaxed lately? Is a close friend blooming with health — and it has nothing to do with love? Is a business colleague who used to have aches and pains all day long now practically skipping? If so, find out their secrets quick! Chances are, they're getting regular massages, taking a great yoga class (or following some other type of regular exercise regimen), eating healthy, or seeing a terrific chiropractor whom they'd love to recommend.

You can find no better credential than a good friend who looks and feels great. But beware: What works for one person may not work for you. And don't forget to look at the source. If the friend who's doing well is a drama queen or a hypochondriac, the alternative therapy she's using may be more hype than hope. And if she tries to sell you vitamins? Run for the hills! Profit is more on her mind than health.

Relaxing Your Way to Relief

You may think that with CFS the last thing you need is something that can make you tired. But the fatigue that erodes your spirit in CFS and the calm, peaceful fatigue you may feel after a relaxing massage are quite different. In fact, many of the methods that relax you — from yoga to massage, from aromatherapy to meditation and hypnosis — can actually invigorate you! They've been known to give people *more* energy and can also go far in helping you quiet your mind. This section goes into detail on some of the most effective ways to help you relax.

Stretching out with yoga

The word *yoga* means "union," and the goal of yoga practice is to form a union, if you will, between your mind, body, and spirit. The series of postures that make up a yoga session are all designed to improve your mental clarity, muscle tone, posture, and sense of well-being. The calm you can experience when doing yoga has been found to help reduce pain in people with CFS.

Did you know that yoga started in India more than 5,000 years ago? It's that ancient! These ancient yogis must have known what they were talking about, because yoga continues to be a popular form of exercise and stress reduction.

I'm not talking power yoga here, the kind you do in 102 degrees Fahrenheit with the same pace as a jog. I'm talking about the pleasure of the stretching-your-body-and-easing-your-mind kind of yoga. You can find classes in relaxation yoga throughout the United States at adult ed schools, YM-YWCAs, community centers, colleges, and neighborhood dance studios — you name it.

Although yoga isn't supposed to get your heart pumping, it is still exercise. Make sure you check with your doctor to see whether you can do the yoga poses. You don't want to overexert yourself. And remember that yoga is supposed to feel *good*. If a certain pose gives you a sharp pain or if you can't hold a particular pose, stop! Lie down with your head up or go into Child's Pose (see the instructions for this pose later in this section). Continuing the exercise when you're feeling pain can exacerbate your symptoms instead of helping you.

Having someone with you when you try any yoga movements or exercise is a good idea, in the event that you get dizzy or weak. The head movements may be problematic for CFS patients who get dizzy or woozy easily. These exercises may be doable for CFS patients *without* orthostatic instability or those with mild to moderate symptoms, but not for everyone. If you have orthostatic problems with poor blood pressure control, you want to avoid any heads-down poses.

In order to get a better idea of what yoga is all about, check out the instructions for the relaxing Child's Pose illustrated in Figure 9-1 (remember to check with your doctor first before doing this or any other yoga pose):

1. **Sit on your knees with your feet together and buttocks resting on your heels (your knees should be slightly separated); place your hands, palms down, on your thighs.**

   If you feel any pain, or can't reach your heels, use a folded pillow underneath your thighs.

2. **Inhale deeply, and as you exhale, bring your chest as close to your knees as you can without straining and reach your arms in front of you.**

   If you aren't too uncomfortable, proceed to step three.

3. **Bring your hands palms up to the sides of your body, as if you were a cocoon.**

4. **Hold this position for 20 to 30 seconds, or as long as you comfortably can, and then slowly come up to the starting point (from Step 1).**

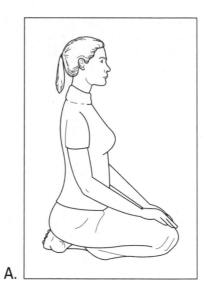

A.

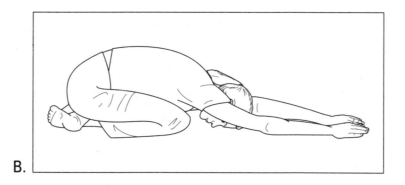

B.

Figure 9-1:
The Child's
Pose is an
excellent
way to
stretch and
soothe your
back and
arms.

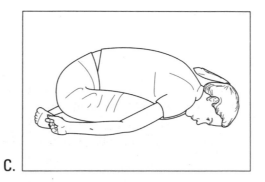

C.

Tai chi anyone?

Tai chi chuan, usually called *tai chi,* is an ancient Chinese form of mind-body exercise that looks like a slow dance from afar. Because physical exercise can create even more pain in people with CFS, a gentle form of exercise such as tai chi may give you some relief. Utilizing specific, concentrated motions aligned with your breath, tai chi is almost a form of meditation, a way of combining the physical with the mental, that may alleviate some of your symptoms, such as dizziness, loss of energy, and pain.

For more on tai chi and other forms of holistic fitness, you can check out *Mind-Body Fitness For Dummies* by Therese Iknoian (Wiley). And remember to check with your physician before starting any type of physical exercise to avoid the risk of hurting yourself and aggravating your CFS.

Figure 9-2 shows another relaxing yoga pose — the Cat-Dog Pose. Here are the steps for doing it properly:

1. **Start on all fours on your mat (hands and knees) and make sure that your hands are parallel to your shoulders and not stretched in front of you; your back should be straight and parallel to the floor, and your head should be in line with your back — not looking up or down (no straining!).**

   Spread your fingers to help with balance. If your knees are uncomfortable, place a folded blanket underneath them.

2. **Inhale and slowly move your head down, and as you do, pull your stomach in towards your back so that your back is rounded; gently move your head down.**

   This position is the Cat Pose. Think of a cat as she stretches her back, and you will have the right move.

3. **Exhale and slowly move your head up; your back should follow and be slightly arched.**

   Don't hold in your stomach. Your shoulders should round. This position is the Dog Pose.

4. **Move from Cat to Dog slowly, inhaling on the Cat Pose and exhaling on the Dog Pose without arching or straining your shoulders; do this movement 10 or 15 times, or as many times as you can and still feel comfortable.**

   You should feel the stretch in your back, neck, and pelvis as an excellent way to relax.

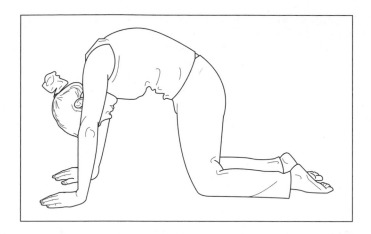

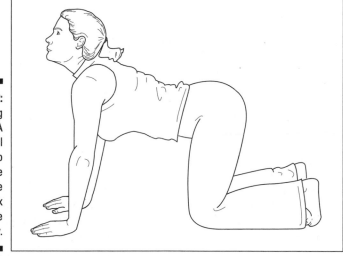

Figure 9-2:
The Cat-Dog
Pose: A
wonderful
way to
elongate
your spine
and relax
your whole
body.

See the book *Yoga For Dummies* by Georg Feuerstein and Larry Payne (Wiley) for more information.

Massaging the stress out of your body

Almost everyone has heard about the benefits of massage — the way it helps you relax, soothe sore muscles, and stretch out all your tension. For people with CFS, gentle massage can be an excellent way to ease anxiety and give you a feeling of well-being.

The form of massage that may help you with your CFS symptoms (not to mention that can probably get your insurance company's thumbs-up) is called *therapeutic massage*. In a therapeutic massage, your masseuse literally rubs the area of soft tissue that's in pain, thereby releasing some of your discomfort. Massages have even been found to ease some irritable bowel symptoms for some people.

To discover more about massage, you can check out the book *Massage For Dummies* by Steve Capellini and Michel Van Welden (Wiley).

Soothing your body with aromatherapy

Aromatherapy works on your senses, specifically your sense of smell. Certain aromas can calm you, and other can make you more alert. If you find scents soothing or relaxing, aromatherapy can be just the thing to help supplement your traditional therapies.

If one of your CFS symptoms is a sensitivity to chemicals, chances are aromatherapy isn't for you. The smell of lavender or peppermint oil may be all you need to start experiencing achier, itchier, and worse flu-like symptoms. As always, check with your doctor before dabbling in aromatherapy.

The most important thing to remember about aromatherapy is to not use it undiluted. Only a few of the essential oils, such as lavender and tea tree, used in aromatherapy can be applied directly from the vial. In most cases, you should add a few drops of scent to bath water, along with a neutral, no-scent oil base, such as grapeseed oil. Try to make your bath as comfortable as possible, with a bath pillow, a candle, and a washcloth over your eyes. Hmmm. . .

Make sure that you use real essential oils and not a fake oil or perfume oil. Fake essential oils don't carry the same benefits as real ones and may even do more harm than good!

You can look over Table 9-1 to see the more common essential oils and how they may help some symptoms associated with CFS.

Table 9-1	Some Common Aromatherapy Essential Oils	
Essential Oil	*What It Is*	*Symptoms*
Lavender	From a shrub native to the Mediterranean, especiallyProvence; grown in America, too.	Anxiety, insomnia, and headaches
Tea Tree	Native to Australia and used for thousands of years by the Aborigine tribes.	Bacterial infections, colds, and flu-like symptoms
Geranium	Extracted from the leaves of the flowering plant. Grown in China and Egypt.	Anxiety, depression, and irritable bowels
Eucalyptus	Indigenous to Australia and brought to Europe by a botanist in the 19th century.	Flu-like symptoms, rheumatoid arthritis, and infection
Rose	Extracted from the leaves. Primarily grown as essential oil in Bulgaria.	Depression, inflammation, and cramps

Rose essential oil is often very expensive, but rosewood oil is a good and inexpensive substitute that carries many of the same benefits.

Aromatherapy isn't just about the bath if you have CFS. Yes, you want to relax, soothe aching muscles, and feel less anxious. But too hot of a bath may tip you over to the other side, making your symptoms worse instead of better. If you want to try an aromatherapy bath, think tepid water — not too hot, not too cold. Or, you may decide to use essential oils in a diffuser that releases the scent into the air, which can be very soothing.

What if you love lemon, lavender, geranium, and jasmine? If you can't decide on what scent to use in the bath, use them all! Just put in one or two drops first to make sure that together they don't smell like, well, dirt.

For more on this subject, you may want to invest in *Aromatherapy For Dummies* by Kathi Keville (Wiley).

Harnessing the power of prayer and meditation

Yes, you do have an illness, and maybe you're even thinking that your body is failing you. Your mind is strong, but your body is weak. Meditation can help ease the panic and fear. Prayer can give you an inner strength. Both provide relaxation and a chance to forget those negative thoughts, those fears about your body, and those beliefs about yourself. Anxiety and chronic pain can disappear for a moment.

With meditation or prayer, you don't have to be in a church or synagogue. You don't need an altar or a few dozen candles. All you need is some quiet — that's it. You can be lying on a couch or sitting in a chair. You can sit on a yoga mat or lean against a pillow — whatever makes you comfortable.

In the following sections, I go into more detail about how meditation and prayer can help you deal with your CFS.

Mellowing out through meditation

If you're looking for a way to calm your mind, you may want to try meditation. By focusing on a word, a sound, or an image, you can literally "let go" of your stress during meditation. You can reduce anxiety, ease fatigue, and become more focused to go on with your day.

Here's a step-by-step guide to meditation — and a sense of calm:

1. **Find a comfortable place to sit, recline, or lie down.**

   Make sure your clothes are loose, your feet are warm, and your phone is off. You can cover yourself with a blanket, if you'd like, and you can put a rolled towel over your eyes to keep your environment nice and dark. Feel free to put on some quiet, soothing music.

2. **Close your eyes and take three deep breaths (in through your nose, out through your mouth); work up to a count of eight on the inhalation, hold for a count of eight, and then exhale for a count of eight.**

   Eventually try to double your exhalation count.

3. **Concentrate on a sound or on a quiet, peaceful place as you breathe in and out (continuing Step 2).**

The "om" sound is commonly used during meditation. Examples of a peaceful place on which you can meditate include a forest with sun glinting through the trees or a beach with gently rolling waves.

4. **Try to be as still as possible while meditating.**

   If you get an itch on your nose, try to draw your attention to it and make it stop without moving. If thoughts start flowing into your head — and they will — don't fight them. Let them in, and then let them out.

5. **Try to meditate for five minutes, slowly working up to a full half hour or ten minutes three times a day.**

   You will open your eyes feeling refreshed, revived, and calm.

You don't have to go it alone when it comes to meditation. You can find books (such as *Meditation For Dummies* by Stephan Bodian [Wiley]), CDs, and DVDs that can instruct you. Many CDs and DVDs also provide gentle, soothing music. To find these meditation tools, type the word *meditation* into an Internet search engine and check what's out there. One caveat: Make sure a money-back guarantee comes with your purchase. You should be able to return the material for a full refund if it doesn't do as promised.

Reaching a state of ah-hhh

Deep relaxation. A feeling of calm that isn't filled with pain. A pleasant tiredness. Who wouldn't want that — especially if you have CFS. One of the best ways to relax is by doing this brief exercise right before you're ready to go to sleep (this exercise is done best while lying down):

1. Close your eyes and take three deep breaths in and out.

2. Clench your toes as best you can, and then let go.

3. Move to your legs; contract them, and then let go.

4. Tighten your stomach, and then let go.

5. Do the same clenching and unclenching with your chest, shoulders, arms, hands, and jaw.

6. When you get to your head, stick out your tongue and make every feature clench, and then let go.

7. Imagine a white light moving up your legs to your head, a white light that heals as it moves up to your head and then away into the sky.

That's it. By now, you have fallen asleep or, at the very least, may feel a little less achy and a bit more relaxed, which may make it easier to fall asleep.

Finding peace with prayer

In many religions, prayer is an essential part of the spiritual tapestry. While Christians, Hindus, Muslims, or people of other faiths may not be able to agree why or to whom they pray, you may want to try prayer as a source of calm from your life with CFS. Whether you choose to pray in the quiet of your own home or at a place of worship, prayer can provide relief, hope, and a strength of purpose. You may find that prayer is a way to communicate with a higher power — and perhaps to let go of your struggles with CFS to something or someone greater than yourself.

Mesmerizing CFS symptoms through hypnosis

Hypnosis has come a long way since those days of clucking like a chicken while under the influence. It's no longer an entertainment or spectacle. Hypnosis has been found to be very successful in helping to alleviate various ailments and bad habits, from quitting smoking to losing weight, from feeling pain to feeling nauseated.

Hypnosis can also be effective if you do it yourself. No need to spend a fortune on a doctor or travel miles away — both potential hardships if you have CFS. Self-hypnosis to alleviate your pain and help you sleep, as well as feel more hopeful, is simple. You can find CDs and DVDs that teach you the steps of self-hypnosis, as well as take you on a guided imagery journey to where your pain is gone.

Not everyone is a good subject for hypnosis, however. Take this simple test to see whether self-hypnosis can help you:

1. **Sit up in a chair with a good back so you are comfortable.**

2. **Take three deep breaths, and as you breathe, focus on something on the wall — a painting, a spot, a line, or on a burning candle; try not to blink.**

3. **Count backwards from ten to one, keeping your eyes open until you have no choice but to close them.**

4. **Raise your right arm, which should feel light, almost as if it were rising by itself.**

5. Tell yourself to lower your arm.

If you have hypnotized yourself, you should experience resistance, eventually lowering it, but not right away. If you haven't, you can move your arm at will.

If you're able to hypnotize yourself by using these steps, you may want to check out a CD or DVD on self-hypnosis or seek out a professional. If you weren't successful in hypnotizing yourself, you can try again, proceed as if it had worked, or choose to give up on this alternative therapy. Not everyone is susceptible to hypnosis.

Don't be afraid of hypnosis. You can get out of a trance any time you want by just opening your eyes.

Many people choose to light a candle to set a mood for self-hypnosis. If you're using a candle, make sure it is in a well-ventilated place, on a fireproof dish, and away from the curtains, just to keep everything safe.

Relieving Your Symptoms with Herbs and Supplements

The use of supplements and herbs is becoming so legitimate that the National Institutes of Health (NIH) has established a division to study the effects of them. Can they help? The studies are still ongoing, but some of the herb and supplement regimens nutritionists have recommended for people with CFS include the following:

- **Alpha-lipoic acid** is a supplement that works as an antioxidant, fighting off those "free radicals," or reactive electrons, that attack your immune system.

- **Coenzyme Q10** is a supplement that may help give you more energy and create a healthier cell structure.

- **Essential fatty acids (EFA)** are supplements intended to help make your immune system stronger.

- **Evening primrose oil**, found in capsules, is supposed to help soothe aches and pains and give you more energy (sounds great to a person with CFS, right?).

- ✔ **Ginseng** is an herb used extensively in Europe and China to promote energy and zest.

- ✔ **Probiotics** are the "good" bacteria that help you stave off infection. You can find them either in the form of a dietary supplement (in capsule, tablet, or powder form) or in certain foods (like yogurt or fermented and unfermented milk).

- ✔ **Magnesium** may give you more energy, help you build stronger muscles, lift your spirits, and pep up your circulation. Some people with CFS have been found, in small studies, to have a deficiency in this mineral.

- ✔ **St. John's wort** is an herb that works as a natural antidepressant for some people.

Consult your doctor before taking St. John's wort because combining this herb with other medications, herbs, or supplements you're currently taking can be hazardous to your health.

- ✔ **Vitamin C** is supposed to strengthen your immune system and help your liver in the detoxification process.

- ✔ **Zinc** may help with your fatigue. This mineral is also a powerful agent to ward off infection.

Be careful: Too much zinc can actually have the opposite effect — making you *more* susceptible to illness! Other side effects include sores in the mouth or throat, fever, indigestion, nausea, heartburn, and increased tiredness or weakness. Be sure to talk to your doctor about the amount of zinc you should be taking.

You can find these herbs and supplements in health food stores as well as some large discount stores and drug stores. If you're having a difficult time locating a specific herb or supplement, be sure to ask someone in that store or department for help.

Always tell your doctor about any herbs or supplements you want to take *before* going out and buying them. Some supplements can interfere with the work of your traditional medicine, and some can cause life-threatening problems.

For more information on herbs and vitamin supplements, you can read *Vitamins For Dummies* by Christopher Hobbs and Elson Haas (Wiley) or Christopher Hobb's other book, *Herbal Remedies For Dummies* (Wiley).

Lining Up Your Bones with Chiropractic Care

Chiropractic medicine is fairly new in medical terms. A healer named Daniel David Palmer founded it in 1895 when he discovered that aligning the spine was able to help people with acute and chronic back pain. Today, the same philosophy still holds: Illness is caused by abnormal nerve transmission through the spinal cord. If one vertebra is out of whack, then the health of your whole body could be affected, so chiropractors believe.

Although no clinical studies on the role of chiropractic care in people with CFS have been conducted, scientific studies have shown that chiropractic adjustments can be effective for low-back pain and tension headaches. Some people have also said that the spinal manipulation they received gave them more energy.

As with many fields of medicine, some "bone-chilling" stories of chiropractic fraud are out there. To make sure you're in good hands, check out the organizations I list in the section "Using licensing associations" earlier in this chapter and see who the organizations recommend in your area.

Chapter 10

Exorcising CFS Symptoms with Sensible Exercise

*P*eople who don't know better may suggest that you get off your duff and start working the CFS out of your system with a strenuous exercise program. With CFS, strenuous exercise programs not only don't work, but they can also trigger an ugly push-crash cycle with increased symptoms As a person with CFS, you must redefine exercise compared to what you may have done before you were ill. Some exercise can make you feel better and stronger, give you a sense of well-being, pump up your energy level, and help you avoid atrophying muscles. In this chapter, I lead you through the process of assessing your energy level and your ability to exercise, assist you in developing a sensible exercise program, and reveal some mild to moderate exercises clinically proven to help CFS patients.

Only you and your doctor know for sure whether exercise is right for you. You can find over 30 studies researching exercise on people with CFS (and fibromyalgia) — and no common consensus. Some studies suggest that aerobic exercise is vitally important to your health. Others say that limited, chunks of exercise combined with rest can give you excellent benefits. And still others say that exercise could cause a viral infection in the heart, and you should stay away from it. In short, you and your doctor have to decide what's best for you and your CFS. But if you can create an exercise regimen that works for you, without overexerting yourself, most experts agree you should go for it!

Plugging Into the Rationale Behind Exercise Therapy

What you may have heard is true. If you have CFS, exercise isn't going to have the same results as it does for someone who simply wants to lose weight or get toned. If you have CFS, you have to figure out what your limits are and what you can and can't do. But limits don't mean anything — zilch. Having limitations just means that you have to adapt. Studies show that the most benefits from exercise occur in the first ten minutes of leaving the couch and going out the door. You can still get benefits from exercise despite your illness. In this section, you can discover what exercise can specifically do for you if you have CFS.

Exercise isn't "for everyone else." You may think it's crazy to even try because whenever you've tried to take a walk or do some arm lifts, your symptoms have come back tenfold. But that's only because you didn't understand your limits. You need to pace yourself. With the right attitude, a doctor or therapist's guiding hand, and a knowledge of what you can do and what you can't, you can get benefits of exercise despite your CFS.

If you've recently been diagnosed with CFS, exercise isn't as important as treating your pain or your fatigue. But the longer you have the condition, the more important it becomes. If your CFS isn't getting better in a few weeks, then the kind of gentle exercise that I describe in this chapter can very well be just what you need to make you feel better physically and mentally.

Preventing muscular atrophy and bedsores

If you have had CFS for several months or more, exercise is vital to avoiding muscles that *atrophy* (slacken and foreshorten) and bed sores and skin breakdown. Atrophying muscles can be very painful, so you want to avoid it at all costs.

Walking away the stress

Whether you're worried about your job, your relationship, or your chronic illness, exercise can help. I'm not talking about training for a marathon here. I'm talking about nonstrenuous, gentle exercise that improves blood flow and keeps you from becoming completely deconditioned without bringing you down.

Walking is the most beneficial exercise you can do because all you need is a pair of sneakers. You don't have to worry about the cost for a fancy gym membership. You need no special skill. And people of all shapes, sizes, and conditions can do it.

You can start out with a walk around the block — or even to the next room if your fatigue is too severe. Just the act of moving for *one minute* can improve your circulation and reduce your stress.

Reducing fatigue

This idea almost sounds like a contradiction — exert yourself and feel *less* tired? If you have CFS, remembering that you aren't an athlete, or even someone who wants to get in shape, is important. What you're striving for is feeling better, and that means a slow start, frequent rests, and simple moves.

Just because you feel good one day doesn't mean you should start training for the Ironman. Yes, seize that opportunity with perhaps a five- or ten-minute walk at a slow pace, or some stretches. (Check out some gentle yoga moves in Chapter 9.) But don't push. You'll end up in the *push-crash cycle* and feeling even more tired and even achier. Even worse, you may decide to forget about exercise completely — which could mean losing a chance to feel better about yourself, losing the opportunity to overcome deconditioning (which has its own negative effects), and loosing the chance to gain some control over your life.

Improving your sense of well-being

Think endorphins, those pleasure-enhancing chemicals released by the brain when you're happy, eating chocolate (yum!), or, yes, exercising. Most people need to exercise regularly and "feel the burn" in order for those endorphins to kick in. But people with CFS have had endorphin highs by just plain walking. They start out very slowly and work their way up.

Use common sense. If you've spent the day dealing with a crisis at home, or if you went to the supermarket and brought home a bunch of bags, you've probably done enough for one day.

Discovering Your Optimum Exercise Activity Level

Be realistic. If you have severe CFS symptoms, and are so tired you can barely lift yourself out of bed, you aren't going to think about exercise. Exercise is more for people who have had CFS for some time and need to prevent their muscles from slacking and their joints from getting stiff.

Always discuss exercise with your health care professional first. She may help create an exercise program for you, or she can help monitor your progress. She may also suggest another health care professional who is more of an expert in the role of exercise in illness, such as an occupational or physical therapist. But whether you have someone motivating you or you're doing it solo, some smart moves can guarantee success — and destroy the exercise myth, "No pain, no gain." This section details the who, what, where, and when of exercise if you have CFS.

Post-exertional malaise is a fancy name for a phenomenon that isn't unusual in people with CFS. The term refers to the acceleration of symptoms following even mild physical (or mental) exercise, usually beginning between 12 and 48 hours after the exertion. This malaise can last for days — even weeks — and it is one characteristic of CFS that separates it from other conditions.

Beware of the "push-crash" cycle. Because the symptoms of CFS vary in severity, a person with CFS may get up one day and feel unusually good, and they "push" themselves far over their tolerable limit. This is followed, usually on the next day, by a "crash" in which symptoms increase significantly, and may last for weeks. It sometimes takes time to find a tolerable limit that helps the person avoid overactivity and conserves energy.

You can read everything out there about activity levels and exercise and CFS, but when it comes right down to it, *you* are the deciding factor: your likes and dislikes, your capabilities and disabilities, your time constraints and daily routines. Customize your ideal exercise activity routine through trial and error, and the following section can help get you started. You may also want to consider putting yourself in the capable hands of an expert (see "Finding the Right Personal Trainer for You" later in the chapter).

Journaling your exercise journey

One way you can keep track of your progress and help customize an activity pattern for yourself is by using a very simple tool: an exercise log. In the log, be sure to keep track of the time of day you exercised, what you did, how long you exercised, and how it made you feel. Keep the log for a week or two — or longer, and check it often to ensure it helps keep you on track. Here is a sample of how you should set up your log:

Date:

Time:

Workout

    Cardiovascular:

        What I did: _____

        Heart rate: _____

        For how long? _____

    Strength-training:

        What I did: _____

        For how long? _____

    Flexibility:

        What I did: _____

        For how long? _____

Comments:

Here's an example of a filled-in Exercise Log:

Date: October 30, 2006

Time: 9:30 a.m.

Workout

    Cardiovascular:

        What I did: Walking in place

        Heart rate: 95

        For how long? 3 minutes, 3 times, with 5-minute rests in between

Strength-training:

> **What I did:** Bicep curls and leg lifts
>
> **For how long?** 30 seconds, 2 times, with 1 minute rests in between

Flexibility:

> **What I did:** Yoga Cat-Dog Pose
>
> **For how long?** Three minutes continuous

Comments: Used a 2-pound weight for the first time with my bicep curls! Only for my second repetition. Will try to use weights for both repetitions next time.

Starting off slowly

Graded activity is the rule for people with CFS. Start slowly, both in exertion and duration, and increase slowly. The tortoise does win the race.

Here are some "make sure" suggestions to ensure your workout doesn't work you out:

- ✔ Make sure you can get out of bed easily, and that moving around isn't a chore.

- ✔ Make sure you can pretty much do all your daily activities without having a relapse of worsening symptoms.

- ✔ Make sure you haven't been having a stressful day.

- ✔ Make sure you aren't feeling too tired (and don't fool yourself).

- ✔ Make sure you start with something really simple: arm stretches over your head, a slow walk around the block, or floating on your back in the water, propelling yourself every so often with either your arms or legs.

- ✔ Make sure you remember the 3:1 ratio — three minutes of rest for every one minute of exercise.

- ✔ Make sure you don't exercise more than **three times** a week at the start.

- ✔ Make sure you're feeling good enough doing the very basic exercises before moving on to more moderate steps — and in no circumstances should you start something more intense until you've been doing light exercise for a few weeks first.

- ✔ Make sure that if you find yourself "crashing" within 24 to 48 hours after your exercise session, you go much, much slower the next time around and stay at that level until you can do it safely without provoking symptoms.

To help you determine what activities you should pursue when you're starting out, here is a list of minimum to light physical activities to consider. These may not seem like "real" exercises, but they certainly help you get moving:

✔ Arm stretches

✔ Brushing the dog

✔ Drying your hair with a hair dryer, head bent down

✔ Gathering ingredients for cooking

✔ Gentle yoga

✔ Grocery shopping

✔ Minor household chores, such as dusting or cleaning the sink

✔ Packing a suitcase

✔ Putting dry clothes away

✔ Putting groceries away at home

✔ Scrubbing your body in the shower

✔ Setting the table

✔ Shampooing and rinsing your hair

✔ Slow dancing in place

✔ Slow leg lifts

✔ Strolling in a mall with frequent stops

✔ Sweeping a floor

✔ Using a computer (hand movements)

✔ Using a vacuum cleaner

✔ Utilizing a hand-held mixer for two or more minutes

✔ Walking from room to room, without stairs

Embracing moderation

After you can manage getting out of bed, washing up, doing a few errands, or getting some work done, you can then think about developing some exercises that can help build stamina as well as increase and improve muscle strength and joint flexibility. But even then, yes, I'll say it again: Easy does it.

After you're making good progress on your light activities, you can move on to what you may consider to be actual exercises. Professionals suggest that exercise should be at a three to one ratio (3:1), with rest periods of three minutes between every one minute of exercise. For some people with CFS, this method can mean only two or three minutes of exercise — and that's okay. Just make sure that you follow the exercise with six to nine minutes of rest. You don't want to relapse. Easy does it.

An exercise program may be the thing that actually enables people with CFS to meet activities of daily living or even to be able to get out of bed; exercises can be done in bed or sitting in a chair — even squeezing a "stress ball" or doing arm and leg lifts can help reverse deconditioned muscles and joints.

Some suggestions for starting your exercise regimen in earnest include the following:

- ✔ **Think activity management.** Your goal is to find a balance between rest and exertion. This balance will ensure the optimum benefits of exercise. Your mood will be better, your pain less, and your sleep improved. How do you do this? With a little bit of exercise at a time. Remember the 3:1 ratio: three minutes of rest for every one minute of exercise.

- ✔ **Create realistic goals.** Maybe you'd like to walk for 20 minutes without causing post-exertional malaise. Or maybe you're just looking for a little bit of independence. Whatever it is, keep your goal simple and easy to manage.

- ✔ **Be flexible.** With CFS, you're going to have some days that are better than others. You need to be a barometer, gauging how tired you are, whether you've had a stressful day, and whether you need to rest.

- ✔ **Do your exercise in chunks.** You can't do a step class or hip-hop dance — not only in terms of exertion (I've never taken a hip-hop class!), but in terms of time. With CFS, doing five minutes of exercise in the morning, then doing another five minutes in the afternoon, and maybe another five in early evening is better for you. (This exact plan, of course, depends on how long you've been exercising and how you feel. If you're just starting out, even this schedule may be too much.) Studies show that people who divide their exercise time throughout the day get the same benefits as people who go for the burn in a 45-minute class.

- ✔ **Combine your exercise with stretching and toning.** Strengthening your muscles and keeping flexible can build your stamina, help your ability to move your body, and may reduce pain. (See the section later in this chapter on strengthening exercises.)

> ✔ **Accept who you are and what you can do.** CFS is a debilitating illness —
> there's no doubt about it. And, yes, some people get more severe symp-
> toms than others. Don't try to keep up with the CFS Joneses. They may be
> able to walk around the block, but you're barely handling picking up and
> grasping objects. That's okay. Eventually, you'll be able to do more — on
> your own schedule. Doing too much too soon can create that push-crash
> situation (emphasis on the crash), and you can feel worse than ever.

Exercise doesn't necessarily mean hitting the gym, however. If you're CFS
symptoms are mild or moderate, here is a list of activities you might pursue
during the course of the day that certainly count as moderate exercise.
Please note that some people may be able to do a few of these, but only after
building up to this level and only if they have mild CFS symptoms:

✔ Ballroom dancing

✔ Bicycling 5 to 9 mph on level terrain

✔ Calisthenics (light)

✔ Coaching children's or adults' sports

✔ Dancing (ballroom, folk, line dancing, and so on)

✔ General home exercises, light or moderate in effort, such as getting up
  and down from the floor

✔ Golf (with a cart)

✔ Hiking on slightly hilly terrain

✔ Line dancing

✔ Modern dancing, disco

✔ Race walking (less than 5 mph)

✔ Roller skating or in-line skating at a leisurely pace

✔ Softball (slow pitch)

✔ Stationary bicycling (using moderate effort)

✔ Table tennis (competitive)

✔ Using crutches

✔ Using a rowing machine (with moderate effort)

✔ Using a stair climber machine at a light-to-moderate pace

- ✔ Walking at a moderate or brisk pace of 3 to 4.5 mph on a level surface inside or outside, such as

    • Walking to class, work, or the store

    • Walking for pleasure

    • Walking the dog

    • Walking as a break from work

- ✔ Walking downstairs or down a hill

- ✔ Water aerobics

- ✔ Weight training and bodybuilding using free weights, Nautilus- or Universal-type weights

- ✔ Yoga

Ramping it up — Something to work up to

Instead of a "lean, mean machine," think of yourself as a swimming pool. You have to check a pool's levels every day before you can swim. The same goes with your body. Ask yourself whether you're feeling up to exercising today. Check your stress, fatigue, and activity levels each day before you start.

Here is a list of vigorous activities for you to consider:

- ✔ Backpacking

- ✔ Basketball game

- ✔ Bicycling more than 10 mph or on steep uphill terrain

- ✔ Boxing (in the ring, sparring)

- ✔ Calisthenics (push-ups, pull-ups, vigorous effort)

- ✔ Circuit weight training

- ✔ Dancing energetically or competitively (any form of dance)

- ✔ Field or rollerblade hockey

- ✔ Football game

- ✔ Jogging or running

- ✔ Jumping rope

- Karate, judo, tae kwon do, or jujitsu
- Kickball
- Lacrosse
- Mountain climbing, rock climbing, or rappelling
- Performing rapid jumping jacks
- Race walking and aerobic walking (5 mph or faster)
- Roller-skating or inline skating at a brisk pace
- Rugby
- Soccer
- Stationary bicycling (using vigorous effort)
- Step aerobics
- Teaching an aerobic dance class
- Tennis
- Using an arm-cycling machine (with vigorous effort)
- Using a rowing machine (with vigorous effort)
- Using a stair climber machine at a fast pace
- Walking and climbing briskly up a hill
- Water jogging
- Wheelchair basketball
- Wheelchair tennis
- Wheeling your wheelchair
- Wrestling (competitive)

Working Out with Specific Exercises and Toning Moves

Just because you have CFS doesn't mean that you can't do exercises like everyone else. You may not be able to do them at the same intensity or duration, but you can still make the "right moves" for better health. This section shows you how.

Getting pumped up with cardiovascular exercise

CFS and cardiovascular exercise both begin with *c,* but other than that, you don't see these two phrases together most of the time. But you can find ways of combining aerobics with your condition, and reaping successful results.

Cardiovascular exercise involves your heart. It gets your heart pumping, your circulation flowing, and your body moving. Getting your cardio is beneficial on so many levels: for your heart, for your weight, and for your attitude. But, by its very nature, cardiovascular is more intense than, say, meditation. You have to move. And with CFS, that can be tough. However, getting a good cardio workout may not be impossible for some people with CFS.

Cardiovascular exercise is all about energy management — via what health care professionals call the *pacing and envelope theory,* which I describe in the following:

- ✔ **Pacing** means moderating your exercise to minimize a push-crash episode. Your doctor may suggest you try something specific, and divide the activity up into small, manageable amounts, with plenty of rest in between.

  For example, your doctor suggests you clean your bedroom. You may make the bed, then rest. Dust your night table. Rest. Clean the full-length mirror. Rest. Vacuum the rug. Rest. Small chunks ensure you won't overextend yourself. They can also help you gauge how much you can do. It may take all day — or more — to clean your room, but that's okay.

  When your activity level is stabilized, and you aren't overextending yourself to the point where your symptoms get worse, your doctor may up the ante, adding another room, or combining making the bed and the dusting. In small increments, your activity level increases.

- ✔ **Envelope** has nothing to do with mailing yourself a letter or watching an award show. Envelope theory has to do with monitoring your energy. Like a bank account, if you're overdrawn one day, you have to replenish your account the next day. If you have $10.00, you know you can't spend $11.00, or a check will bounce. The same holds true for energy. Small increments means your account stays in the black. But it also means that using up your energy stores puts your account at zero — and you need to spend the next day or days putting energy back in. How do you do that? By resting.

  Eventually, you'll figure out how much you have to spend on a given day or week, and then you can spend your energy wisely, with no "symptom fees."

Check with your doctor to find the right cardiovascular exercise for you, your CFS, and your heart.

Sitting up and pushing up

If you have CFS, just the act of sitting up in bed can be difficult, let alone doing stomach crunches on the floor. But if you've figured out your exercise limits and have gradually built your tolerance, modified sit-ups and push-ups can become a part of your routine. They just have to be modified to accommodate your energy stores and CFS symptoms.

Check out the following sections for some ways to make sit-ups and push-ups a part of your routine.

Think big green (or blue, yellow, or red) ball

You can purchase these balls (sometimes called *balance balls*) at any sporting goods store or online. And any gym worth its treadmill has them. These balls, ranging in pressure from soft to hard, can help cushion your body so you avoid strain.

People with orthostatic or balance problems should not try these without someone assisting.

The first exercise you may want to try with your ball is the *sit-up curl,* described in the following steps (pictured in Figure 10-1):

1. **Lie on your back on a soft mat; put your hands behind your head, fingers interlocked, but not holding up your head.**

2. **Place the exercise ball under your legs, so your knees are draped over it.**

3. **Inhale and position your head so you're looking up at the upper wall in front of you.**

   Don't strain by pulling your head up with your fingers. Let your abs do the work. The first few times you may even want to keep your shoulders on the floor.

4. **Inhale as you slowly move down to starting position.**

5. **Rest for at least a count of 20.**

6. **Repeat if possible, but do no more than eight total.**

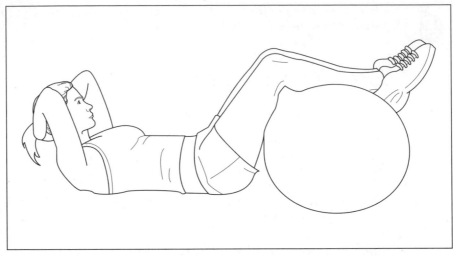

Figure 10-1:
Sit-up curl.

Another exercise to help strengthen your abdominal muscles is the *sit-up crunch*. To do this exercise, you must following these steps (the exercise is illustrated in Figure 10-2):

1. **Lie on your back over the exercise ball, so that your center is firmly on it.**

2. **Interlock your fingers and place them behind your head; put your feet firmly on the ground and position your head so you're comfortable, not straining.**

3. **Inhale.**

4. **Exhale and slowly move up as far as you can, using your abs to pull you up.**

   Don't strain! Only go as far as you can. Your mid-back should *always* be on the ball. If you have orthostatic problems, make sure someone is with you to help prevent a fall if you get lightheaded or weak.

5. **Inhale and slowly move back to your starting position.**

6. **Rest for at least a count of 20.**

7. **Repeat, if comfortable and able.**

   Build up to only eight over time.

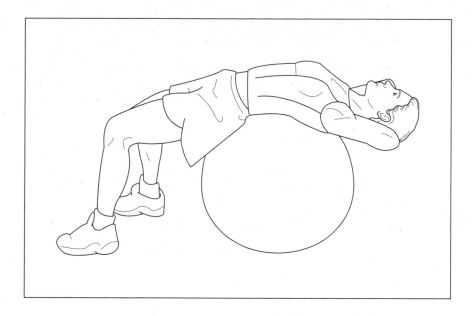

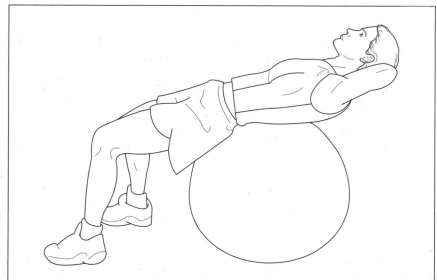

Figure 10-2:
Sit-up
crunch.

For one more exercise with the ball, try the following *lower-ab lift* (check out the picture in Figure 10-3):

1. **Lie down on your back on your soft mat and place your hands about shoulder width apart.**

2. **Place the exercise ball under your knees, so your body is perpendicular.**

3. **Inhale.**

4. **Exhale and very slowly lift your buttocks off the mat; keep your knees soft!**

Don't attempt to do more than slightly raising your buttocks until you see how you feel. If you stay stable, you can try to lift your whole hip area completely off the mat, but only if you're comfortable! Remember not to strain.

5. **Inhale and gently lower yourself back to the mat.**

6. **Rest for a count of at least 20.**

You can build up to eight repetitions, if able and comfortable, with rests in between.

Use a mat

There are mats (like the ones you wipe your feet on daily), and then there are *mats*. A mat can help cushion your body as you do your moves. A mat is vital for yoga to help prevent you from slipping. Yoga mats are made to prevent feet and hands from slipping in some of the postures.

Many people use hard Styrofoam-like mats in gyms for floor work, but they are too hard if you have CFS symptoms because they are like an extra, extra, extra firm mattress and accentuate any of your aches and pains. The ideal version is like a mini-mattress. This type of mat has some stuffing in it so that you aren't flat on the floor like a pancake, and you can feel more comfortable.

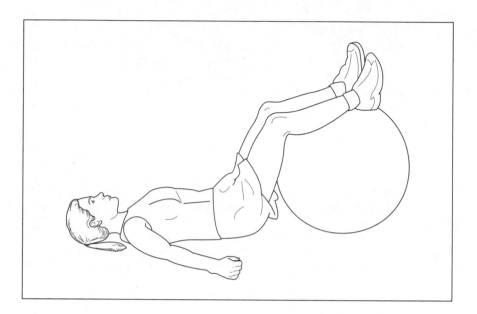

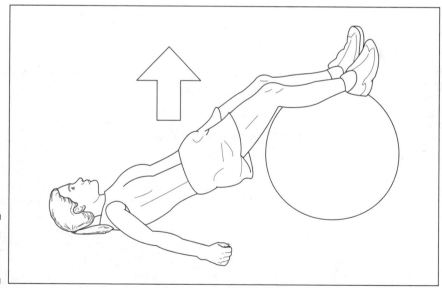

Figure 10-3:
Lower-ab
lift.

Rest, rest, rest

Yes, when an exercise teacher tells you to crunch quickly 30 times before stopping, she calls it "working the abs." But for someone with CFS, you may call it *wrong!* Do your sit-ups slowly, resting in between each one for a count of 20. If you experience no after-burn, then you can rest for 15 seconds instead, and so on.

Push-up soft

Push-ups aren't the exercise of choice for people with CFS, because they put too much strain on the arms and shoulders. However, if you're starting to feel better, or if your energy is strong enough, you can try doing a few. But make sure you use a soft mat and keep your feet up (see Figure 10-4).

You may want to try a modified push-up. This form of push-up is often a smarter choice for someone with CFS. You can do this modified push-up by doing the following (and check out Figure 10-4 for a visual example):

1. **Lie on your stomach on a soft mat — your hands on either side of you and elbows out.**

2. **Lift and cross your feet.**

   Keep them crossed during this exercise.

3. **Inhale.**

4. **Exhale and very, very slowly lift your arms up; start with a very small lift, lifting your head and upper chest, with your elbows still bent.**

   Be very careful not to strain yourself.

5. **Inhale and come back to starting position.**

6. **Rest for at least a count of 20.**

Gradually build up to the point where your elbows are straight (but not locked) when you're pushing up — if you can. Stay with the small lift for the first few weeks or so. If you feel stable, and are comfortable and able, try moving up a little bit, in increments, until you're in full push-up mode. (But always keep your feet crossed and up.)

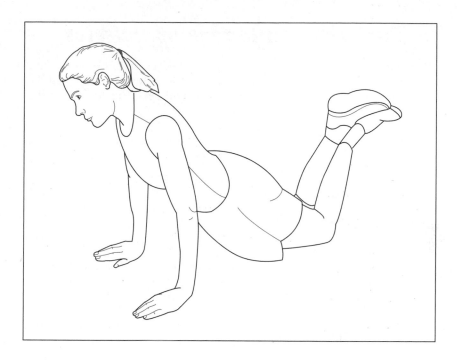

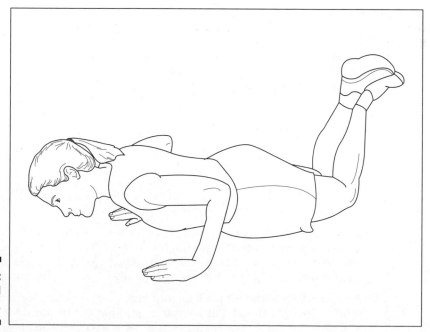

Figure 10-4:
Modified
push-up.

Pumping iron to tone up muscles

Cardiovascular activity is only one part of a sensible exercise routine. Strength-training and toning your muscles is just as important. Here, as with cardio, you need to know your limits. You need to pace yourself and conserve your energy.

Pumping iron is especially good for people with CFS because it can

- Reduce muscle and joint pain
- Improve strength
- Improve flexibility
- Increase stamina

In the beginning, leave the dumbbells to the gym rats and use only your body for resistance. Remember the motto: Easy does it. Here are some simple strength-training exercises to try when you're starting out:

- **Shoulder moves:** Sit in a chair, back straight and feet on the floor. Look straight ahead. For a count of eight, move your arms up to your shoulders (or as far as you can comfortably do). Hold for a count of eight (only if comfortable), then lower for a count of eight. Rest for 20 seconds, and then repeat.

- **Leg lifter:** In the same chair, arms holding the sides, lift the right leg for a count of eight. Your goal is to have your leg go out straight, parallel to the floor, but go easy! (It may take several weeks to reach this.) Hold for a count of eight, and then lower for a count of eight. Rest for 30 seconds. Then do the same exercise with your left leg. Repeat the whole sequence, but do no more than five repetitions to ensure your energy isn't depleted.

- **Wall hugger:** Stand in a doorway. Put your arm out and hold the side of the door frame. Then move your body out — except for the arm. This move gives you a nice stretch in your shoulders and upper arms. Hold for a count of 12, and then step back. Rest for 30 seconds (sit, if necessary). Repeat the same exercise with the other arm.

- **Thigh squeeze:** Sit back in your chair, feet on the floor, head looking straight ahead. Contract your thigh muscles and hold for 20 seconds. The movement should be barely visible. Then rest for 40 seconds and repeat. Do this exercise up to five times — but only if your body feels stable.

- **Bicep curls:** Sit straight back in your chair, feet on the floor and head looking straight ahead. Put your arms straight out at shoulder length, and then, for a count of 8, curl your arms in and out. You should feel this movement in your fingers, wrists, lower and upper arms, and shoulders. Put your arms back to your sides and rest for 30 seconds. Repeat. Do this exercise up to five times — but only if you feel stable.

Up against the wall

If you feel strong enough, you may want to try using the wall to provide resistance instead of using weights (which may still be too difficult to manage at first). Stand arm's length away from the wall, with your palms secure on it. Keeping your feet in place, slowly lean in towards the wall by bending your elbows. Then slowly straighten your elbows, pushing yourself back out. This movement can help you gain strength in your arms.

You can also use the wall to work your lower half, if you're strong enough. Stand with your against the wall. Then slowly sink down about half way, so that your knees are bent and your thighs have the weight. (This position resembles someone sitting in a chair — without the chair.) Count to eight, then slowly move back up to a standing position. This exercise can help tone your buttocks, hips, and thighs.

As with any exercise, wall or no wall, *always* check with your health care professional before attempting to do it! And, if you have orthostatic problems (get easily lightheaded or weak, it's a good idea to have someone nearby should you need help.

Think of these fabulous five exercises as a goal, but not a regular habit – once or twice a week, if tolerated, may be a realistic goal You don't want to overdo it and exacerbate your CFS symptoms. Always remember to consult with your doctor before starting a strength-training program or if you find a particular exercise to be too much for you.

When you've begun to build up your strength, pacing yourself and conserving your energy, you may want to try doing some exercises with weights. But keep to the 2-pound weights in the beginning. Studies show that using 2-pound weights also tones those biceps and triceps!

The first exercise with weights that you may want to try is the *sitting bicep curl,* which I explain in the following steps (see Figure 10-5 for an example):

1. **Sit on a chair or bench, feet on the floor.**

2. **Grasp your weight, palm in; balance your elbow on your knee for support.**

3. **Inhale and slowly move your right arm out until your arm is level with your knee (or as far as you can easily go).**

4. **Exhale and slowly move your arm up to your chest to a count of eight.**

   CFS patients may need to start with a lower count when beginning.

5. **Inhale and lower your arm to a count of eight.**

6. **Rest for at least 20 seconds, and then repeat the same exercise, using your left arm, if you're able and comfortable.**

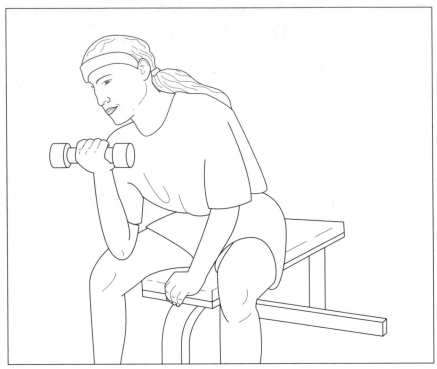

Figure 10-5:
Sitting bicep
curl.

To tone a different muscle in your arms, you can try the *tricep fly*:

1. **Lie on your back on a soft mat, a 2-pound weight in each hand.**

   It may be a good idea for CFS patients to start with no weights and then add something less than 2 pounds; for instance, start with a small (8-ounce) food can, and then increase to a large (16-ounce) food can before moving forward with 2-pound weights, as able.

2. **Put your arms straight up in the air, about parallel to your chin; your palms should be facing each other.**

   See Figure 10-6 for an example of this position.

3. **Inhale.**

4. **Exhale and slowly move your arms down as far as you can comfortably go towards the floor, as if you were unfurling a cape; hold for a count of five.**

   People with CFS may need to start with a lower count.

5. **Inhale and move your arms back to the starting position (from Step 2).**

6. **Put your arms down, let go of the weights, and rest for a count of at least 20 seconds.**

7. **Repeat this exercise up to five times as able and comfortable.**

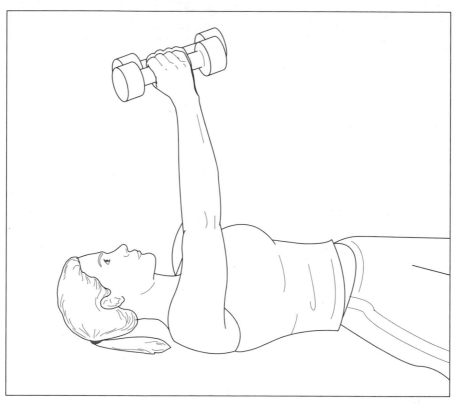

Figure 10-6:
Tricep fly.

Last but not least, you can try the *shoulder fly*. You can do this exercise by following these steps (see Figure 10-7 for an example):

1. **Stand straight up — stomach in, head level; put your weights in each hand, arms at your side and palms facing in.**

2. **Inhale.**

3. **With palms facing the floor, exhale and move your whole right arm up as high as it can comfortably go (about head level or lower) for a count of eight.**

4. **Inhale and lower your arm back down to your side for a count of eight (may need to be lower for CFS patients).**

5. **Rest for at least a count of 20.**

6. **Repeat the same exercise with the left arm.**

7. **Rest for a count of at least 60 — sit, weights removed, if necessary.**

8. **Repeat this exercise on both arms up to five times (but only if comfortable!).**

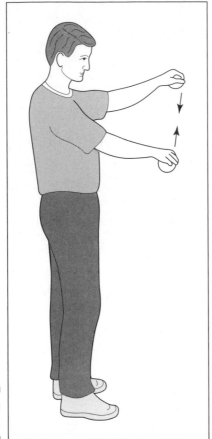
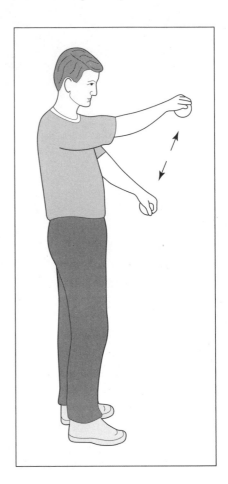

Figure 10-7: Shoulder fly.

Working your core muscles with Pilates

Although similar to yoga, Pilates (pronounced pih-LAH-teez) doesn't go as far back as ancient India. Pilates was invented by Joseph Pilates (hence the name) in 1880. As a youth, Pilates was very sickly and weak, and, unwilling to stay that way, he created a unique exercise regimen that focuses on one body part and, at the same time, works the *core* — that area between your chest and your hips (think of it as your body's center). When your core is strong, it helps relieve back pain and improve your circulation. Mr. Pilates also invented a series of apparatuses to go with his program, but you can still get a Pilates workout with a mat.

These exercises may be too much for the person with CFS when first beginning to exercise. It's critically important that you start slowly and increase any reps or durations *very* gradually. And as always, consult with your doctor before starting any exercise program.

If your condition warrants, you can adapt some of the following moves:

- **Half-flutter:** Get your core going with a half-flutter. Hold in your stomach and lie flat, face up, on your mat. Bring your legs up and flip them up and down like a scissor while holding in your stomach.

- **Circles:** Lie on your side, your bottom arm stretched out above your head. Move the leg on top in a giant circle, front to back, and then a medium-sized circle, and then a small one. Then reverse the circle, and go through the circles again from large to small. Rest for one minute, then turn over on to your other side and repeat the exercise with the other leg.

- **Rocking horse:** Do a gentle rocking motion, which will strengthen your core with a minimum of effort. Lie on your mat face up, hands around your bent knees, and your head tucked down, as if you were a cocoon. Then rock back and forth, as if you were a rocking chair. You should feel your back easing, but you shouldn't feel strained. Rock 10 to 15 times, and then rest for one minute before repeating.

If your rocking is getting too intense, stop and go back to a slower motion.

For more in-depth information on Pilates, you can check out *Pilates For Dummies* by Ellie Herman (Wiley).

Going nowhere fast: Walking in place

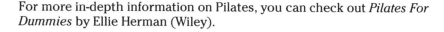

Let's say you're not sure about your energy quotient. You're afraid to take a walk outside. What if you fall? Or find out that you can't go another step a half a block away? Being unable to help yourself is a terrible thought. Sure, you can walk with a buddy. But what if no one is available?

The best solution is walking at home. Better yet, walk in place while you watch television, or listen to music, or talk on your hands-free cell phone. How do you actually walk in place? Think of a soft march — lifting your legs up slightly (even just to your ankle) and moving slowly. Some suggestions for walking in place:

- **Wear walking shoes or sneakers.** Even though you're not hitting the pavement, you're still technically walking. And that means having the right equipment — in this case, good, comfortable walking shoes.

- **Think "chunks."** Start out by walking in place for a minute (yes, only a minute), then resting for three minutes. Feel okay? Walk in place another minute. Rest for three minutes. If you're still doing fine, tack on another minute, and so on. But don't do more than ten minutes — you don't want to push and crash.

✔ **Occupy your mind.** Make sure you're watching a show on TV that you like, or maybe listening to a book on tape while you walk. Going nowhere won't seem as tedious, and you won't get bored.

✔ **Try varying rhythms and styles.** If you're finding that you can handle walking in place without danger of depleting your energy, try changing your walking pattern. Maybe you can march for 30 seconds, lifting up those knees. Perhaps you can swing your arms. Or maybe you can speed it up for 15-second intervals.

Finding the Right Personal Trainer for You

A big part of any exercise program is motivation, especially if you're fatigued and not feeling well. A personal trainer can provide that motivation: making you accountable once or twice a week, giving you pep talks and inspiration, and watching your moves and making sure you're doing things correctly.

Your best option is to find a personal trainer (or perhaps a physical or occupational therapist) who has an understanding of CFS, so he doesn't try to push you too hard with a go-for-the-burn mentality. If the trainer doesn't already know about CFS, you may need to provide educational materials (this book!) to help him have a solid understanding of your CFS and what you need from him as a trainer.

Because of your condition, your insurance company may possibly help pay the costs of either a personal trainer, a physical therapist, or an occupational therapist. Be sure to check with your insurance company before hiring a personal trainer so you can count the costs.

If you decide that a personal trainer could help you, remember: He isn't a luxury. He's an integral part of your treatment and recovery. He can help you reap the full benefits of an exercise program without the dangers of overexertion. In this section, you discover how to get a personal trainer who's right for you.

Searching for just the right fitness guru

After you've decided you want to go the personal trainer route, what next? The best experts are those referred by your health care professional. You may also want to check out the following resources:

✔ **Sport rehabilitation facility:** These centers have trainers working with people with a variety of injuries and conditions.

✔ **Health club or gym:** As long as the gym has good credentials, you should be okay.

✔ **YMCA or YWCA:** These organizations' trainers are all required to have certification before they can work. Also, you can get a personal training session at a much better price here than at an exclusive club.

Like a physician, personal trainers have to have their credentials accessible. You have every right to know where a trainer has been certified and how much experience she has. Two associations that provide certification are the American Fitness Professionals & Associates (AFPA) and the American Council on Exercise (ACE). The gold standard of professional training credentials is the American College of Sports Medicine (ACSM).

After you're confident in your trainer's experience and ability, you're ready to see whether your personalities mesh. Are you the quiet type, but the trainer talks a mile a minute? Do you like to keep your distance? Finding someone you like and who can motivate you is just as important as credentials. If you don't like a particular personal trainer, don't be shy. Ask for someone else. Trainers are used to changing partners and won't take it personally.

Conversing with your trainer: It's not just chit-chat

You have to face it: CFS is serious. And the dangers of push-crash are very real. You don't want to start an exercise regimen only to have your symptoms worsen a day or two later.

A certified personal trainer familiar with your condition is ideal. But whomever you find, talking to her about your CFS is crucial. Let her know if you're feeling tired or straining too much. It can mean the difference between improvement and moving backwards.

Part III

Living and Working Well with Chronic Fatigue Syndrome

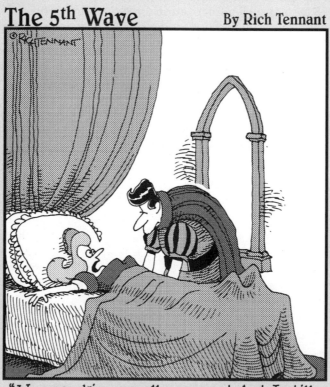

The 5th Wave   By Rich Tennant

"You can kiss me all you want, but I still don't think it's going to cure my CFS."

In this part . . .

CFS not only messes with your health, it messes with your life! That includes your work, your relationships, and your ability to just go out and have a good time.

In this part, I show you how to reclaim your life when CFS tries to steal it from you and from your loved ones. I reveal strategies and tips for developing a healthier, more productive work schedule. I present therapies and techniques to assist you and your loved ones in removing relationship stressors that often aggravate symptoms. I provide practical advice on what you can do to support a loved one who has CFS and to aid children who either have the illness or are living with a family member who does. Finally, I pull back the curtains to reveal ongoing research that holds out hope for improved treatments and perhaps even a future cure.

Chapter 11

Setting Up a Healthy Daily Routine

. . . .

In This Chapter

▶ Choosing foods that help ease your CFS

▶ Finding a healthy weight that works for you

▶ Figuring out how to get a good night's sleep

. . . .

*F*ocusing on pharmaceutical and therapeutic treatments for CFS can often distract from the importance of daily routines and nutrition. However, you need to be paying attention to how you're living as well as how your CFS symptoms are being treated.

Why is healthy living so important when you have CFS? Healthy eating patterns may help alleviate your CFS symptoms, from fatigue to pain to irritability. Sleep is also an important part of healthy living. If you have CFS, you know that fatigue and feeling sleepy are two very different things. You need to establish a daily rhythm, a daily routine, to ensure that you sleep well and deep. (In Chapter 10, I discuss the benefits of exercise, and having a better night's sleep is one of the biggest benefits.)

In this chapter, I encourage you to develop a custom daily routine that often assists in regulating your system and lessening the frequency and severity of your symptoms.

Tailoring Your Menu for CFS-Friendly Foods

Food and mood go together like blue suede and shoes. When you drink too much coffee (or any caffeinated drink), you get jittery. When you eat too much of anything, you feel uncomfortably stuffed (and with CFS, you don't need the added discomfort).

Food can also affect any chronic condition you may have, and that includes CFS. You can't find any "CFS foods" per say, but if you suffer from CFS symptoms, improving your diet is a good way to start helping yourself stay on an even keel.

Your body and your emotions will thank you if you commit to eating right. In this section, I offer up some suggestions that can make healthy food your CFS best friend.

Taking advantage of nutritional information

So much information is out there in the public arena telling you what you should and shouldn't eat that you may have a hard time deciding where to start looking for nutritional information. One way to get a good start on healthy eating is to follow the United States Department of Agriculture (USDA) MyPyramid Plan, represented by the food pyramid illustration shown in Figure 11-1.

You can also get into a good habit of looking at the nutritional information on the labels of the food you buy (before you buy it). Making sure you buy the right kinds of food can help you avoid getting unhealthy food into your house and most likely into your stomach. For more details on these healthy-eating strategies, keep reading.

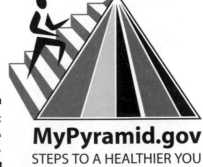

Figure 11-1:
The USDA
MyPyramid.

MyPyramid.gov
STEPS TO A HEALTHIER YOU

Following nutritional guidelines

Basically, the MyPyramid Plan represents nutritional guidelines recommended by the USDA. Those guidelines are divided into six different food categories and provide an idea of what you should (and shouldn't) eat and how much each day. (You can check out the visual representation of this pyramid in Figure 11-1.)

The *amount* of each food group you should eat depends on your age, sex, and level of physical activity. To get the specifics on how much of each food group you should be eating, check out the USDA MyPyramid Web site at www.mypyramid.gov. This site has many ways for you to find the info you're seeking. You can also request information via the following: USDA Center for Nutrition Policy and Promotion, 3101 Park Center Drive, Room 1034, Alexandria, VA 22302-1594; phone 888-7PYRAMID (888-779-7264).

The MyPyramid guidelines outline the six major food groups, and I've included some basic info on each category in the following:

✔ **Grains:** Foods made from wheat, rice, oats, cornmeal, barley, or any other cereal grain product is considered a grain. Pasta, bread and cereal are just a few examples of foods that are considered grains. The types of grains that you want to focus on include whole grains, because they add healthy fiber to your diet. Stay away from regular pasta, which is a refined grain, not a whole grain , and (this one you probably already know) cake.

Starchy, refined carbohydrates can be hazardous to your health. Not only can a giant bowl of spaghetti pack on the pounds, but it can make you even more lethargic than you already are. The combination of refined carbs and refined sugar can be deadly to your blood sugar balance. Try exotic types of rice, couscous, or whole-wheat pasta for a change of pace.

✔ **Vegetables:** Yes, you've had broccoli coming out of your ears. And don't even mention Brussels sprouts! But you can find some delicious veggies out there, and many supermarkets even have them precleaned, precut, and microwave ready. Veggies are chock-full of antioxidants, vitamins, minerals, and fiber. Try string beans, cauliflower, yellow and red sweet peppers, and any other rainbow variety. Eat fewer starchy vegetables, such as potatoes, green peas, lima beans and corn.

Because roughage can cause gastrointestinal distress (a common CFS symptom), try cooking vegetables in the microwave for 30 seconds or in boiling water for 3 minutes, which will make them softer and easier to digest.

✔ **Fruits:** This food group is like veggies — full of vitamins, minerals, and antioxidants. You have more exotic choices than ever when it comes to fruits — from passion fruit to kumquats to over ten types of apples!

citrus fruits, such as grapefruits and oranges are highly acidic and may irritate the stomach of someone with CFS. It may be necessary to limit these types of fruits if they cause heartburn or stomach distress.

✔ **Milk products:** These dairy products include foods such as milk, cottage cheese, and yogurt. However, lactose intolerance is a pitfall for many people, including people with CFS. But you can find products that are soothing to your stomach and can help you avoid gas and bloating common with irritable bowel syndrome (IBS), which can be a by-product of your CFS. Everything from milk and yogurt to cottage cheese now has lactose-free options. Cheese has good proteins as well, but it also contains a lot of fat. Choose low-fat cheeses.

✔ **Proteins:** You may be surprised that proteins include more than just beef. This food group includes chicken, pork, and beans. However, you may find that beans cause bloating and other intestinal problems. If they cause you problems, it's a good idea to limit the amount in your diet. The same goes for fatty steaks and ribs. But lean meats (such as skinless chicken or ground turkey), fish, and pork chops add needed protein for energy, as well as other nutrients to build up your strength.

✔ **Fats and oils:** You may have heard that fats will make you fat, but that way of thinking is an old saw and not always true! Everyone needs fat to live, for certain hormonal and digestive processes, for your skin and hair and nails, and even for energy. But stick to unsaturated fats or monosaturated fats — olive, canola, or peanut oil — to ensure that cholesterol doesn't build up in your body. Saturated fats, such as butter and lard, are made from meat by-products (such as butter), and can clog up those arteries fast. And trans fat (trans fatty acids), the newest enemy, is even deadlier. Trans fats are man-made or processed fats, which are made from a liquid oil. When the oil goes through a hydrogenation process, it becomes solid. A good rule of thumb when considering adding fat to your diet is to stay away from fats that are solid or firm at room temperature.

Moderation is key when it comes to fats and oils. Try sprinkling some olive oil and wine vinegar over a mixed green salad instead of pouring on the dressing. Use a no-stick cooking spray (with little to no fat) or chicken broth for sautéing, and bake instead of fry.

Stick to these guidelines and, like the fellow walking up the pyramid stairs in the MyPyramid figure, you can feel healthier and calmer. Maybe you can't walk as fast as him, but adding mild exercise that fits your abilities can give you an even healthier boost. (See Chapter 10 for information on exercise.)

Although not an official slice of the MyPyramid, you should try to avoid sugars as much as possible. However, no one lives in a vacuum, and you will have times when you have to have that chocolate ice cream or that banana cream pie. But beware: People with CFS appear to be much more sensitive to food chemicals, and that means sugar and substitute sugars. Try to stick with honey or stevia, a natural sweetener made from the bark of a South American tree, to sweeten up your foods.

Interpreting food labels

After you're armed with basic nutritional guidelines (from the preceding section), you can put them to good use by carefully examining the food labels before you buy, to make sure you're getting what you pay for. Figure 11-2 shows a basic food label.

Figure 11-2:
Reading your food labels is important to healthy living.

Nutrition Facts

Serving Size 1 Cup (240mL)
Servings Per Container 2

Amount Per Serving

Calories 120	Calories from Fat 45

	% Daily Value*
Total Fat 5g	8%
Saturated Fat 3.5g	18%
Trans Fat 0g	
Cholesterol 25mg	8%
Sodium 120mg	5%
Total Carbohydrate 11g	4%
Dietary Fiber 0g	0%
Sugars 11g	
Protein 8g	16%

Vitamin A 10%	•	Vitamin C 2%
Calcium 30%	• Iron 0% •	Vitamin D 25%

* Percent Daily Values are based on a 2,000 calorie diet. Your daily values may be higher or lower depending on your caloric needs.

Serving size: This varies from package to package. Serving sizes don't always reflect the typical amount that an adult may eat. In some cases, the serving size may be a very small amount.

Calories: The calories contained in a single serving.

% daily values: The percentage of nutrients that one serving contributes to a 2,000-calorie diet. Parents or children may need more or less than 2,000 calories per day.

Nutrient amounts: The nutritional values of the most important, but not all, vitamins and other nutrients in the product.

So what do the different parts of a food label mean? Generally, you can interpret a food label like this:

- ✔ **Serving Size:** Reading the serving size properly is important, because people mistakenly believe that a whole package is a serving. Identifying the serving size is important because all the nutrient information on the label is specifically for just one serving.

- ✔ **Number of Servings:** This section tells you just what it appears to — how many servings are in one package. In the example in Figure 11-2, the box contains two servings, which means you have to double the calories, fat, and all the other ingredients to get the totals for the entire package. And, if you're trying to lose weight, you may be biting off more than you *should* chew.

✔ **Calories:** The official definition of a *calorie* is the amount of energy you get from food. But for most people, the thing that's important is the number of calories: Is it high or low? If you have CFS, you're most likely more sedentary than other folks, so you want to keep your calories lower to avoid gaining weight. An ideal daily amount of calories is anywhere from 1,500 to 2,000. Weigh yourself after a few days of mindful eating, and if you've gained weight, lower the number of calories you digest each day (for example, switch from 1,800 to 1,500).

Never go below 1,200 calories a day, because anything lower and you may not be getting the nutrients your body needs. On the label in Figure 11-2, you'll see that there are 120 calories in one serving (240 if you ate the whole box!).

✔ **Calories from Fat:** This part of the food label shows you how much of the total calories of a serving is derived from fat. Ideally, that number should be low (about one third or less of the calories), except for salad dressings, which you can expect to be rich in oils.

✔ **Fats, Cholesterol, and Sodium:** Read these numbers carefully. Eating too much fat, especially saturated fat and trans fatty acids (trans fat), cholesterol, and sodium can be hazardous to your health, increasing your risk of certain chronic illnesses like heart disease, some cancers, or high blood pressure.

When reading these three sections of the food label, keep the following guidelines in mind:

- **Eat foods that are low in fat.** A really quick and easy way to calculate the general low-fat versus high-fat content in a food is to use the ratio of 3 grams of fat per 100 calories. You can consider anything at or below this ratio low fat, and anything above it to be a higher fat. For example, any food with 250 calories should have no more than 7 grams of fat.

- **Know the difference between good fats and bad fats.** Look at the label closely: Under the Total Fat row is the amount of saturated fat (which means it comes from animals or palm or coconut oil). Saturated fats can clog arteries, but unsaturated fats can be good for you, because they decrease the bad cholesterol in your bloodstream.

  Trans fats are also listed on the label because they're as bad as saturated fats and have been found to increase the bad cholesterol, or LDL, in your arteries, which can cause heart disease. Delete this sentence if you use the description in the above section: "fat" bullet point. For example, margarine is made from trans fatty acids, which is just as bad for your health as pure, unadulterated butter. You want to look for a food label that has 0g in the Trans Fat row. Many food manufacturers are reducing trans fats in their foods – you may have already seen the bright labels that say "No Trans Fat"

✔ **Dietary Fiber:** Fiber helps your digestive system work right. Eating fiber has been found to help prevent certain cancers. Normally, people are encouraged to eat as much fiber as possible. But if you have CFS, you may very well also experience gastrointestinal distress. In this case, too much fiber can make you gassy and bloated — and more uncomfortable.

Each person is different. What's too much for one person can be too little for another. Experiment and see how much fiber helps you feel good without the bloat. Start with small amounts and then increase slowly in small amounts. And it's important that you increase fluid intake whenever you increase fiber intake to keep the fiber soft and moving quickly through your intestinal tract. In the sample in Figure 11-2, zero fiber is in a serving — not a good choice for anyone!

✔ **Carbohydrate, Sugar, and Protein:** These could be considered fuel for your body. Sugar gives you short-lived energy that wears off pretty quickly, leaving you de-energized. Some carbohydrates can do the same, while others don't wear off as quickly. Proteins are a longer lasting fuel. In fact, everything you eat is separated — carbs, sugar, fat, and protein — and pared down to the tiniest amounts of nutrients in the intestinal tract (with a little help from the liver), so that the macaroni and cheese you just digested can feed hungry cells.

✔ **Daily Values (and the bottom of the label):** The daily value is the recommended dietary guidelines for everyone, not for a specific product. The numbers in the Daily Value column pertain to the percentage of each ingredient in a 2,000-calorie diet. Remember that the daily value percentages are based on only *one* serving. The info on the bottom of the label shows you the total daily values, and it never changes.

Finding what foods work best for you

Instead of only arming yourself with nutritional information that can help you get a handle on your CFS symptoms (see preceding section), the best way for many people to see what pushes their CFS symptoms' buttons is through an elimination diet.

An elimination diet isn't a surf-and-turf dinner, but it's not a starvation diet either. An elimination diet is basically as it sounds. You start with a very sparse diet, adding foods daily. If you feel fine, then you keep adding. If you start having an allergic reaction (bloatedness, sensitivity, gassiness, or more CFS symptoms, such as fatigue), then you know that food is bad for you and you eliminate it from your diet! An elimination diet lasts only five to ten days.

By eliminating certain foods from your diet, you may be able to avoid aggravating or adding to your CFS symptoms. In this section, I go into more detail on the elimination diet to help you pinpoint what you can eat and what you can't.

Making sure you're ready for the diet

Before you begin an elimination diet, check with your doctor about setting up an elimination diet plan. Always make sure you get your doctor's okay — especially if you have existing allergies!

In addition to checking with your doctor, here are some other tips to consider before starting an elimination diet:

- **Don't try to begin your diet during any holidays or upcoming celebrations.** Who wants to be on a diet at a wedding?

- **Get your family's cooperation so they can give you support.**

- **Keep a food and symptom diary.** Jotting down what you eat in a small notebook can help determine what foods are good for you and which ones aren't. Noting any symptoms that occur (up to 24 hours after eating) when you eat specific foods helps you analyze your diet.

- **Figure out how to separate detox from decline.** If you've been drinking coffee, say, or having sugary desserts, stopping cold turkey isn't a good idea. Allow three to five days for withdrawal before starting the elimination diet. You don't want a caffeine-deprived headache that may look like a CFS symptom trigger.

Discovering foods you can eat

After you have your doctor's go-ahead to start your elimination diet, your future menu plans for the next few days probably look a bit bleak, right? Luckily, you can always eat certain foods while on the elimination diet — in moderation, of course, - and unless you're allergic to them.

Those foods you can eat during an elimination diet generally include the following:

- Vegetables (except corn, peas, and any type of bean)

- Meats (except bacon, hot dogs, deli, sausages, and other processed meat products)

- Rice, oats, and barley

- Alternative grains (like amaranth, quinoa, and buckwheat that are in any health food store)

- Fruit (except citrus and any that you consume more than once a week)

- Water (bottled, spring, or distilled)

- Herbal tea

Pinpointing foods to avoid

During the elimination diet, you need to avoid certain types of food because many people have sensitivities and allergies to them. The foods that you absolutely shouldn't consume during this time (at least temporarily) include the following:

- Chocolate
- Milk
- Processed foods
- Sugar
- Wheat
- Food coloring and/or dyes
- Sodas and flavored drinks
- Eggs
- Bacon and sausages
- Luncheon (deli) meat
- Peanuts
- Frankfurters
- Peas of any type
- Beans of any type
- Corn
- Citrus fruit
- Any type of fruit you usually eat more than once a week
- Tea (except for herbal kinds)
- Coffee (both decaffeinated and caffeinated)
- Flavor enhancers (such as MSG)
- Sugar substitutes

Starting the elimination diet

Keeping in mind what you should eat and shouldn't eat, a standard elimination diet usually follows this criteria:

1. **Eat only foods on the allowed list for the first two days.**

2. **Each subsequent day (after the first two days), add one food to avoid (from the avoid list).**

For example, if you had eggs one day and felt okay, then you can add fruit, so the next day you're eating vegetables and fruit.

3. **As you add each food to your diet, monitor your symptoms in your food and symptom diary.**

   Ask yourself: "Today I added chocolate. Did I feel more tired? Did I feel pain?" Jot down any reactions, which can occur anywhere from one minute to 24 hours after eating the food to avoid.

   If you experience any of the following symptoms, you may have food sensitivity, which can exacerbate your CFS:

   - Inability to concentrate and focus
   - Memory loss
   - Hyperactivity
   - Anxiety
   - Stomach pain
   - Muscle aches and pains
   - Irritability
   - Pounding headaches
   - Nasal congestion
   - Fatigue
   - Dark circles under your eyes

   Note that several of these symptoms are very similar to those of classic CFS (for more info, see Chapter 2) — which can also mean that food sensitivity could be at the root of your problems, not CFS! Always check in with your doctor.

4. **Stay on the diet for five to ten days.**

   If you aren't able to pinpoint the exact foods that are bad for you, start over for another five to ten days after one week.

5. **Eliminate those foods to which you reacted from your regular diet.**

   Cutting these foods should help alleviate, or at least avoid exacerbating, your CFS symptoms. You can also add any food to avoid to your foods-you-can-eat list if, in the first go-around, you had no reaction. I also suggest that you talk to your doctor, telling him about your reactions and how you plan on cutting certain foods from your diet, to get his opinion.

Pass the sugar

Does your sugary cereal make you more tired? Don't despair. You can find delicious whole-grain cereals that can help you eat healthy without putting on the pounds. Look at the labels and try to choose cereals that are high in fiber (2g or more) and low in sugar. A small amount of nuts and honey are okay if you need a sweet boost.

Avoiding the junk-food jitters

Junk food is just that: junk. The powers that be are cracking down on fast-food restaurants and food companies all the time, always pushing for healthier foods or (at least) the availability of food information. As a person with CFS, you should strive to keep your body as healthy as possible — and that means avoiding junk food as much as possible.

Fast food is loaded with chemicals, from preservatives to flavor enhancers, that can create havoc in your already-sensitive system. Your best bet is to stay away from fast food as much as possible. If you're on the road and the only choice is a "golden arch," choose one of the healthier menu options: salads, yogurt, and fruit.

Junk food addict? Don't despair. Healthy alternatives to the chips and dips and cookies are out there. Look for baked potato chips, whole-grain crackers, and fat-free popcorn. Purchase cookies that come individually wrapped in small snack packs, so you're less likely to overdo it. But remember: Even so-called natural and healthy options may contain chemicals that can help to set off symptoms. Make food labels your best friend (see the section "Taking advantage of nutritional information")!

Still having a hard time giving up certain foods that you know are bad for you? Consider looking for healthier substitutions. Table 11-1 provides you with a list of healthier, lower-fat food choices that you can substitute for your favorite bad ones.

Table 11-1	Good Food Substitutes for Junk Foods
Instead of:	*Enjoy:*
Fried foods	Lightly sautéed, baked, or grilled foods
Butter or margarine (with trans fats)	Light butter and olive or canola oil
Coffee	Herbal tea
White bread	Whole-grain bread
Semolina pastas	Whole-wheat pasta
Soda and ice-tea drinks	Sparkling water or flavored water
Cream soups	Broth-based soups
Chocolate bars and candy	A piece of real dark chocolate
Mashed potatoes	A baked potato or yam
Jelly and jams	Real-fruit spreads
Regular yogurt	Lactose-free and low-fat yogurt
Bologna or ham	Sliced turkey
Canned fruit	Fresh melon chunks

Alcohol and CFS don't mix. Many people with CFS report that they are alcohol intolerant — even a few sips of beer or wine bring on symptoms or feelings of being tipsy. Not only can alcohol make you sleepier, but any medications you're taking may make it downright dangerous to imbibe. If you want an alternative to alcoholic beverages, you can choose a nonalcoholic drink, like a nonalcoholic strawberry daiquiri or a seltzer with lemon or lime.

Keeping your cuisine a calming experience

Unfortunately, the weakness and fatigue that comes from your CFS makes it difficult to eat right. How can you go grocery shopping and fix a meal if you can't even get out of bed? But if you don't eat right, you face the danger of becoming malnourished — which can only make your symptoms worse!

How do you deal with this Catch-22? You need food, sure, but you don't need to be stressed out about it. Here are some tips for calm and healthy eating.

✔ Ask your support team — family, friends, and/or visiting therapists — to help you with buying and cooking your meals.

✔ Take advantage of online grocery shopping, such as www.peapod.com.

✔ Make the natural frozen dinner your friend. You really can find frozen dishes out there that aren't chock-full of preservatives. Amy's and Kashi have delicious meals and are preservative free.

✔ Use your microwave (instead of your oven or stovetop) to bake yams, cook plain, frozen vegetables, and even cook fresh fruit to use as a topping.

✔ Create an eating schedule, with your meals at regular hours and a few snacks added in. A schedule can help you be as consistent as possible and help calm frazzled nerves. A meal plan also gives your digestive system a break (which is important for folks with CFS).

✔ Stay as close as possible to healthy, whole foods, such as chicken and fish, whole grains, fruits, and vegetables (except citrus fruit, peas, and corn).

Certain kinds of fish may contain mercury, which may cause increased problems for people with CFS. Search the Web to find information on fish varieties that are less likely to contain mercury.

✔ Ask your doctor about nutritional supplements, such as Ensure, to make sure you're getting the nutrients you need every day. (For more on supplements, see Chapter 9.)

✔ Drink bottled water to stay hydrated and herbal tea (without caffeine) to stay calm.

✔ Take a page from the people who brought you the food pyramid (see the section "Taking advantage of nutritional information"). Take the MyPyramid allotments to heart: eating plenty of whole grains, fruits, vegetables, and chicken and fish for protein, and keeping fats and sugars to a minimum. (See Figure 11-1 for the actual chart.)

Cooking up a few tasty CFS-friendly dishes

What's a CFS-friendly menu? Anything that's not "too" spicy, greasy, oily, full of sugar, or salty. The Greeks had it right: moderation in all things. If it was good for an entire civilization, it's probably good for you, and the other members of your family to boot!

The important thing to remember if you have CFS is to eat. Sometimes you may feel so tired and achy that the last thing on your mind is food. But try, really try, to have three solids a day to keep your moods balanced and your body nourished. Also try to be consistent. Have your meals at regular times during the week as much as possible.

The following sections give you some advice on what meals you should be eating on a daily basis as well as what you should be eating when.

Breaking your fast

Breakfast is important because it starts your day out right. If you have a complex carb and a protein (say whole-grain bread and low-fat cheese), you can help stabilize your blood sugar and get some energy to avoid the mid-morning slump. Try to eat breakfast within an hour of waking up. Any more and you'll be starving and weak — and reaching for that danish or cream-cheese-filled everything bagel.

 Thank goodness for instant oatmeal. Instead of the need to stir and stir and stir the pot, you can make a delicious, warm breakfast in a minute. Have peaches, berries, or a banana instead of orange juice, and enjoy eggs (if your elimination diet shows it's okay), –whole-grain toast, and fruit spread.

Dining in versus dining out

For people with CFS, dining out isn't just a question of finances. You must ask yourself how you're feeling — and if you think you can spend a night out. But just because you have CFS, it doesn't mean you can't enjoy yourself once in a while. If you want a way to make dining out fun and healthy without exacerbating your symptoms, I suggest the following:

- **Make reservations at a nearby restaurant so you can get home in a pinch.**

- **Keep your dining plans informal.** Plan for a cup of tea at the local diner, so if your symptoms flare up, you can easily cancel.

- **Stick with places that offer seafood and chicken.** Leave the steakhouses for another time.

- **Order healthy items from the menu.** Look for food that is grilled, baked, or sautéed — not fried.

- **Eat little or none of the bread that comes with your meal.** Eating bread is considered eating empty calories. Take one slice of bread if you must, but then ask the server to take away the bread basket. If your companions are eating bread, put the basket on the farthest end of the table from your seat.

- **Avoid overeating.** Soup or salad can fill you up without any dangerous overeating. Avoid cream soups, and ask for the salad dressing on the side.

- **Enjoy a decaffeinated cappuccino for dessert.** This option has less calories than most desserts and doesn't give you the jitters of caffeine.

- **If you really, really want a glass of wine, opt for a wine spritzer instead.** A wine spritzer is less potent if you don't want a lot of alcohol.

Eating a light lunch

A light lunch keeps your energy up and stops you from feeling sluggish. You should eat lunch no more than four hours after breakfast — and a light repast doesn't mean one shrimp or a butter plate filled with greens. A light lunch means a yogurt and fruit; a sliced turkey sandwich with tomatoes and lettuce; vegetable soup and a whole-grain roll; or a salad with feta cheese and olives, strawberries, and walnuts, or three different types of greens.

Don't forget about the "4 o'clock slump." If you're at work, brown bag some nonfat mozzarella sticks, celery, baby carrots, or an apple. If you're at home, keep these healthy treats in full view in your refrigerator.

Sometimes the simple things are what keep you on course. A fat-free, diet hot chocolate has only about 25 calories, but mixed with hot water, it tastes like a mouth-watering treat — filling and satisfying.

Sitting down for a sensible dinner

Try to eat dinner no more than six hours after lunch (or a little later if you have a late afternoon snack). For dinner, think of a trilogy of foods, a three-part harmony of eating — a three-colored platter. In other words, think of dinner in threes: one starch, one protein, and one vegetable.

The following are some healthy dinner hints:

- The more colorful your foods, the more nutrients they have. Think of a yam, some wild salmon, and green beans. Bellissimo!
- Make vegetables your largest portion.
- Protein portions should be about the size of your palm or a deck of cards.
- One cup of starchy foods (like potatoes, rice, and couscous) is about the size of a tennis ball.
- Save a piece of fruit for dessert — when you're watching television or as a late-night snack.

Try to avoid eating after 8:00 p.m. (or three hours before going to bed). You don't want to go to sleep on a full stomach, because you will be uncomfortable and getting sleep will be that much harder.

Reaching and Maintaining Your Optimum Weight

One of the side-effects of CFS is, I'm sad to report, weight gain. Some reasons why include the following:

- Restricted exercise
- Lack of mobility
- Lack of energy
- Medications, such as some antidepressants
- Poor sleep
- Changes in brain chemistry and/or metabolism

If you don't change your eating habits and restrict calories, you will gain weight. Period. But too much restriction, and you won't get the nutrition you need — which spells increased fatigue and decreased energy. In this section, I detail how to find — and stay with — a weight that works for you.

Calculating a healthy weight for you

As long as you're eating healthy and getting the nutrients you need, losing weight can help you regain some of your lost zest. Researchers have found that if you lose 10 percent of your body weight, you will achieve the health benefits of someone who loses 20 percent or more. In other words, lower blood pressure, better blood sugar levels (which keep your moods on an even keel), diabetes prevention, and less risk of heart disease all occur with just a loss of 10 percent of your current weight.

Today, more and more doctors are using body mass index (BMI) instead of pounds to determine whether you're in good health. Your *body mass index* is the amount of fat versus muscle. Using Figure 11-3, move up the left side of the chart to find your height, and then move across to your current weight. If you have a BMI between 18 and 24, you can consider yourself at a healthy weight. You're considered overweight if you have a BMI of 25 to 29. You're considered obese if your BMI is 30 or more.

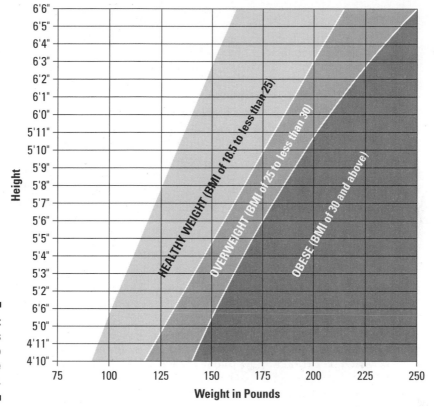

Figure 11-3: Use this chart to calculate your BMI.

Knowing your BMI can help you see if you need to lose weight and adjust your calories per day accordingly. Exercising, if you're able, can help turn fat into muscle. But *only* if you can! Your CFS can make that hard. (For more on CFS and exercise, check out Chapter 10.)

Shedding pounds: The stress-free way

Losing weight always comes down to this: Expend more energy than you put in. That translates into the following weight-loss guidelines:

- ✔ Exercise to use up more energy and burn up those calories.
- ✔ Eat fewer calories so that your body must eat up your fat reserves.

Because you have CFS, exercising more isn't an option — you may not be able to exercise at all because it can exacerbate your symptoms. So the only option you're left with is eating less food. Here's where it gets tricky: You need to eat enough so that you keep up your energy and get the right amount of nutrients, but less than you have in the past so you can lose weight.

To lose weight, I suggest sticking with a 1,200-calories-a-day diet if you weigh less than 180 pounds and a 1,400-calories-a-day diet if you weigh more than 180 pounds. You should lose about 1 pound a week. Stay on this diet only until you reach a healthy BMI; after that, you can add some calories back into your diet.

You can find many healthy diet programs on the Internet that allow you to also participate at home on your computer, which include the following:

✔ Weight Watchers (www.weightwatchers.com)

✔ e-Diets (www.ediets.com)

✔ French Women Don't Get Fat (www.frenchwomendontgetfat.com)

These diets all consist of a healthy variety of foods and steady-but-sure weight loss. However, these programs do cost some money.

If you'd rather go it solo, purchase a calorie-counter book and keep a running tab each day. (Don't forget to count each serving!) Dieticians and nutritionists all agree: Keeping a food log can help you shed your pounds easier. Sometimes people eat unconsciously and you may not be aware of how much you're actually putting in your mouth. By writing down your foods — and servings — you're not only keeping an accurate account, but you may just stop and say, "Do I really want that cookie?" Further, a food log is a good reference tool in case you aren't losing weight and you need to see what you've been eating.

It would be great if everyone could pop a pill and lose ten pounds fast. Unfortunately, it doesn't work that way. Even the fat absorption-reducing medications out there now can only go so far — about three or four more pounds, if at all. Plus you have to deal with a big drawback: oily stool and diarrhea, neither of which helps with your fatigue, energy, or well-being.

Getting a Good Night's Sleep

You can find nothing like a solid eight hours of sleep to give you more energy, a fresh outlook on life, and a positive way to start the day. Unfortunately, if you have CFS, getting a good night's sleep can seem like finding the Holy Grail. In fact, 70–95 percent of people with CFS have trouble sleeping.

What came first? The chicken or the egg?

Everything from infection to immunological disorders, neural and endocrine malfunctions, and stress (all possibly related to CFS) can keep you up at night — not to mention your CFS symptoms, such as pain, muscle aches, and headaches.

On the other hand, if you aren't sleeping well, your lack of sleep is going to affect you — making you more vulnerable to infection, immune disorders, neural and endocrine malfunctions, and stress. Bad sleep is also going to make any existing CFS symptoms worse, whether it be pain, cognitive dysfunction, memory loss, or fatigue.

Some people with CFS have disrupted tossing-and-turning sleep patterns. Others are tired but wired, unable to go to sleep no matter how tired they are. Still others have *hypersomnia* (sleeping too much), in which they can sleep 12 to 14 hours a day but still wake up exhausted!

Your sleep cycles are divided into four stages, and each cycle lasts about 90 minutes. The first stage is those first few moments when you transition from wakefulness to sleep. Stage two is a little deeper, where you go back and forth through the night, from deeper stage-three and stage-four sleep, back to stage two, and so on. Stages three and four are called *delta sleep,* which is when you have your *REM* (rapid eye movement) dream sleep. If your sleep patterns are interrupted, you can wake up cranky and foggy.

In this section, I go over some suggestions that may help you *really* sleep — not just toss and turn all night.

Establishing a healthy sleep schedule

Before you can create a consistent sleep schedule, you need to determine whether you have a sleeping problem. Chances are, if you have CFS, you have some sort of sleep-related complaint, whether it be difficulty getting to sleep or staying asleep, tossing and turning (restless sleep), or unrefreshing sleep.

Some medications can play havoc on your sleep, and specialists recommend that if you have CFS you should start at ¼ or ½ the usual prescribed dosage, particularly for medicines that have sedating effects. Consult with your doctor before discontinuing or changing any medication doses.

To help create a sleep routine, follow these suggestions from the experts:

- ✔ **Develop a sleep schedule that is realistic — and stick to it.** If you find that your day ends around 8:00 p.m., plan on going to sleep at 9:30 p.m. If you're a night owl, up until midnight, make sure you wind down around 11:00 p.m. and are into bed at the stroke of midnight (and no later, sleeping beauty!).

    Make sure you give yourself enough time to have eight hours of sleep when you create your sleep schedule.

- ✔ **Wake at the same time every day — whether or not it's a work day.** Try to get out of bed and start your day on a consistent basis. A consistent sleep routine is more likely to help you get a solid eight hours!

- ✔ **Avoid daytime naps.** Little cat naps will make it harder for you to fall asleep at night.

- ✔ **Make time for an extended wind-down period before you go to bed.** Take some time when you're finished with the day and all you have to do is relax; watch some unexciting television or read (but not a thriller!). For more tips on how to relax at the end of your day, check out a later section in this chapter, "Falling asleep by reading some sleep tips."

- ✔ **Don't do even light exercise before going to sleep!** In fact, make sure you exercise at least four hours before hitting the sack.

- ✔ **Don't get into bed until you're ready to sleep.** Use your bed for sleep and intimacy only.

- ✔ **Avoid eating anything right before you go to sleep, especially a big dinner!** Feeling stuffed and uncomfortable isn't the best way to try to have a good night's sleep!

Falling asleep by reading some sleep tips

Hmm . . . what would you do for a good night's sleep? If you have CFS, you'd probably give a cash reward! To help make the end of day blissful instead of "blast-ful," try some of the following tips:

- ✔ Drink some herbal tea without caffeine. One particular brand, Celestial Seasonings Sleepytime Herb Tea, really does help you fall asleep.

- ✔ Listen to a deep-relaxation CD, a creative visualization journey, or even a meditation CD.

✔ Try the following deep-relaxation method:

- Lay on your back, your arms and legs in a comfortable position. Your head should be resting comfortably on the pillow.

- Starting with your feet, squeeze your toes together, then your legs, buttocks, arms, chest, and finally your head.

- Don't forget your face. Grimace. Open your mouth and stick out your tongue. Squint. Then give a great big breath out.

✔ Self-hypnosis has come a long way. You can find many CDs and audio tapes to help you enter a sleep state.

✔ Millions of Americans fall asleep listening to Jay Leno. I can't think of a reason why you can't do the same with the late-night talk show of your choice.

✔ Start reading something bland, like a cookbook or a lifestyle magazine. Reading something that doesn't cause you any stress can help you relax.

Lock-Stepping with a Daily Routine

Controlling your CFS takes a daily routine that encompasses everything that you do, every day (as you probably already guessed if you've flipped through the previous sections of this chapter). Yes, you must be flexible and allow for symptom flare-ups, but, on the whole, keeping to a realistic schedule and tailoring your eating and resting habits accordingly can help you cope much better. In this section, I give you the information you need to form your own, individual routine.

Establishing a healthy schedule

Okay, some people out there schedule everything — from brushing their teeth to shampooing their hair. I don't want you to feel like you have to do that (and, I suspect, neither do you). But I do want you to think of your day in blocks of time, each block representing a different activity. Remember, you usually need more time to do things than other people, so I would suggest that each block be at least two hours.

Always plan in periods of rest and recovery from activity. Pushing all day until evening time only incites a push-crash cycle, spiraling into relapse.

Be sure to show your health care professional the schedule you've created before starting it. He may be able to give you some suggestions based on his observations.

A schedule is flexible and can always be moved around. If the schedule doesn't work, change it slightly and keep changing it until it does work or ask your doctor for some advice. For example, if you find that you get more fatigued later in the day, plan more in the morning. If you find that you can't get out of bed one day, let that be your daily activity! Don't do too much — you can always add something later.

Be sure to stick with your schedule because it gives you consistency, which can help with less stress and better sleep.

Encouraging your family to cooperate

As with anything else in life, you may be able to go it alone, but it sure does help to have support. Enlist your family to help get you moving if you need some motivation. Put a copy of your daily schedule on the refrigerator or in the bathroom. Let everyone know what you're doing so they can check on you and offer help if need be. And who knows? You may inspire your loved ones to make their own blocks of time, thanks to your newfound efficiency!

If you're the caregiver, check out Chapter 14 for more tips on how to cooperate with the needs of your loved one with CFS.

Chapter 12

Working When You Have CFS

Chronic fatigue syndrome (CFS) is a condition that can be as debilitating as clinical depression or multiple sclerosis. It can compromise your job performance, stir up conflicts with colleagues, and even have you demoted or fired for poor job performance. Problems at work can lead to further emotional, psychological, and financial stresses, which can worsen your condition.

Taking steps to reduce worksite stress, modifying your work schedule, and picking up some coping skills can dramatically improve your productivity, reversing the downward spiral. In this chapter, I show you how to manage your workday world to cope more effectively with CFS.

Disclosing Your Condition: To Tell or Not to Tell?

When you're newly diagnosed with a condition that has no cure and an uncertain course with no predictable end, you face a daunting set of challenges — medical, emotional, social, and professional — as you figure out how to manage your life with a chronic illness. For those in the midst of building careers, one of the toughest challenges is deciding whether to disclose your condition to supervisors and colleagues.

You may be concerned about how others will react. And with a diagnosis of CFS, where the symptoms are vague and still not fully accepted by some in the medical community, perhaps you're worried that your bosses won't take your diagnosis seriously. You may become anxious, even depressed at concealing your "secret"; you know that you may not be able to carry your normal workload, so you feel the need to come clean. You may also be worried about your medical insurance. If you're unable to work, how will you pay for your medical care?

If you're looking for a job, you may feel even more vulnerable. If you tell a prospective employer about your CFS, will she be okay with any special accommodations that you may need? You may feel that you need to disclose your illness in order to even get a job.

The decision to tell others about your CFS is highly personal, one that *you* will live with, whatever you decide. After you tell, the genie is out of the bottle so to speak, and you can't take it back. For some, honesty is the best policy. They feel being open and forthright will reduce their level of stress and let them know exactly where they stand. For others, the risk of disclosure is too great; they fear embarrassment, loss of status, and the stress of knowing that others know. So should you tell? The decision really is up to you. In this section, I help you make the right choice for *you*.

Weighing your options

The consequences of telling or not telling can seem damning either way. Of course, you can't be fired for being sick, but your hours, and consequently your salary and benefits, may be greatly reduced. You can try to work through your illness, using sick time and vacation to rest on those days when your symptoms are particularly debilitating, but what do you do when you run out of sick or vacation days and still need to take time off? You don't want to risk being fired, because you need your insurance. You can't find an easy answer to this dilemma, but this section can help you weigh your options.

Considering your work situation

The only way to make the decision about whether to tell is to dispassionately review your situation, taking the following factors into account:

- ✔ **Your work culture:** Is your work environment one where the nose-to-the-grindstone mentality is the ideal? You may consider disclosing your condition and seeing whether you can work from home more often. In other cases, you may want to look into changing jobs.

- ✔ **Your supervisors:** Are they open and receptive, or are they the crack-the-whip types who look down on you for going home "early" at 5:00 p.m.? Hopefully, they're the former, but if they aren't, you have to bite the bullet and tell them if your symptoms are getting in the way of your work. If your symptoms are interfering, you may need to take time off and get disability — not go to the office. (See the later section titled "Filing for Disability" for details on this process.)

✔ **Your colleagues:** Are your co-workers supportive or super-competitive, always looking for a weak spot? If they're supportive, you may want to go ahead and tell them. If they're not, confide in a colleague you consider a friend and try to work out a strategy. Perhaps your co-workers will be more accepting if they understand that you're not simply slacking off or out partying all night. Of course, you may want to look for another job if your co-workers would consider you "soft" for having CFS. Besides, who'd want to work with a bunch of people who feel that way?

✔ **Your human resources (HR) department:** Will HR back you up and let you keep your insurance if you need to reduce your hours? Only you can decide how much to tell your employer about your CFS status. On the plus side, telling her about your diagnosis is the only way to protect your legal right to any accommodations you may need to keep your job.

Your HR department has the information you need to file for disability (see the later "Filing for Disability" section). It can be very helpful in answering any questions you may have about the law.

Looking at the benefits and advantages

This decision is complex, and you shouldn't make it until you've thought it through. First, as you decide what to do, consider some of the following positive results that could happen after you tell your employer and colleagues about your CFS:

✔ **Gaining empathy:** In the ideal situation, your supervisors are understanding, your colleagues are sensitive, and everyone makes an effort to accommodate your medical needs. By telling your boss and your colleagues, you may increase your support circle. People understand that you have a valid reason for your fatigue.

✔ **Obtaining worksite modifications:** If you don't tell your boss, you can't expect any accommodations for your illness. If you explain that you have CFS, your employer makes the necessary work schedule changes you need. You may get the freedom to take the time you need to rest during the day; your work week may be reorganized. You may even be given tools, such as a computer, so you can work at home when commuting to work is too difficult. See "Flexing your workplace and schedule" later in this chapter for more information.

✔ **Reducing the stress of keeping secrets:** Coming out of the CFS closet takes a great burden off your shoulders. You can concentrate on dealing with the illness rather than spending your energy trying to hide it.

- **Protecting your legal position:** By telling your employer about your CFS, you are, by law, allowed to keep your job. You get to keep your full insurance benefits, including any family benefits, and aren't required to pay a bigger share of your insurance premium. You also can't be demoted or forced to accept a lower salary.

  Legally, you can be fired only if your boss has given you enough warnings about your work habits and you haven't made the effort to explain and fix them. By disclosing your condition, you protect yourself and give your boss the opportunity to help your job responsibilities better align with your current abilities, which can also boost your confidence.

Now here are things to think about when you take the worst-case scenario into consideration:

- **Colleague backlash:** Your work mates may have to take on your workload when you can't make it to the office — with no added compensation. You may not look that sick to them, so they don't quite believe that you're as sick as you say. Your colleagues may begin to edge you out of the work group and no longer include you in the office gossip — you may even become the subject of the office gossip and hear about the bowling party only *after* it has taken place.

- **Loss of status:** You can't be fired, but you know that you're no longer viewed as the rising star. You don't get the promotions you were in line for, and you can tell by the subtle hints that there won't be any more promotions in the near future.

- **Increased stress of wondering what others may think:** Is the colleague in the next cubicle suddenly getting frosty? Are people stopping a conversation as you walk to the coffee machine? Does your boss's closed door mean he's on the phone with HR? Stress can feed paranoia and anxiety like nothing else — and unfortunately, stress can lead to less efficient work and more mistakes on the job.

- **Job discrimination:** Even though it's not supposed to happen, being honest about your condition can leave you open to discrimination, limiting your prospects for advancement if you're already employed, and it may preclude you from getting hired if you're looking for a job. Proving discrimination can be difficult when companies say that you're simply "not the right candidate for the job."

- **Job loss:** Yes, you know you can't be fired for being sick, but your boss may find a way to fire you without using illness as the prevailing reason, blaming it on poor job performance or the like. You know the illness is likely the cause, but you can't prove it.

  The law is with you, regardless of whether you've officially filed for disability. A company can't fire you or decide not to hire you because of CFS — it falls under the Americans with Disabilities Act (ADA). See the nearby sidebar for details.

Researching your rights

If you live in the United States and have CFS, the good news is that you're protected by the Americans with Disabilities Act (ADA). You can't be summarily dismissed from your job because you have a medical disability, and your employer must provide "reasonable accommodations" or "modifications," as the ADA specifies, "to enable people with disabilities to enjoy equal employment opportunities." For more about your rights as an employee with a disability, contact the United States Equal Employment Opportunity Commission (EEOC) or visit the Americans with Disabilities Act Web site, `www.usdoj.gov/crt/ada/adahom1.htm`, where you can find a wealth of information about your rights.

Many people with CFS and other chronic conditions attempt to work a part-time schedule as a means of maintaining income while adjusting to the limits of their condition. However, if you later have to go on full disability, most companies don't provide long-term disability benefits to part-time workers, and depending on the employer or policy, the position you last had (not the one you may have had for years before) determines benefits eligibility. So before you cut back your full-time job to part-time hours and benefits, be sure to investigate how your benefits are impacted and whether you can afford to do it. Some people, however, may not have the luxury of making a choice; their illness will force them to make one, and then they are without a job.

Breaking the bad news (diplomatically speaking)

If you decide to disclose your medical condition, you need a strategy to ensure that you'll still have your job (even with modifications), your medical benefits, and the respect of your colleagues.

You may want to tell your boss directly about your CFS. Before you do, get a letter or statement from your doctor stating that you have CFS, what your symptoms are, and what accommodations you're likely to need to continue working. As further evidence that CFS is a real medical condition, you may even want to take in some brochures or information fact sheets from the Chronic Fatigue and Immune Dysfunction Syndrome (CFIDS) Association of America or the Centers for Disease Control and Prevention (CDC).

You also want to ensure that any information you disclose to your boss and human resources (HR) is held in strict confidence. Most HR departments in larger companies are aware of this and may even have forms that you can fill out that clearly state the company's responsibilities and your right to privacy. Smaller businesses may not have these safeguards, but your rights are still protected under the Americans with Disabilities Act (ADA) if the business has 15 or more employees. If your firm has fewer than 15 employees, you may be entitled to similar protections under state and local laws. (For more on the ADA, check out the sidebar "Researching your rights.")

Before you meet with your boss or the HR department, you need to face your own concerns. Putting them in writing can help you to get a clearer picture of what you really feel, and it's the first step in devising a strategy to deal with them. First, jot down worst-case scenarios that you think could happen if you disclose your CFS, such as the following:

- I'll lose my job.
- I'll have to cut back on my hours, and therefore my salary will be significantly lower.
- I'll miss out on promotions, or I may even be demoted.
- My colleagues will treat me differently. They may resent that I get more time off or more accommodations and privileges than they do.
- I may lose my insurance coverage or have to pay higher premiums.

Then write down what you need to manage your CFS and maintain your work status:

- I need to keep my job and all its benefits.
- I need to have my medical insurance remain at its current level of coverage.
- I need to rearrange my work schedule — perhaps working fewer hours in the office and some from home.
- I need to know that any information I provide will be kept strictly confidential and not used against me.
- I can't work at all right now, so I need to proceed with the instructions of the disability act laws to get disability (see "Filing for Disability" later in this chapter").

Writing things down gives you a sense of control over something that seems to come to you at its whim. And that control, that mastery, may give you the self-confidence you need to do what needs to be done, reducing your anxiety and depression. Another plus: what you need to do gets done!

Generally, your boss and HR are the first people who need to know. Set up an appointment, bring your doctor's statement and brochures, and come prepared to discuss your needs and concerns.

The best way to deal with your co-workers is to really determine who truly is a friend. If there's no one you can trust, don't tell anyone until you and your boss and HR have come up with a plan. If you can trust some co-workers, you can tell them after you tell your boss — the last thing you want is for your boss to hear last.

Calculating the Possible Personal Financial Costs

The Centers for Disease Control and Prevention (CDC) reported on a 2004 study that estimated the economic cost of CFS. The annual loss was about $20,000 per household, which is half the average household's mean income.

A loss of $20,000 is a dramatic cut for most United States households and may threaten the loss of the family's home if the working partner's income isn't sufficient to cover the household expenses. If you're single, having CFS could mean that you have to move in with relatives or even apply for public assistance as well as disability benefits.

And the losses aren't just in salary. If you contribute to your medical plan, you may have to contribute a larger percentage of your reduced salary relative to what you earned before. Your future income and retirement are also impacted. If you contribute to your 401k or pension plan, you may have to reduce the amount you put into the plan, and if your employer offers a matching contribution, the financial burden over the course of your anticipated work life can be substantial.

Costs for services you may not have had to think about may now be essential additions to the family budget, such as babysitting services or household help. You may even have more expenses for medical services not covered by your insurance.

Depending on your severance agreement, you may have to pay your own insurance premiums. You're entitled under COBRA (the Consolidated Budget Reconciliation Act) to keep your insurance under your company's plan, but now you may have to pick up the full tab yourself.

Over time, these costs in terms of added expenses, unearned income, and reduced benefits can add up to hundreds of thousands of dollars. In this section, I discuss some of these visible and invisible costs directly related to your job so you can avoid being shocked by the possible financial changes in your life.

Earning less by producing less

It's a fact of life: If you don't keep up your work, you'll earn less — either in the present or in terms of future raises. If you're forced to cut back on your work hours, you'll probably earn less. Period.

You can find ways to adjust your work so that your production isn't decreased. Here are some ways around the produce-less, earn-less rule:

- ✔ Work from home.
- ✔ Work a shorter amount of time but spread it out over seven days.
- ✔ Work on some freelance work to make up for the lost income (see the later section "Freelancing from your home").

For more tips on how to be more productive as a worker with CFS, check out the section "Pumping Up Your Productivity" later in this chapter.

Taking a pass on promotions

Passing up that promotion you worked so hard for may be tough, but if the promotion means longer hours, increased workload, and more responsibility, you may just have to. Your natural impulse may be to test the waters to see whether more and better sleep at night can get you through the day. But as much as the added money is helpful, especially if you have added expenses, you can't do yourself and your loved ones any good by taking on too much. In the worst case, you may accept the promotion and realize you can't do the job; the result may mean losing your job altogether, along with your income and benefits, or seeing your health decline.

However, if you can negotiate your work situation in such a way that your needs are taken care of and you can alter or modify it as your needs change, then go for that promotion! Otherwise, as much as the prospect of more money and prestige appeals to you, you may just have to say *no*.

Getting demoted or fired

You can't be fired just for being sick. Although most people know that, it still happens. Of course, the illness is never the stated reason for termination, but your employer couldn't very well tell you that you're being fired because you have CFS, now could she?

If you've been an exemplary employee and you have proof — performance evaluations, complimentary e-mails, and letters from satisfied clients —

you can certainly pursue a discrimination case if you choose to go that route. If so, you need to go to human resources.

Demotion is somewhat less clear cut than being fired. If you can't do your job at the level that you're expected to, your employer has the right to offer you a job or a schedule more suited to your current abilities. Unfortunately, a drop in income may also come with that assignment. Not many employers are willing to pay an employee more for doing less.

If you've been fired or demoted for legitimate reasons, all is not lost. You can check into disability benefits (see "Filing for Disability") or look for a job that allows you to work at home or that is slower-paced. And always apply for unemployment: That's what that money is there for!

The company isn't always your enemy. Remember that you shouldn't always go to the discrimination line. Sometimes a person is fired because she can no longer do her job well, even after the employer has made modifications.

Paying the doctor bills

If you have insurance, most of your bills should be covered. Depending on your medical plan, you may still have a high deductible or high copays. If your income is lowered because of a cutback in your hours, your doctor bills may take a larger chunk of your diminished income. If you decide to try any alternative therapies or agree to special medical tests or medications that aren't generally approved for CFS, you may have to pay those bills out of pocket.

How can you manage all your bills, plus the added doctor bills? Here are some tips for managing and prioritizing your bills and lowering your medical costs:

- ✔ **If your medical plan is a health maintenance organization (HMO) with a roster of in-plan doctors, try to find a specialist in the plan.** In some HMO plans, you don't have an additional copay for in-plan doctors.

- ✔ **Review bills from your doctor or the hospital.** Make sure you understand all the items listed. Most items are listed by code numbers, so if you don't understand a specific charge, call the number on the bill and ask for an explanation.

- ✔ **If you can't afford the full payment, call your provider and ask whether you can make arrangements to pay a regular amount each month to pay off the charge.** The good news is that late charges are rarely tacked on to medical bills, so you may be able to stretch out your payments without having to worry about finance charges.

✔ **Prioritize your bills.** Your medical team will be a big part of your life from now on, so try to pay your medical bills. List all the bills and the amounts you owe and draw up what financial planners call an *FPLP:* first-pay/last-pay schedule. Along with rent, mortgage, insurance, and basic necessities, put your medical bills near the top of the list.

✔ **Contact your creditors to see whether you can work out a payment plan with them.** Making small payments on each bill rather than paying some bills in full and postponing others may be a better option for you.

Note: Some premium credit cards and mortgage loans come with disability coverage so that the finance charges are suspended and longer payment plans are possible if the cardholder becomes disabled. Definitely check with your creditors to see whether this clause is in your contract. And if you apply for new credit, make sure you check for such policies before you sign on the dotted line.

✔ **If you incur a lot of bills and have claim denials that you can't resolve on your own, consider hiring a professional billing and claims specialist to resolve your disputes for you.** Hiring a professional can cost you between $50 and $250 per hour, but such services can save you up to 40 percent on your bills. Check out the Medical Billing Advocates of America (www.billadvocates.com) or the Alliance of Claims Assistance Professionals (www.claims.org) to find a specialist in your area.

✔ **If you have a high deductible and you can afford it, you may consider opening a health savings account (HSA) or flex plan.** If you can afford to put away money into an HSA, you can save on taxes. For every $5,000 you put into an HSA, you can save about $1,500 a year, and any funds you don't use grow tax-free and roll over from year to year. For more information on health savings accounts, visit the United States Department of the Treasury at www.ustreas.gov/offices/public-affairs/hsa.

Flex plans, which are similar to HSAs, are another option. You can put in $5,000 per year in pre-tax dollars. It must be used in full by the end of the year, or the remaining money is forfeited.

✔ **Claim your excess bills on your taxes.** The IRS allows you to deduct the amount of medical expenses for you and your dependents that exceed 7.5 percent of your gross income. The list of eligible expenses is quite extensive and includes things you may not expect, such as transportation to and from medical appointments and modifications that may need to be made to your home to accommodate your disability. For more information, see www.irs.gov/publications/p502.

Incurring additional expenses at work

If you require services or assistance outside of the normal work parameters that incur additional expenses, you can ask your employer to pick up the tab. In most cases, if you're valued enough, they try to accommodate you. If they don't, try to work out a payment plan with the creditors. You may also want to consider finding other work at this point, too.

Take Elena for instance. She was recently diagnosed with CFS. Her physical symptoms are relatively mild, but she discovered that occasional brain fog would cloud her judgment and make thinking difficult, especially in the afternoon. Determined to continue working, both as a matter of pride and as the single parent of three children, Elena approached her boss to ask for special accommodations that would allow her to keep her job as a senior accountant of the mid-sized firm. Not trusting herself to drive when her brain was cloudy, she requested that her firm pay for a car service to take her home in the evenings after work. Luckily for Elena, her firm agreed that this was a reasonable accommodation and paid for the service.

Making it through the lean times

The consequences of a sudden drop in income can be enormous. Combine it with a debilitating condition, such as CFS, and you can feel as if you just fell into the moneyless pit. You want to make sure that you can continue to pay your bills and enjoy a decent standard of living. You need to find ways to help you when things get too tight. Here are some suggestions:

- ✔ **Seek help from other sources.** Churches, synagogues, mosques, and other houses of worship can be a great source of monetary and nonmonetary support, and most have an outreach program to help members in need. For example, they may be able to pay a bill for you for several months or gather volunteers to help with tasks such as shopping, cooking, or driving the kids to school. Just make sure you don't become completely dependent on these resources. When you can get back on your feet financially, do so.

- ✔ **Look around the house for stuff you can sell.** If you're homebound, set up an online account with an online merchandising company such as eBay. You can manage your sales while lying in bed if you have to and get a family member to do the shipping and handling for you.

- ✔ **Sell your services as a telephone consultant.** If you have an expertise that you can talk to others about, tell family and friends to get you referrals. Here's your chance to make some money from your in-depth knowledge of computer software or stamps! You could even parlay your obsession with, say, 18th-century English literature into tutoring.

Pumping Up Your Productivity

Before you decide to quit your day job, you can do a few things to make the most of the time you spend at work. Even if you have a modified workday, you can still be productive. The key is to make a plan, get organized, stay focused, and make it happen. In this section, I give you suggestions on getting the most out of your efforts.

Energizing yourself throughout the workday

Sustaining sufficient energy to function productively while at work is very important. However, finding that energy can be a challenge. You need to gauge your energy level on a day-to-day basis to set your goals each day and ultimately be more productive.

The first rule of conserving energy is to pace yourself. Reserve the more difficult jobs for the part of the day when you feel most energetic. Think of your tasks as primarily mental or physical. Avoid scheduling too many physical tasks in succession.

Set an amount of time for a task that you feel you can manage energywise. When that time is up, stop to relax or turn to a much easier activity. Take regular rests, even when you feel okay. You need breaks from both prolonged sitting and standing. During your breaks, try careful stretching, meditation, and relaxation exercises to revitalize yourself (for more on exercise tips, see Chapter 10).

Consider some of these other useful tips for conserving your energy at work:

- **If you're taking medication, stick with it.** For example, if you're on sleep medications, taking them as prescribed can help you get back to a normal sleep pattern. More rested at night means more energy during the day.

- **Pay attention to your body.** Make note of when and under what circumstances your symptoms worsen, and take steps to avoid them. For example, your energy may be lowest in the afternoon, which may be the best time for a short nap to recharge your batteries.

- **Watch what you eat and drink.** Now is not the time to diet or skip meals. Put yourself on a regular eating schedule, eating nutritious, whole foods that keep your energy level high. Stay away from the doughnuts, cookies, and other empty-calorie, sugary foods. Make sure you also drink plenty of fluids, which is particularly important for people with CFS who have problems with orthostatic instability (dizziness at certain postures due to variations in blood pressure).

✔ **Ask your doctor about vitamins.** Vitamins may strengthen your immune system, provide important antioxidants and other nutrients, and give you more energy. If you get the go-ahead, include them in your eating schedule.

✔ **Watch out for over-the-counter medications (OTCs) for conditions other than pain.** You may be tempted to reach for an over-the-counter medicine to calm a cough or give you a quick pick-me-up, but be careful. Even an innocent cough suppressant can have ingredients that can make you feel sleepy. Ask your doctor or pharmacist to recommend a cough suppressant or similar medication that's less likely to make you drowsy.

Staying focused

Slipping into a mental fog is common when you have such a debilitating illness as CFS. In fact, memory, concentration problems, and feeling like your brain is in a fog are common symptoms of CFS.

CFS patients have used the following strategies to combat brain fog (and I recommend you do the same):

✔ **Organize your workspace.** Clutter can slow you down and make you feel even more tired or overwhelmed.

✔ **Plan out your day.** Try to get in the habit of keeping a daily to-do list to help keep you focused on the tasks at hand. Use that calendar your employer provides! If you work on a computer as many people do, you may consider using calendar programs that are installed in your computer, such as Microsoft Outlook, that you can use to set up appointments, create task lists, and even set audible reminders.

✔ **Delegate some of your responsibilities or ask your boss to arrange for some help.** If you can give away some tasks to someone else, grab the chance so you can focus on what you do best. Set reminders for yourself to follow up. Again, your calendar program can help you keep track of assigned tasks and their progress.

When you do encounter a task you can do and do well, take the opportunity to do it yourself. You don't want to take advantage of others or show that you aren't up for the job, and doing what you can helps keep you in good spirits.

✔ **Arrange the tasks that require concentration and focus for early in the day.** If you're more alert in the morning, schedule your most important tasks and appointments before noon. Many people with CFS feel lethargic toward the end of the day. Leaving less important tasks for later frees you up to focus on the major tasks in the morning.

✔ **Do one task at a time.** Multitasking is the expected norm for most workers today, but try to limit yourself to doing one task at a time. Trying to eat, surf the Web, and talk on the phone not only makes you inefficient, but it may also serve to make you feel even foggier. If you have a major project with many component parts, break down the job into smaller tasks.

✔ **Repeat directives to yourself several times to make them stick in your mind.** The more you hear an instruction, the more likely you are to remember it.

✔ **Take notes.** Write things down or enter them into your electronic reminder. You may even want to purchase one of those tiny electronic recorders you can carry with you to dictate notes to yourself and then play them back later.

✔ **Keep your brain limber.** Crosswords, jigsaw puzzles, Sudoku, and brain-teasers can help you focus your thoughts. The focus required in "training to train your brain" in this way can help you to focus on other tasks as well.

✔ **Keep distractions at a minimum.** For some people, TV or a radio blaring nearby can compete for attention. Others claim it helps them focus. Discover what works best for you. If your co-workers' conversations bother you, try using earplugs. If that doesn't work, politely explain that you need more quiet. If that still doesn't work, request to move your desk to a quieter location. Also, set official times for appointments, even with your co-workers. Constant interruptions can cause you to lose your focus.

If you find that you're still struggling, a good professional organizer or motivational coach can teach you how to change your thinking so you can better plan and manage your activities. An occupational therapist (OT) who's trained in energy-conservation techniques may also be able to help. You can find a licensed OT from your local hospital or rehabilitation center. For coaches and organizers, let your fingers do the walking and find some local people online or in the yellow pages. Ask for references — and call them — before going ahead and meeting with any professional. One note: Health insurance may pay for OT, so check with your insurance company. Your employer may pay for an organizer or OT person as well, so you may want to ask your HR department.

Flexing your workplace and schedule

The Americans with Disabilities Act (ADA) provides you with the right to request that your employers provide reasonable accommodations to help you perform your job to the extent that you're able. To figure out what kind of modifications may need to be made to help you do your job, take an inventory of your symptoms and then see whether you can rearrange your schedule and your work environment to meet your needs.

You may want to keep a journal while you're at work to take note of when you do things well, when you struggle, what you struggle with, and possible solutions. That way, you can be prepared when you meet with your boss to discuss accommodations.

Possible solutions to consider include the following:

- **Job restructuring.** Depending on your job, you may be able to redefine the tasks that would normally fall under your job description.

- **Accepting a less-taxing position.** Changing positions may mean a loss of status and salary, but it may also mean staying employed and keeping your benefits.

- **Doing part of your job from home or getting on a part-time schedule.**

- **Taking unpaid leave with the promise of being able to return when you're able.**

- **Doing all your work from home.** You may try all these modifications and still find that you still don't have the energy to get to work and put in a full day. Your last resort may well be that you need to ask your employer to give you the equipment and the communication tools enabling you to work from home.

If you're too ill to even work at home, make sure you register for disability insurance.

Freelancing from your home

If you've had to leave your job and are stuck at home, you can find many things you can do from the comfort of your own home to earn an income and keep you occupied without overtaxing yourself.

If you have an area of expertise, you can become a consultant and sell your advice. Even if your job is physical, such as an auto mechanic or short-order cook, you can still answer questions from those who know less about the subject than you do.

Striking out on your own is challenging for anyone, and as appealing as being your own boss is, it can present an even greater challenge for someone with CFS. But with a bit of planning and help from others, freelancing is possible. Here are some tips for successful freelancing:

- **Define your area of expertise.** Identifying that skill where you have a network intact, one where you can use your contacts to get work, is usually best. Regardless of what skill you want to use, do some homework — make sure you're capable of doing the work and that there's a market for it!

- **Develop a portfolio that demonstrates your skill.** For example, if you were a staff writer, put some of your published articles in a portfolio book to show prospective clients.

- **Build your client base.** Call all your friends, family, and former colleagues and let them know about your new business.

- **Join a professional organization in your field.** By joining an organization, you can network with people who are really in a position to help. You can also build up contacts. Also look into local business groups, such as the Chamber of Commerce, in your area.

One of joys of freelancing is that you can decide what work you can and can't do. Just remember not to take on more work than you can handle in light of your CFS. You don't want to risk falling even more ill or losing clientele when you can't follow through on a job.

Filing for Disability

Many people resist filing for disability for several reasons. First, they may not want to admit that they're unable to work. People in the U.S. have a strong work ethic and admire hard work. However, you shouldn't let your work ethic cloud your judgment. Waiting to see whether you'll feel better only delays your claim.

Another reason people delay filing for disability is that they feel they'll be living off the system and don't want to be dependent. Remember that you paid into the system for precisely this reason — help for when you need it. You earned the right to be disabled; now is the time to take advantage of this right.

The Social Security Administration (SSA) has several publications that can guide you through the filing process. You can also apply for disability online at www.ssa.gov or call toll-free at 800-772-1213. Automated information is also available 24 hours a day. If you're deaf or hard of hearing, call the TTY (telephone typewriter) number at 800-325-0778.

 Know upfront a cold but true reality: CFS claims are actually rarely approved on the first try, and the resulting appeal process can go on for years. Sobering, yes, but not impossible. With more and more research out on CFS today, it's becoming more "legitimate" — which will hopefully make it easier to get benefits in the future.

In this section, I go over some of the particulars of disability benefits.

Weighing the pros and cons of disability

Deciding whether to file for disability is an intensely personal one. For some people, it means finally accepting that they have an incurable medical condition — a hard prospect to face. For others, the decision means liberation from the denial of the illness and the freedom to relax and face the illness once and for all.

Before you apply for disability, you need to consider both the positive and negative results of receiving it. First, consider the following pros:

✔ No more nine-to-five workdays . . . yeah!

✔ You can focus on getting better.

✔ Your work schedule can be more flexible.

✔ You eliminate a major chunk of work stress.

You also have to consider the possible cons of receiving disability:

✔ Salary reduction

✔ Loss of camaraderie with your colleagues and co-workers

✔ Loss of job status

✔ Possible increase in stress at home and in relationships

✔ Loss of benefits, including medical insurance coverage (for you and other family members), that may be part of your compensation package

If you make the decision to file, you should do so right away. Processing your claim can take three to four months. You also want to make sure that you have enough resources to live on until your payments begin.

Hedging your bets on whether you qualify

The Social Security Administration (SSA) has two programs under which you may qualify for disability payments: the Social Security Disability Insurance (SSDI) program and the Supplemental Security Income (SSI) program. Both programs have detailed and specific guidelines about who qualifies and for which program.

Under the SSDI guidelines, a person qualifies for disability payments if he or she "cannot work because they have a medical condition that is expected to last at least one year or result in death." You should be aware before you file that Social Security doesn't cover partial or short-term disability.

The Social Security Administration applies two earnings tests to see whether you qualify for benefits under its programs:

- ✔ A recent-work test based on your age when you became disabled
- ✔ A duration-of-work test to show that you worked long enough under the established guidelines

You may also qualify for short- and long-term disability insurance under your company's ERISA (Employee Retirement Income Security Act). Check with your plan administrator's human resources department to find out whether you qualify.

Long-term disability (LTD) is difficult for people with CFS to obtain. The diagnosis of depression and some other mental health disorders almost always has a two-year payment limit in LTD plans. If your doctor uses depression as part or all of your diagnosis when filing an LTD claim, the benefits will end after two years — and you may need assistance for many more.

Filing the essential paperwork

Whether you decide to file under ERISA (Employee Retirement Income Security Act) or with the Social Security Administration (see preceding section), be prepared to fill out a lot of forms! The information required can be quite extensive, and if you neglect to answer all the questions or leave out information, your claim may be delayed. You can expedite the process if you gather all your medical information before you start.

Considering temporary disability

Five states (Rhode Island, California, New Jersey, New York, and Hawaii) and Puerto Rico offer short-term disability insurance. This program offers partial compensation for loss of wages to workers for temporary nonoccupational disability. If you live in one of these states, you can check with your plan administrator or the human resources department to see whether you qualify and to help you through the application process.

Short-term disability coverage can begin as quickly as eight days after you've been out of work. Plans vary, but you may receive a portion of your salary for a maximum of 180 days of continuous disability.

The items you need to provide when filing include the following:

✔ Your Social Security number

✔ The names, addresses, and phone numbers of doctors, caseworkers, hospitals, and clinics involved in your care as well as the dates of your visits

✔ The names and dosages of any medication you take for your condition

✔ Additional lab reports and medical records from your doctors, therapists, and other health care professionals

✔ Work information, including the type of work you did and length of employment

✔ A copy of your most recent tax return or W-2 Form (Wage and Tax Statement); you can get copies of your most recent tax returns and W-2 forms from your accountant or HR department.

Hiring a disability attorney

Even if you provide all the information requested, your claim for disability may be denied. The process of filing and appealing can be quite intense, so trying to navigate by yourself can be exhausting. If you can afford it, get an attorney from the get-go so you don't have to go it alone and deal with the frustration and stress that comes from bureaucracy — and the fact that your CFS may not be recognized at first. Look for an attorney who specializes in disability cases.

The benefit of having an attorney handle your claim is that he or she can get copies of all the notices and requests the Social Security Administration sends you. An attorney can properly interpret the requests and take care of them efficiently and quickly.

The attorney becomes responsible for following up, thus relieving you of the stress of having to keep up with the paperwork. He or she may also be able to spot errors much more quickly than you would.

Chapter 13

CFS and Relationships: How to Stabilize the Rocking Boat

* *

In This Chapter

▶ Finding and giving the support you and your loved ones need

▶ Exploring relationship therapy and maximizing its benefits

▶ Discovering help that's right for you and your loved one

* *

Many of the best relationships come equipped with stress — and rocky relationships can make you feel like you're in a pressure cooker. Having CFS applies even more pressure to the relationship. As soon as you recognize fissures in your fragile relationships, I encourage you and your significant others to seek help.

Some patients and their loved ones discover that determination combined with the right relationship therapy often leads to deeper, more intimate relationships than they've ever experienced — even before CFS reared its ugly head. In this chapter, I offer you advice and strategies for mending scarred relationships and helping everyone involved better cope with the ravages of CFS.

Rounding Up and Arming the Troops to Battle CFS

Living with CFS brings with it inevitable challenges in your relationships with family, friends, and intimate partners. Before you became ill, you may have invested a lot of time and energy into your relationships. When you have a chronic illness like CFS, your priorities require an adjustment. The nature of the illness forces you take care of yourself first; you must dismiss accusations that you're being selfish and try to garner as much support as you can. While you don't want to appear needy, you can cope with your CFS better with a strong support system, so you have every right to assemble your team.

You can't do it all by yourself! If you have CFS, you're going to have limits. You aren't going to be capable, physically or mentally, of doing things the way you have in the past. Figuring out how and when to ask for help isn't just a convenience — it becomes a way to survive. Give the ones you love a chance to help — just as you would do if *they* were sick!

Your support system can be as narrow and as far ranging as you feel comfortable. You may feel comfortable asking for support from immediate family and friends, or you may not. But your support system isn't limited to that small group; others you may tap for support include neighbors, people from your religious affiliation, your health care team, therapists or other mental health professionals, and other people living with CFS. In this section, I help you find out whom you can trust and why.

Recognizing that ignorance is enemy number one

When it comes to CFS, ignorance is definitely not bliss. So many people with CFS have a hard time convincing others that CFS isn't just an excuse to get away with doing nothing, that you may find yourself having to educate your loved ones about the illness at every turn. Yes, it's tiring, but the more they know, the more they'll understand.

You can help your family members and loved ones gain an understanding of your condition by being patient with yourself and them. You can further encourage your loved ones' CFS education by doing the following:

- ✔ **If you have brochures from your doctor or any CFS organizations, you can distribute them among your loved ones.** Information is power — and the more your loved ones know about your illness, the more understanding they will be.

- ✔ **Encourage your close friends and family members to go on the Internet and do some research.** Send them e-mails with links to reputable Web sites such as the Centers for Disease Control and Prevention (CDC), the National Institutes of Health (NIH), and the CFIDS Association of America (see the appendix in the back of this book for theses organizations' Web sites and phone numbers).

- ✔ **If you have a spouse or a partner, ask him to meet with your doctor or health care practitioner.** Have the doctor explain CFS thoroughly. Take a list of questions that you have gone over with your loved one. Make sure your partner asks the doctor questions and feels comfortable with the answers.

> ✔ **Read books and articles on CFS together.** Read about safe exercise, healthy diets and nutrition, the right medications, and possible alternative therapies. Credible Web sites, such as www.cfids.org, can be great sources of information.

No matter how well you explain CFS, some members of your family may still have difficulty accepting your limits. Your natural impulse may be to set out to prove that your CFS is real, pointing out each symptom (perhaps with a bit of added drama). Resist the urge. Be patient, loving, and understanding, and do what you can to help them with their thoughts and feelings. You can only provide the information about CFS; choosing whether to believe you is up to them.

Friends are family, too. Take the time to educate them about your condition. Sometimes friends are hesitant to ask questions that need to be asked. Tell them to ask away — and be very direct with what CFS is and how it makes you feel. Some of your friendships may not be able to survive this major life change, which can be painful for the both of you. On the other hand, other friends can become very close — closer than before you had CFS.

Opening up to your loved ones

People with chronic illnesses like CFS experience a wide range of conflicting emotions. For various reasons, many CFS patients may tend to bottle up their emotions or express their emotions in less-than-constructive ways. These behaviors add to the feeling of isolation that a chronically ill patient already endures.

Through thick and thin

Maria's friendship with Silvia was, in a word, volatile. Best friends since third grade, they were always competitive with each other but seemed to thrive on it. The more accommodating of the two, Maria would give in when Silvia became intractable, which was most of the time.

But Silvia was also the friend you could always depend on, so when Maria was diagnosed with CFS, Maria immediately called her friend for a shoulder to lean on. Silvia didn't disappoint. After listening carefully to all Maria's symptoms and educating herself by researching CFS on the Internet, Silvia helped Maria make a list of all her friends and colleagues, what skills they had, and ways they could be of support to her. Maria was lucky. She had someone to help her through the initial rough waters of CFS. CFS can test the limits of friendship and quickly separate the true friends from the fair-weather ones.

The lines of communication absolutely must be kept open! Statistics indicate that up to 85 percent of marriages in which one partner has or develops a chronic illness eventually fails. I say this many times in this book, but I have to say it again because it's so important: Keep the lines of communication open!

Easier said than done, though, right? What can you do to keep the lines of communication open and try to beat the statistics? Here are some suggestions:

✔ **Talk about problems as they arise.** Don't hold back. Withholding can lead to resentment and anger that may explode into open conflict.

✔ **Keep your conversations positive.** While communicating your concerns honestly, try not to dump. You don't want to blame each other or make your partner feel guilty or inadequate. Use positive terms.

✔ **Get emotional support.** Tap other family members and friends for support, but bear in mind that they have their limits too and often can't separate their emotions enough to provide objective input. You may need to see a counselor to help you sort out the new family dynamics, so you should leave this option open.

✔ **Renegotiate intimacy.** CFS makes the sufferer feel tired and unable to engage in physical intimacy like before. Decide how you can achieve physical intimacy that affirms your commitment to each other, but that allows for the CFS partner's limitations.

✔ **Be flexible.** You may need to swap roles and responsibilities.

✔ **Face money problems head on.** Be realistic about finances. You may need to adjust the family's budget and cut expenses. Get the help of a financial advisor, if necessary.

✔ **Make sure you're *both* getting the care you need.** The well spouse needs help too! If you're the partner of someone with CFS, try to get away for a while to spend time with friends. Look at it as respite care for you, to replenish your spirits so you can continue to be the supportive partner you want to be. (For more on ways you can meet your own needs as a CFS caregiver, check out Chapter 14.)

✔ **Get a spiritual boost.** If spirituality is a part of your daily life, seek to restore yourself through your spiritual practice. It can make you feel stronger and more resilient.

Keeping the lines of communication open, where everyone is honest and forthcoming, is the best way to build a strong support system. See Chapter 14 about keeping the lines of communication open if you're the caregiver for someone with CFS.

Being diplomatic: How to ask for the help you need

For some of you, admitting that you need support may make you feel weak or vulnerable. But think about it: If your friend were sick and needed your help, you would gladly jump in, wouldn't you? More than likely, your friends feel the same way and are willing to help if you ask.

Think about how you want to tell them about your CFS and what you want to ask them to do. Here's a list of "don'ts" when communicating with loved ones:

- ✔ **Don't dump.** Don't hit them with the worst of the possible symptoms you may develop. You can let your friends and family know that your condition is chronic, but don't present them with a worst-case scenario.

- ✔ **Don't minimize.** While you don't want to lay it on thick, you also don't want to make light of your condition. CFS can wax and wane, so make sure your loved ones know that you will have bad times and relatively good times.

- ✔ **Don't make your CFS seem worse than it really is.** Save the drama. Your change in health status is dramatic enough.

- ✔ **Don't focus on your illness all the time.** Find other things to talk about — just like you did before you were ill. Don't let your CFS become the only focus of your discussions. Otherwise, your illness will soon consume the relationship, and the common bonds of friendship will disappear.

Other than just trying to avoid saying the wrong thing when asking your friends for help or talking about your CFS, you can follow this list of communication "do's":

- ✔ **Do tell your loved ones exactly what you need.** Be specific. You may need help with shopping for your groceries, housecleaning, or just simply having them listen to you for a while.

- ✔ **Do encourage them to ask questions.** The more questions your loved ones ask, the more they can understand your CFS and what you're going through. And be sure to answer their questions honestly.

- ✔ **Do let them know that your needs may change.** Because your CFS can flare up and subside, you may not need the same level of help all the time.

- ✔ **Do thank them.** Every time. *A lot.* Everyone likes to feel appreciated. Make sure your loved ones know that you treasure their support and that you're grateful for all the help they give you.

- ✔ **Do be considerate of their time and their feelings.** Avoid the tendency to overload your friends and family with requests for help and ask from them only what they're able to give in return — keep expectations realistic.

If you have kids . . .

Honesty is always the best possible policy — even if you have very young children. But you don't have to go into detail. Be frank, but use simple language. Make sure your kids understand that they can't catch your illness — even though CFS is not considered fatal, it's not prudent to make such an assurance with any chronic illness.! And be sure to give them hope: Tell them you and your doctor are working hard to make sure the family can do some of the fun things they've done in the past.

If your kids are in their teens, they may resent the fact that your illness takes you away from them. If you think that's happening with your kids, arrange for them to meet with your doctor or find an outside expert who can help them understand and cope. And take time to listen — you can do that even when you must lie down. Your teen needs to know you hear what she feels.

If your kids are young adults either in college or in a career, or even older, they may worry excessively about you or feel guilty that they can't make you feel better. Help them understand that your CFS isn't their fault by talking to them, listening to them, and seeking outside help, if necessary. Make sure you tell your kids how much you love them and how much you appreciate their love and concern. See Chapters 14 and 15 for information on helping children with the issues surrounding CFS.

Not everyone has a way with words — and when words are needed to express emotions, people may become literally speechless. Many people also have trouble asking for help; they don't want to inconvenience anyone and they don't want to lose your love. If this sounds like you, remember that the ones you love may know you really, really well, but they aren't psychics. They need to know what you want. Speak up, speak clearly, and say *please.* And be sure to show your appreciation with a thank you and a hug.

Empathizing with their pain

Your loved ones feel your pain — and you have to feel theirs as well. If those people closest to you seem to have trouble understanding what's going on or are unable to give you the support you need, put yourself in their shoes for a minute. CFS affects not just you, but your family and loved ones as well. Your diagnosis meant a life change for them, too. Your loved ones may be experiencing the same emotions as you're feeling, even though you have different perspectives.

Like you, your loved ones are likely to go through the same emotions as you did when you were first diagnosed: the denial, fear, anger, and guilt that comes before acceptance. Each person goes through these stages at their own pace and may even swing back and forth among them. It may feel unfair that you have to take care of your loved ones when you are so sick, but remember that illness creates a complex dynamic in relationships; hidden feelings emerge and roles change. A breadwinner may become a dependent. A child may have to discover how to be an adult. A carefree teen may have to learn that he has to make some sacrifices, too. Even though you're the one who is ill, you still have a responsibility to consider the other person's feelings and understand that they also hurt for you.

Your loved ones have to face the outside world, too — which means that those around them may be skeptical, unsympathetic, or put off. This lack of understanding puts a strain on them as well. Coupled with their worry over you, you can see why arguments can occur, and why, in their frustration, they may even lash out at you. Be sure to remember that an argument is just that — and that your loved ones still love you.

Considering Relationship Therapy

A good relationship therapist can help you and your partner navigate the ups and downs of your CFS diagnosis as well as help you reframe and incorporate the changes CFS makes in your lives.

Hidden pressures, angry triggers, boiling-over stress — these problems will come out one way or another. Better they come out with an objective, professional therapist as a referee than at home where the china closet is ten yards away.

Evaluating a relationship therapist

Finding a relationship therapist is easy — hundreds are listed in the phone book. But finding a *good* therapist can be a tricky and prolonged endeavor. In your search, you may notice many kinds of therapists are out there, practicing different types of psychotherapy. From Freud to Jung, primal screams to the social worker at your HMO, you have many therapeutic disciplines to choose from.

Often people unconsciously seek out the therapist that will tell them just what they want to hear. People are incredibly, and often unconsciously, self-protective. After all, who wants to expose herself and risk the chance of getting hurt? But seeking a therapist already indicates that something is wrong in your relationship that you need to expose and explore. Yes, you may be afraid of what you may find — but not finding it is worse. You need to find a relationship therapist that you're comfortable with, but who will also tell both of you the truth.

So do you choose to see a psychiatrist who can prescribe medication or one that can't? What about a psychologist or a psychoanalyst, a social worker or a nurse practitioner, a counselor or a new-age type of therapist? And then you have to consider the difference between someone who is licensed as opposed to someone who is certified or registered. What does it all mean??

Choosing the right therapist all boils down to one question: Is he right for *you?* Remember, you both may need to see a therapist, but you're still a team. After you are in the therapist's office, here are some questions to help you both decide if he's right for you:

- **How much experience do you have with the problems that CFS or other chronic illnesses present in a relationship?** Even if the therapist doesn't have exact experience with CFS, it would be helpful if he understands how a chronic illness can alter the dynamics in a relationship.

- **How do you help your patients? Do you have a particular therapeutic approach?** The therapist can't claim a 100 percent improvement (if he does, it's time to leave!), but understanding his therapeutic approach can help you decide if you feel this approach can work for your relationship.

- **What is your fee?** If you have insurance, it most likely covers only a number of sessions per year, and most plans have a lifetime cap. You need to know the therapist's fee outside of your insurance to see whether you can continue after your insurance coverage ends or if you don't have insurance at all.

- **How often do we need to see you?** If the number of times seems excessive to you, ask why. Once per week or every other week is about average.

In addition to your prepared questions, take note of the nonverbal communication going on. How well does the therapist listen to you? To your partner? Did he interrupt you when one of you spoke? Did he take a phone call or look at his e-mail during your appointment? Is the office pleasant and neat, or is there clutter everywhere? Is the consultation room private?

After that first meeting, both of you need to decide *together* whether the therapist feels right. Talk openly and honestly over coffee after that initial visit with the therapist or on the ride home. For relationship therapy to work, you both have to feel comfortable.

If you feel that the therapist meets your criteria for professional competence and you both get a good feeling, you're ready to set up your initial therapeutic appointment. (For more on taking steps to set up the appointment, see Chapter 8.)

You are interviewing the therapist. You don't have to convince him to see you. Even though you may feel vulnerable, you're in control. You get to decide whether you want to continue with this therapist or not.

Teaming up with your therapist for optimum outcomes

If you've sought out a relationship therapist, you and your loved one have most likely realized that you can't wade through the CFS mess on your own. One you've made a decision on a therapist, you need to know what to expect — and this section helps you decide just that.

Knowing what to expect

Going into a relationship therapy session for the first time and not knowing what's going to happen can be an intimidating experience. Your best bet to eliminate some of the initial reluctance you may feel is to get an idea of what's in store for you at your therapy sessions. If you can ease some of the first-session jitters, you and your therapist can optimize the time you have together, without having to spend added time making you or your loved one feel more comfortable.

So what happens at your first appointment? Generally, therapists see each partner separately first before seeing them as a couple, so your first sessions may be just you and the therapist. (Even though you're seeing a relationship therapist, not all your sessions will be together.) In that first session, you most likely do all the talking, because you need to explain what the problem is. Your therapist should be actively listening, taking notes, and asking you questions for clarification. He may also ask you about what you want to accomplish in therapy.

You and your therapist can then work out a therapeutic structure that includes a schedule of appointments for you and your partner, whether you and your partner will have separate visits, any additional fees outside of insurance, and other pertinent details.

Preparing for therapy sessions

You don't have to come in to the relationship therapist's office with your full biography from birth to the present prepared, but you do need to come prepared to talk. You may feel the problem you're having in your relationship is huge and all-encompassing, but if you focus on a specific aspect of the problem, such as your inability to do anything around your home, you can begin to chip away at the mountain.

Before you and your loved one go to your sessions, you need to decide the following:

- ✔ Which aspect of the problem do you want to address in this session?
- ✔ What steps have you taken to solve this problem on your own, and what was the outcome?
- ✔ What do you want this session to accomplish?

You may find it helpful to jot down some notes as you both discuss these questions, so you can bear these questions in mind as you go through the therapy session. The more actively you're involved, the more successful your treatment will be.

Shifting into problem-solving mode

When CFS presents you with its myriad problems, you may feel like you will never be able to successfully deal with them all, so you shut down or give up. But this all-or-nothing mindset is not only false, it is also counterproductive. You've probably heard the saying, "If you're not part of the solution, you're part of the problem." The same is true when it comes to you and your loved one dealing with the changes CFS brings. You both need to be committed to solving the problems CFS created in your life and your relationship. That's where a therapist can be helpful. He can help you focus on your problems and provide insight. He can offer some suggestions and exercises for you to work on.

Trying to find a solution to your problems may take a mighty effort on your part, but the sooner you and your partner decide to find ways of dealing with CFS and your altered circumstances, the better you can feel about yourself and your situation.

When you find yourself lacking the resolve to be a problem solver, remember that ignoring problems doesn't make them go away. Sometimes you need to talk about the elephant in the room, no matter how difficult or awkward it may seem at first.

Chapter 14

When Someone You Love Has Chronic Fatigue Syndrome

. . . .

In This Chapter

▶ Caring for someone with CFS

▶ Keeping the lines of communication open

▶ Remembering to take care of yourself, too!

. . . .

*G*iving support to someone you love that has CFS can be very difficult, especially if that loved one is your mate. You may not know what to say or what to do. You may lose the support you've come to rely on for your own mental and emotional health.

Concerns about what others think of you and your family can add additional stress. And you may have to take on more responsibility in earning enough money to survive, in managing and maintaining your house, and raising the kids. Frustration and stress can often turn normal, insignificant issues into huge disagreements.

In this chapter, I provide strategies and tips to help you cope with and assist your loved one in more effectively dealing with this often debilitating condition. I tell you how you can maintain helpful and loving communication with your friends and loved ones while treating CFS. I also discuss some ways in which you can deal with the emotional pain that comes from having to help someone with CFS.

Living with a Spouse or Partner with CFS

Living with someone with a chronic, sometimes debilitating, illness can be difficult, and you need to adjust the way you do things and the way you feel. Not only do living arrangements, division of household duties, and child-care responsibilities need to be renegotiated, career and financial goals may also have to be adjusted, postponed, or even abandoned altogether. Coming to this realization can take time and may cause underlying resentments to surface.

Your role as supporter may be markedly different depending on whether you're a man or a woman. In society, men are taught to be tough when faced with pain or discomfort. As a result, some men may display this attitude toward their loved ones who have CFS, expecting them to suck it up and not complain. They may resent becoming both the breadwinner and the caretaker. Women, on the other hand, are usually expected to be nurturing and understanding, and, if the husband is sick, he may expect his wife to take care of him, and she may begin to resent this expectation.

To help you and your loved one avoid feelings of bitterness and, in turn, to cultivate your relationship, keep reading.

Recognizing emotional responses to common CFS issues

CFS can be fraught with emotion for the caregiver. Not only is the person you love no longer herself, but also, she may not be able to even care for herself. She can't shoulder her usual responsibility. But if recognized up front, emotion doesn't have to destroy your relationship.

Following are some emotional hot buttons where CFS often has an impact. If you and your partner keep an eye out for these issues and are prepared to handle them as they arise, you have a better chance of preventing them from exploding into greater problems than they need to be:

- ✔ **Money:** If your family has had two incomes and one spouse is suddenly unable to work because of CFS, this unexpected change will impact your budget. You may need to reassess your financial goals and cut back on luxuries such as entertaining or eating out. Expenses that may not have been relevant or a problem in the past, such as household help or child care, may now be a necessary part of the family budget.

    Money woes are notorious for causing problems in many marriages. With the added stress of CFS, financial concerns can wreak havoc with your relationship. It may be helpful to consult with a financial planner to find ways to readjust the budget to make room for covering new expenses that may be incurred as a result of adjusting to the realities of the illness.

- **Anger:** Feelings of frustration, anger, and resentment at the roles you may no longer be able to fulfill or the new ones you may have to play are common in relationships when one partner becomes ill. This problem is compounded by the fact that your loved one with CFS is well aware of the changes that have to take place within the family. He may feel guilty about not being able to pull his own weight.

- **Guilt:** If someone you love has CFS, you may very well feel angry that that person isn't "trying hard enough" — even though you know it's not her fault. The anger you feel can make guilt descend like a ton of bricks.

- **Resentment:** Go ahead and face it — CFS changes things. Your loved one with CFS may feel as if she is holding you back from moving forward in your life. If you're a caregiver, putting your needs on hold to help your partner through her illness may be something that you want to do because you love her, you may still feel a deep sense of loss or even bitterness. Even if you don't feel resentful, your sick partner may feel you are — no matter how many reassurances you give.

All these emotions are very real — and they need to be addressed. The best way to deal with CFS within the family is to bring these feelings out into the open; encourage your partner and other family members to honestly express their true feelings — the good, the bad, and the ugly. In doing so, you and your family can find new ways to communicate, to reassign family responsibilities, and to relate to each other in ways that are both healthy and supportive.

If you are the loved one of a person who has CFS, remember that your sick partner needs a lot of reassurance. You need to make it perfectly clear that the changes the family must make is not her fault, that, despite all the new stress, she isn't to blame. Reassurance alone isn't enough. You need to let your loved one express her feelings, so that your relationship isn't damaged.

Love in the sick lane

It probably goes without saying that if your partner has CFS, your sex life is also affected. If she is so tired that she can't get out of bed, it follows that she just won't be in the mood at times — and neither will you. Talk to your partner. Confiding in her can go a long way in alleviating your fears and can actually deepen intimacy and your commitment to each other.

If you or your loved one with CFS is having sexual difficulties, talk to your doctor to rule out physical problems, and then talk to your counselor. Your relationship requires love and patience to live through the CFS sexual minefield, but it can be done. Be proactive, communicate with one another, seek help, and take action.

Sharing parental duties

CFS can impact more than your relationship with your spouse or partner. Whether your loved one is a man or a woman with CFS, your partner can feel guilty about not being able to handle all the household responsibilities he or she used to shoulder with ease before becoming ill. And if you have children, things can get more complicated fast.

As with everything else, the important thing is to keep the lines of communication open! (I give you tips on how you can do that later in this chapter.)

Perfecting your problem-solving skills

You may not be aware of it, but one of the most important tasks in a partnership or family is to solve problems. Problem solving encompasses the ability to plan, think critically and creatively, be resourceful in seeking out unique solutions, be flexible (allowing for change and trying out alternate solutions), and seek help from others when necessary.

To be an effective problem solver, you need to be able to assess the issues or situation, and devise strategies for overcoming them in a way that benefits everyone.

You want to avoid stressing out your partner who has CFS, but involving her ensures that she feels loved, accepted, and a decision-maker in your home. Trying to solve problems when the entire family is involved isn't easy. Add CFS to the brew, and it gets even more complicated. But be patient. Finding a solution may take several attempts before something works well for everyone, but keep trying.

Consider some of the following problem-solving suggestions:

- ✔ **Make sure everyone in the family gets to put in his two cents.** Think feedback, feedback, feedback. Don't allow one member to monopolize the meeting. Let each person have a turn by using a talking stick (he who has the stick can talk), or going around the table.

- ✔ **Don't make the family meetings formal — these gatherings should be relaxed and the atmosphere should be loving.** Maybe you choose to meet while eating dessert on Friday night or on a Sunday morning. You can still get everything done without "the tux and gown."

✔ **Have every family member write down one to three things they want to discuss at the meeting and make sure each issue is addressed.** As the primary caregiver, read over the lists before the meeting starts to make sure there's nothing on it to add additional stress. If you see something that may cause tension during a family meeting, try to address it ahead of time with that individual.

✔ **Don't forget to ask for help from a health care professional if you need it.** A professional counselor or therapist has insights into the best way to help solve problems. She is also objective, which means that her emotions don't get in the way.

You can always find a solution to a problem, but it just may take a while. Don't lose heart.

Parenting a Kid Who Has CFS

In a previous section, I talk about handling parental duties if your partner has CFS. But what if your child is the one who has CFS? Being a parent comes with its own set of worries. Being a parent of a child with a chronic illness can feel like a never-ending heartache.

As a parent, you'd prefer to suffer yourself rather than to see your child in pain, or not being "normal" like other children. You may feel that you're somehow responsible — regardless of what the doctors tell you and what you know is true. You may feel helpless that your child has a problem you can't solve.

Maybe it took a while before your child was correctly diagnosed. Statistics show that, as with adults, the symptoms of CFS in children can be vague, and it may have taken many visits to several different doctors before CFS was diagnosed. Also, many children are unable to accurately describe how they are feeling, so it may have taken some time before you knew exactly what was wrong. You may even have suspected that your child's complaints that he was tired were just another tactic to get out of going to school or doing his homework. So now you feel guilty as well as responsible! Don't be so hard on yourself. You can help your child master this illness.

The fact is that intellect and the hard realities have a way of falling by the wayside when it comes to your children. You want to take away their pain and make their lives happy and carefree once again. But, while you may not be able to make CFS go away, you can do a lot to not only make your child feel better, but also give her the tools she needs to understand and manage her illness.

Even though children want to feel special and loved by their parents, they don't want to be different than the other kids, and, you must face it, CFS will make your child feel different. Here are some tips to help your sick kid navigate through life with CFS (for more in-depth information, turn to Chapter 15):

- ✔ **Validate his feelings and ease his fears.** Children internalize just about everything, and your child may feel he did something to cause his CFS. He may feel that the extra cookie he sneaked while you weren't looking or the soda he slipped past you at Johnny's birthday party is the cause.

  Let your child know that this illness isn't his fault. He may even feel that he is being punished by God for all the bad things he's done. You need to let your child talk (without interrupting), and then reassure him (constantly if need be) that getting CFS isn't his fault.

- ✔ **Educate your child about her illness.** Tell your child in terms she can understand what the symptoms are and why she needs to pay attention to them. Explain any hospital procedures she may need to undergo, and prepare her for doctor and hospital visits. Teach her how to ask questions — and encourage her to do so. Your child needs to know that she has a right to ask questions and get answers.

- ✔ **Supervise your child's treatment.** If your child has to follow a specific regimen of rest and healthy eating or if he needs to take prescribed medication, explain the "whys" to him: why he needs to eat differently, why he needs to take medicines, why he needs to rest more frequently.

  Children are remarkably adaptive and will gladly participate in learning about medicines and routines if they're made to feel responsible and grown up. After your child begins to feel better due to following the regimen for a period of time, he will be more likely to comply with the routines in the future.

- ✔ **Help your child explain what CFS is to her friends.** Being able to talk to her friends about her condition is important for your child's development and stability. Help her find the words to assure her friends that CFS isn't contagious and why it prevents her from doing all the normal, everyday things that children and teens do.

  Talking to her friends' parents yourself doesn't hurt either! And, if your child is able to attend school, make sure she knows that it is okay to tell her teacher when she's tired or needs to sit out from an activity. Encourage her friends to come over after school to do homework together or watch TV. Peer relationships are important to maintain for healthy social development.

- ✔ **Recognize malingering.** Once in a while, your kid may want to take advantage. Most people have tried to fake a sore throat or a fever to get out of going to school! Try to remember that just because your child has CFS, it doesn't mean that he is still not a kid. The truth is that he does have a "built-in excuse," and you may be willing at times to let him get away with it, but you may have other times when you want to put your foot down.

Sorting out what is real and what isn't may be difficult, but trust your judgment and keep the lines of communication open. Let your child know that he can talk to you and tell you everything he's feeling, no matter what, even if it means he wants to skip school for the day — and not because he's sick.

✔ **Watch your own emotions.** Resist the tendency to be overprotective or too harsh. Wanting to protect your child from pain is natural and understandable. And the truth is that you do need to be alert and pay attention to your child in a way that you wouldn't feel compelled to do if she didn't have CFS.

But watch that the protecting doesn't become smothering. If your child feels good and wants to go on a field trip, think about saying yes — as long as her teachers and any chaperones know about her condition.

Conversely, you may feel that your child isn't that sick and that your spouse is babying her. Remember to communicate with your spouse. Discover all you can about your child's illness, and involve the entire family in developing strategies to manage it well (see the section "Perfecting your problem-solving skills" earlier in this chapter for more info).

Helping Out a Friend with CFS

If your friend has CFS, you want to be understanding. Offering to help out is the sign of a good friend. However, maybe you want to help, but you're beginning to feel overwhelmed. What do you do if you feel your friend is making too many demands on you? After all, you have your own problems. How do you balance your needs to have your own life while being supportive to your friend?

Finding a balance

If you have other kids in the family, you need to balance giving your sick child the attention she needs without making the well children feel they're being neglected. Sibling rivalry is a problem in most families as children vie for the what they perceive to be the limited time, love, and attention of their parents.

Having the dynamics of a sick child who *does* need more attention and does, at times, need to be favored can compound the problem. Denying to your other children that Susie gets extra attention sometimes doesn't make sense. You need to let all your children know that they're loved — and that just because more of your attention needs to focus on their sick sibling, it doesn't mean that they aren't important members of the family.

You may be wrestling with these questions if you have a friend who has CFS. You want to be supportive, but sometimes *you* feel drained. It can be very difficult being a loving friend to someone who has a chronic illness. Unlike other conditions that are finite, CFS doesn't have a definable end, and you don't know whether you have the stamina to stay with your friend for the long haul.

Friendships normally wax and wane; sometimes you're closer, sometimes you drift apart. How do you maintain a healthy friendship in the wake of one person being constantly ill? How do you know that if you need some space it's a normal part of your relationship and not because your friend has CFS?

To be a good friend without being taken advantage of, try to remember the following suggestions:

✔ **Make sure your friend knows you're there to support her, but *not* to your own detriment; state clearly what you're willing to do.** Know when to help and when to hold back. You may be willing to do your friend's grocery shopping or drive her to medical appointments. Or you may just be able to listen when she needs an ear. A good friend understands and will appreciate your honesty up front. Giving your friend clear guidelines can stop her from second-guessing you.

✔ **Realize that CFS isn't the cause of everything.** Your friend may be needy or selfish *and* have CFS. Having CFS doesn't mean that your friend won't have any of the attributes or personality traits that you found annoying before she got sick. In other words, see your friend as normal. She just occasionally needs special consideration for her very real illness, so don't let her guilt you into doing something.

✔ **If your friend begins to ask too much, step back with love.** In other words, you can explain, clearly and kindly, that you have some chores and social engagements you want to keep. Tell her you want to help, but you also need time for yourself. This may be difficult for the person with CFS to hear at first, but make sure you emphasize that in order for you to help your friend, you have to take care of yourself first. Hopefully, the person with CFS has read her part of this book and will understand how to monitor her expectations.

One issue you may struggle with as a friend is whether tough love is ever okay. We've all seen those television shows and movies in which the strong friend walks into the hospital room and scolds the sick friend for being sick. "If you want to lie there and just give up . . ." the speech usually begins. Invariably, the sick friend realizes the truth of the strong friend's word, and, with a mighty effort, pulls himself from the brink of death to live healthily ever after. CFS isn't a question of will — it's an illness. Your friend can't help feeling fatigued and sick. So, listen and offer suggestions, if asked.

Communicating: A Good Way to Help Everyone

Open, honest, and supportive communication is your greatest tool in helping someone with CFS — and helping yourself. The key to supporting someone who is sick is to be honest and forthright with each other. Be honest about your needs and limitations. And be sure to ask your sick loved one exactly what would help him. You want to be supportive without being smothering or insensitive. If the two of you work together, you can weather any CFS storm!

As much as you want to help, you're not a therapist, unless you have a degree that says so. Know where to draw the line and suggest that your loved one get professional help. But don't play "armchair therapist." Your loved one can be in real emotional danger and need help sooner than later. If that weren't enough, you must also consider the fact that playing therapist is quite a responsibility — and you probably don't have the time or space you need to truly be supportive when necessary.

In this section, I go over some of the ways you can make communication an art form of kind, true, and loving help.

Remaining readily accessible

Communication works best when you make sure you're accessible to the person who needs you. When you are the well person in the relationship, you may feel that you are always on call, and in a sense, you are, but your loved one needs to know that she can call on you when she needs help.

Being accessible doesn't mean just physically being there or just listening and talking. Being accessible also has to do with the *way* you listen and speak. Here are some starting points to help you be accessible for your loved one with CFS:

✔ **Offer empathy, not sympathy:** This guideline can be tricky. You're sympathetic to your loved one's condition, but you don't want him to think that you're feeling sorry for him. The trick is to be understanding, but remain objective. Acknowledge what your loved one says, even by restating his concerns, but don't tell him how bad you feel for him.

✔ **Don't preach and don't compare:** Resist the urge to tell your loved one about all the other people who are worse off than she is. Your loved one probably has enough guilt about CFS without having you suggest that she ought to be grateful or that she is lucky because it "could be worse." Listen, remain open, and try not to judge.

Whether or not you can always be accessible is another story. If you can't be as accessible as you'd like, clearly and compassionately explain why and try to find a solution.

Remembering to listen

Listening is an art. Truly listening means that you can tune in to the other person and hear what they actually say with words as well as with their bodies.

The better you can listen, the better you can support your friend or family member with CFS. Here are some simple ways to hone your listening talents:

- **Concentrate:** Hard to do, but essential. Very often when you listen, your mind drifts to things that you need to do later, what you're going to say next, what's on TV tonight, or any number of things. One way to counteract a wandering mind is to focus on your loved one's face when you find yourself drifting.

- **Pay attention:** Maintain eye contact (but by all means, still blink). Not only does this show empathy, but you can also pick up nonverbal cues. As you watch the eyes and face of your loved one while he speaks, see whether his words match his expression.

  If your friend looks like she's going to cry even though she says everything is fine, tell her that you understand and that everything isn't fine — but you can work around it.

- **Check out the body language.** Leaning forward, touching, or nodding appropriately shows your involvement and concern. Notice if you're beginning to pull back or fold your arms across your chest. These movements, although often unconscious, are easily picked up by the other person as negative, a pushing away of what she is saying, and may lead your loved one to clam up.

Validating your loved one's medical condition

Admit it. You sometimes feel that your partner or friend isn't as sick or fatigued as he purports to be. He doesn't *look* sick, and perhaps, just perhaps, if he tried a little harder, he could probably get those dishes washed, do a load of laundry, or maybe, just maybe, get a job.

ANECDOTE

Asking the right questions

Janice's husband, Sam, really tried to understand what she was going through. He researched CFS on the Web; he asked his doctor, his friends, and his colleagues if they knew about the condition. He even went to a therapist to figure out how to be more supportive.

But weeks turned into months. Sam's patience was starting to wear thin. Instead of listening and paying attention to his wife, he interrupted her or tuned her out. Instead of doing all the household chores, he let the apartment go. Clothes, socks, and dirty dishes littered every surface. Sam didn't care. He wasn't there much these days anyway.

Unfortunately, Janice tried to do the housekeeping herself. She tried to sweep and mop and dust. But after 15 minutes, she had to crawl to the sofa. She cried . . . and cried. But she refused to talk to Sam. She didn't want to tell him how she felt or ask him why he was doing what he was doing. She just retreated more and more inside her illness. Her symptoms only got worse.

Her friends couldn't stand seeing her like this. They all chipped in and hired a cleaning service to get the house in order. Each of her friends also had specific tasks to do to help her. Tina did grocery shopping. Lyle did the wash. Roberta took care of the bills.

Sam started to get jealous. He began to come home straight from work. He started to take back his life. He apologized to Janice and thanked her friends. He realized he'd burned out and needed some time off. He just didn't know how to ask for help.

Don't be a Sam. If you're a caregiver, don't be afraid to ask for help. And don't be afraid to ask for a time out either! No one is perfect. No one is a robot. And no one should feel burdened. If you ask your loved one what she wants, you'll spend a lot less time trying to please her while the resentment grows. You can be much more efficient. The only way to get the right answer is to ask the right questions: "How can I help?" or "What can I do to support you?"

People with CFS often have a hard time convincing the outside world that CFS is a real illness and not an excuse to lay on the couch or in bed all day watching daytime television and eating bonbons. (By the way, if you have CFS, you probably should lay off the bonbons. Too unhealthy!)

The fact is that your partner isn't a malingerer. He isn't pretending: CFS can be debilitating. You can show your support for your partner by acknowledging that CFS has real symptoms and letting him know that you understand that he may not have the energy to do the things he once did.

If you are a woman, you may be disappointed that your partner can no longer be the strong shoulder you used to lean on, that he's not the man he once was. Push these thoughts away. Not only are they unproductive, these thoughts don't mean anything. Your loved one is sick. He has an illness and didn't come with a lifetime guarantee. Turn to family, friends, or a professional therapist to get needed support.

If you' re a man, resist the temptation to fix things by telling your partner what she ought to do. (This advice isn't just about men. If you are a woman, pay attention!) Most of the time, your partner just wants you to listen. The last thing she needs is a pull-yourself-up-by-your-bootstraps lecture or a solution that either has nothing to do with her medical condition or denies it completely. Compassion and listening are key (see "Remembering to listen" for tips on listening strategies).

Wording statements in a less confrontational format

Disagreements are bound to happen in any relationship, and your relationship with your loved one with CFS is no different. As you've probably discovered, having CFS doesn't preclude you from having the normal, everyday problems of life. In fact, they're often compounded. When people feel angry or hurt, they also tend to feel vulnerable, and can react by striking out at the other party, seeking to deflect blame or responsibility from themselves.

Aside from the normal disagreements, you may have times in your relationship when you simply feel overwhelmed. You may need to confront the CFS-affected person. If this happens to be your partner, the rules for fighting fair are even more important.

When it comes to disagreements, try to avoid the following seven deadly statements, guaranteed to escalate tensions and further alienate both of you:

- ✔ You always . . .
- ✔ You never . . .
- ✔ Why can't you be/do . . .
- ✔ It's always about you . . .
- ✔ You make me feel . . . (usually something negative)
- ✔ When do *I* get to . . .
- ✔ What about *me, my* feelings, *my* (fill in the blank)

Instead of them fightin' words, try to remember the rules for successful conflict resolution:

- ✔ **Stay calm.** Hard to do when tensions are mounting, but essential. Keeping calm allows you to evaluate the situation more realistically and reduce any tendency to overreact.
- ✔ **Be respectful.** Avoid name calling, sarcasm, or criticizing your partner.

✔ **Be specific.** Deal with only one issue at a time. This rule can help you to avoid the "kitchen sink" approach to conflict — throwing everything in. Being specific also reduces your tendency to generalize, which usually doesn't arrive at specific solutions to problems you may be having.

✔ **State your feelings, but don't accuse.** Instead of finger-pointing statements such as "you always" or "you never," state your feelings in the matter, such as "I sometimes feel overwhelmed when you get sick and I have to do everything."

✔ **Stay in the present.** Don't bring up every bone of contention that has existed over the past 20 years.

Recognizing Your Own Emotions and Needs

Forgetting yourself when you're caring for someone with CFS is easy. The other person's needs can be so great that taking care of them — plus your household and your work — becomes a full-time job. You have little time to think about caring for yourself. You may even feel guilty for taking time out to enjoy a drink or a movie, or spending time away from your partner when he needs so much.

Being a caregiver *is* stressful. If you're newly thrust into this role, your plans and expectations for the family will undoubtedly change, and with that change may come a whole range of emotions that you didn't think you would have: fear, anxiety, anger, frustration, guilt, resentment, sadness, and even grief.

The golden rule: Don't forget to take care of yourself! If you're caring for a partner or child with CFS, life can become a seemingly endless cycle of flare-ups, doctor visits, and constant giving, giving, giving. Don't be a martyr. You can begin to feel resentful, and your loved one will pick up on it. Make time for yourself. Give yourself a mini-vacation away from the family to restore your spirits. Create a supportive network of people who are positive and who help to uplift your spirits — as well as offer a helping hand when you need some time off.

Taking time for yourself doesn't have to be big or take a long time. Maybe a hot bath filled with lavender can do the trick. Maybe a short trip to the mall with $20 to spend on *you.* Maybe you can catch the early movie at your local theater. A little "you" time can even be a 20-minute power nap. All these suggestions can replenish your giving tank and prevent you from burning out.

In this section, I go over some insights on how to take care of yourself — so you can take care of your loved one.

Keeping tabs on your emotions

One of the first emotions you may feel when faced with a CFS diagnosis in the family is denial. Even though it may seem negative, denial can be viewed as a necessary first step in the process of eventual acceptance and coping.

Fear and anxiety often follow as the reality of the illness and the impact on the family sets in. You can become anxious about how the illness will change the family, about your ability to cope over the long term, and about your loved one's health.

Frustration usually follows close behind — frustration at your loved one's inability to share the load of family responsibilities, the fact that he has CFS, the inability to find a cure for CFS, and the inability of your doctors to have definite answers.

Then comes the anger: anger at your loved one, anger at the doctors, anger at everyone whose life is progressing normally, anger that your life has changed, anger at your loved one's being sick, and even anger at your anger! Don't feel bad; feeling angry is perfectly normal — and even healthy — as long as you acknowledge your anger. Recognizing you're angry is the only way you can ultimately accept the fact that your life has changed, that things aren't as they were. And, if you don't allow yourself to feel that anger, guilt will build up to such a point that it can immobilize you and have potential health consequences for *you*.

Denial. Fear and anxiety. Anger and frustration. Guilt and more guilt. These emotions can get so overwhelming that they can lead to depression — making a difficult situation even worse. After all, how can you take care of someone who has CFS when you can't get out of bed yourself! So be sure to stop, breathe, and give yourself a break. Recognize that all the negative emotions you're experiencing are normal and that you can take steps to deal with them effectively.

If you do feel yourself beginning to be overwhelmed or show signs of depression (such as a weight gain or loss, listlessness, anxiety, inability to concentrate, and feelings of hopelessness and helplessness), see a health care professional as soon as possible (see the section "Pursuing therapy for yourself" for more info).

Your emotions don't have to be all bad. You can have positive ones as well! You may get a feeling of deep satisfaction from caring for a loved one who needs you. Your partner may respond with deep appreciation for the love and commitment you show in the face of this illness. You can feel love and give love. You can gain confidence because of all the things you're now doing. The glass *can* be half full.

Taking care of yourself

Keep saying this over and over again: You can't help your loved one if you don't help yourself. Make it your mantra. Why? Because it's true! If you're burned out, how can you be expected to compassionately and efficiently help someone else? Recognizing that you're an important part of the equation is essential. You need to be sure to do what makes you happy and fulfilled — indulge yourself a little.

In this section, you can find some tips to push that mantra along.

Establishing a healthy routine and diet

Staying healthy and active is important because it can keep you strong. Take care of any underlying health problems; don't put them off until your loved one is better!

Be sure to exercise — working out doesn't have to be in a gym. Walking provides safe, low-impact exercise as well as ample time to think. Even just 10 or 15 minutes of exercise a day (no matter what the format) can help relieve stress.

Also, be sure to eat right. If you consume more protein, fruits, vegetables, and complex carbohydrates, your blood sugar can remain at an even keel. What does this mean for you? More energy, more ability to cope with stress, and a sense of well-being.

You also need to find ways of managing stress. Deep breaths, relaxation exercises, yoga, prayer, a ten-minute nap — all these techniques can help keep the fears and anger at bay. (For more on some ways to work your body and ease your mind, check out *Mind-Body Fitness For Dummies* by Therese Iknoian [Wiley].)

Recharging your batteries

If you don't put gas in your car, it will eventually stop. Similarly, if you don't replenish yourself, you'll soon be driving on empty — and instead of one problem, you'll have two: your loved one's CFS and your burned-out self.

How to recharge those batteries? Find time for your interests. Take some time to do a hobby you enjoy, such as photography, collecting sports memorabilia, or gardening. Take in an early-bird movie. Visit a museum. Go to lunch with a good friend. Walk around the mall. Anything that distracts you from thinking about CFS will work.

Recruiting some help

You may be finding out quickly (or have known for a while) that you just can't do it all on your own — balancing a job, the household chores, the kids, and caring for your loved one who has CFS. Don't feel like you should muster up some superpowers to handle the situation; instead, consider finding some friends or a professional service to help with cleaning the house, buying groceries, or watching the kids from time to time, so you can have a break.

Trade a service you can offer to someone who can offer you something in return, such as coming in to do the laundry or to clean the house. You may also want to check out online grocery shopping (and delivery!) Web sites, like www.peapod.com, or hire a cleaning service. While these options cost money, they may be worth the moolah.

Harnessing the power of positive thinking

Research shows that a positive attitude can help in healing. It strengthens your immune system and helps you stay calm. Optimism is always better than a defeatist attitude! Not only can this positive thinking make the job of caretaker easier, but it can also help with your sick spouse, child, or friend. If your loved one feels hopeful, he just might feel a little better.

Pursuing therapy for yourself

There's no shame in going to therapy. And no excuse is acceptable when you need it. Maybe your spouse is going to a therapist to deal with her CFS-induced depression — and you figure you can't afford two therapists every week. Or maybe you feel there's nothing wrong with you and you don't need a therapist. But, believe me, going to the right therapist can help you better cope with stress, anxiety, fear, and anger.

Talking it out with a trained professional can help you become a better caregiver and help keep your relationship solid. Someone trained to help you cope with a life-altering illness can help you see things from a different vantage point. She can be much more objective. And the best reason? You can cry, stamp your feet, and let it all out in a therapist's office — instead of taking it out on your loved one, the rest of the family, or a good friend. Check with your doctor or a local hospital to find someone who specializes in therapy for caregivers.

You don't have to force yourself to go to a therapist you don't like. It won't work, and continuing to go is a waste of time for both of you. Remember that for the therapeutic process to work, you need rapport. If the first therapist doesn't do it for you, be sure to get a second (or third) name, just in case.

Joining a support group

You don't have to go it alone. Help is out there. Why a support group? You can find nothing like a group of people going through the same thing as you are to offer compassion, understanding, insight, and practical advice. Quite simply, they know what you're going through, and you can help each other cope.

Along with your local hospital (a good source for finding support), you can check out the following resources for finding a support group in your area:

- ✔ National Family Caregivers Association, 10400 Connecticut Avenue, Suite 500, Kensington, MD 20895-3944; phone 800-896-3650 or 301-942-6430, fax 301-942-2302; Web site www.thefamilycaregiver.org

- ✔ National Alliance for Caregiving, 4720 Montgomery Lane, 5th Floor, Bethesda, MD 20814; e-mail info@caregiving.org, Web site www. caregiving.org

Chapter 15

Leading a Child Through the CFS Minefield

. . . .

. . . .

*W*henever children are involved in chronic fatigue syndrome, whether they have CFS or are living with someone who has CFS, parents and caregivers must demonstrate a sensitivity to the child's concerns and needs. They have to provide their children with the coping skills they need to deal with CFS in their lives.

Of course, everyone would rather not have to deal with CFS! But the situation does introduce the child to adult problems. It also provides an opportunity for her to develop problem-solving skills to carry with her throughout her life. In this chapter, I offer medical advice on how to properly care for a child who has CFS and guidance in how to support a child who's living with a loved one who has CFS.

Securing an Accurate Diagnosis for Your Child

When your child exhibits troubling symptoms, it's time to visit the pediatrician. A reduction in activity is the number-one symptom to look for if you suspect your child has CFS. Another common symptom is orthostatic intolerance (OI), in which the child gets very dizzy when sitting or standing up from a seated position.

Symptoms can include listlessness. Your child may not be as social as she was. Her activity level is low. She may also complain about dizziness, and her grades in school can drop. If you suspect your child has CFS, this section tells you how to get a correct diagnosis.

Talking over symptoms with your pediatrician

When your child's symptoms are vague, as they can be with CFS, you may have a hard time convincing your pediatrician that your child is sick. You're convinced something is wrong, because you know your child, but your child's doctor may not be so easily convinced — and with good reason. Doctors still don't have established criteria for diagnosing CFS in children, and some doctors feel that CFS shouldn't be diagnosed in children under 12. So how can you know what ails your child, and how can you know if the pediatrician's diagnosis is correct?

The key to securing the right diagnosis for your child is:

- ✔ **Observe your child.** According to the Centers for Disease Control and Prevention (CDC), diagnosing CFS in children is difficult because children may have difficulty in verbalizing their symptoms, and they're wonderful at getting used to symptoms and adapting themselves. So it's up to you to probe. Observe your child carefully and make a list of the symptoms she displays. Take the list with you when you visit the pediatrician, but be prepared.

- ✔ **Work with an open-minded doctor.** Be prepared not to be taken seriously the first time around at the doctor's office. You may be dismissed as an overprotective parent, or worse, one that is exaggerating or even causing your child's illnesses. If you suspect that your child has CFS, though, seeking out a doctor who is willing to take all the physical symptoms into account — along with any psychiatric symptoms — before making a diagnosis is important. See Chapter 5 for information on how to track down the best doctor.

- ✔ **Trust your gut!** You know your child best.

Although you can't find set diagnostic criteria, you can use a list of symptoms that can lead you to suspect that your child has CFS. The two major criteria of CFS in children, mentioned earlier, are gradual but persistent fatigue that lasts for six months or more, with a significant reduction in activity including things your child enjoys doing.

ANECDOTE

When you know something's wrong

Rita was the first to notice. Her normally active, rambunctious 10-year-old daughter, Kamiah, began complaining about being tired a lot. She said she felt achy, but couldn't pinpoint just where. She also said she had a headache. She said she sometimes felt dizzy and didn't want dinner, but just wanted to go to bed.

Rita checked Kamiah's temperature and found she had a slight fever. Thinking she was coming down with the flu, Rita gave her daughter some over-the-counter cold medicine and sent her to bed. But rather than bouncing back as she normally did in a few days, Kamiah stayed just about the same. After a week of not getting better, Rita took Kamiah to the pediatrician, but he couldn't match Kamiah's symptoms with a specific condition. He took some blood and ran tests, but when Rita checked back for the results, she was told everything was normal.

But Rita knew everything wasn't normal. She knew her child, and she knew that Kamiah's behavior was far from normal. When Kamiah's teacher called Rita in for a conference because Kamiah was falling asleep in class, Rita knew she had to seek a second opinion. After a third and fourth opinion, several medical tests to rule out other conditions, and a lot of research on the Internet, Rita and Kamiah's new pediatrician arrived at the diagnosis of CFS.

If Rita's story sounds familiar, then you know how difficult it can be to get the right diagnosis for your child. CFS isn't the first diagnosis a doctor may come up with when faced with the vague symptoms most children come to the examining room with.

Other potential CFS symptoms in children include the following:

- ✔ Complaints about being tired, accompanied with a reduction of activity
- ✔ Low-grade fever
- ✔ Sore throat
- ✔ Painful lymph nodes
- ✔ Weak-feeling muscles
- ✔ Muscle and joint pain
- ✔ Moping around
- ✔ Extreme fatigue after gym class or on the sports field
- ✔ Headaches
- ✔ Complaints of trouble seeing clearly
- ✔ Sleeping a lot, but still tired

- Difficulty concentrating in school
- Being in a "fog"
- Dizziness or lightheadedness
- Belly pain or stomachaches

Kids' CFS symptoms seem to change more frequently than do adults' CFS symptoms. Sometimes their complaints will vary dramatically from day to day. Watch for any changes in symptoms. This can be an important signal for CFS in children.

These symptoms mimic many other conditions, including fibromyalgia and arthritis, so even if the symptoms are specific, it may still take a while to arrive at the correct diagnosis.

Because doctors don't yet have set diagnostic criteria or diagnostic tests for CFS, a diagnosis is made by observation and eliminating other possible causes of your child's illness. So your doctor may prescribe blood, urine, or other physical tests to rule out other illnesses. He may even recommend neurological tests or psychological assessments to evaluate your child's cognitive skills and to rule out emotional issues, such as depression or anxiety.

Considering the likelihood of mononucleosis in your teen

Mononucleosis, or mono, is often suspected when your teen goes to the doctor with the list of vague symptoms (which I list in the previous section) that characterize CFS. To complicate matters further, some teens develop CFS *after* an attack of mono. So how can you tell whether your child has CFS or mono? And if your child had a bout of mono, can you help to prevent the development of CFS later on?

Mononucleosis, or the "kissing disease" (so-called because it can be spread by kissing), is an infectious disease caused by the Epstein-Barr virus (EBV). Most people (whether they've been kissed or not) have the antibodies to EBV in their systems. Why? Because they were probably exposed as children. The peak time of infection is the teen years from about age 15 to 17, or you may say the time when teenagers are kissing the most.

The difference between CFS and mono is that doctors know that the latter is an infectious disease spread primarily by saliva, the onset of symptoms is generally more rapid than CFS, and the symptoms tend to intensify as the illness progresses. Mono can also be detected via a simple blood test.

If your teen does come down with a case of mono, make sure that he gets plenty of rest, lots of fluids and good nutrition. We don't know if these can prevent the onset of CFS, but it can't hurt to try.

The researchers also looked at other possible contributing factors, such as medications taken, the social life of the subjects (how many friends they had), and if they also were depressed. But none of these factors seemed to make a difference in whether the person was more at risk for CFS. The one contributing factor to whether a person who had mono went on to develop CFS was physical fitness. Those subjects who were more physically fit following the initial mono infection were much less likely to develop CFS. Another reason to get your teen off the couch!

Ruling out drug abuse

If you have a teen — and if the public service announcements are doing their job — you're alert to the signs of drug abuse. Some of the early signs of drug abuse can mimic the symptoms of CFS, so you may have to do a bit of sleuthing. Of course, you trust your teen, but you're also realistic. You've probably discovered long ago that your teen doesn't tell you everything, and that peer pressure may have pushed your child into using drugs.

But while some symptoms such as loss of interest in school, sleeping in class, withdrawing from family activities, or tiredness can mimic CFS symptoms, other clues such as a change in behavior, suddenly hanging out with a different group of friends, and becoming more secretive than usual can clue you in that something pharmaceutical, not physical, is causing the change in your child's behavior.

Eliminating the possibility of other common childhood maladies

One of the reasons CFS is so difficult to diagnose in children is that the symptoms so often mimic common childhood ailments. You wonder if your child's sudden need for more sleep or his vague aches and pains are simply due to growing pains, or any of the following common conditions:

- Allergies
- Anemia
- Depression

✔ Migraine headaches

✔ Phobias

Other less common but possible conditions that may present symptoms similar to CFS are

✔ Anxiety disorders

✔ Rheumatoid arthritis

✔ Fibromyalgia

✔ Hypothyroidism

✔ Learning disabilities

✔ Lupus

The good news is that physical tests can rule out most physical causes, and a psychologist or therapist can assess your child's overall psychological state.

Helping Your Child Cope with CFS Symptoms in Daily Life

For children, daily life is all about routines. In fact, children prefer routines (no matter what they say!). Routines help children feel safe and keep their world predictable. As a parent, you probably have set up a bedtime routine and a daytime routine. And if your child is able to attend school, you may have even more routines set in place. When your child has CFS, you may need to tweak the routine a bit. By including your child in creating a new routine, you can give him a sense of mastery and control over his illness.

You and your child need to set up a routine that sets the right balance between school, exercise, after-school activities, and fun. Here are some suggestions:

✔ Determine how much sleep your child needs to feel rested without over-doing it. Remember that oversleeping doesn't make your child feel better.

✔ Set up a consistent wake-up time and bed time — and stick to it (even on the weekends).

✔ Have scheduled mealtimes and keep your child eating healthy! (For more on healthy eating, see Chapter 11).

✔ If your child needs to rest at school during the day, determine how long this period needs to be, and be sure to work with her teachers as well as the school nurse.

✔ If your child is involved in a group sport, speak with the coach to determine how much time your child should play to minimize a possible increase in symptoms. You just need to balance playing with adequate rest and be very aware of physical limitations.

✔ If you have family or special events, such as a movie night, don't delete these activities altogether. Just schedule down time, as necessary, to compensate for any period of activity.

For more details on how to develop a schedule in general, you can flip over to Chapter 11.

Fielding common childhood CFS complaints

You've probably heard the following complaints in at least one form or another from your CFS child:

"I'm tired."

"I ache all over."

"My head hurts."

"I don't feel like going to school!"

"Why can't I be like all the other kids?"

"Why did this have to happen to me?"

You'd probably tell him to stop whining if he were a "normal" kid, but you also want to be understanding and want your child to know that his feelings are valid. Plus you want the lines of communication to remain open, so your child feels like he can always come to you with his concerns — even if it comes out in a whine.

Complaints about aches and pains are normal — and are often the complaints of children everywhere. If you have other children in the household, most likely they've had the same complaints at one time or another. Deal with your CFS child the same way. Acknowledge that he has legitimate aches and pains. If medications have been prescribed, administer them along with liberal helpings of love.

Remember, faking or exaggerating an ailment is often a good tactic to get out of facing that Algebra test. Just because your kid has CFS doesn't mean he won't behave like kids who don't have a chronic illness. Just be wise enough to tell when the ailment is real and, when necessary, add a bit of tough love: "Yes, I know you ache, but I think that it's important that you go to school anyway."

Dealing with the more philosophical questions, such as "Why can't I be normal?" is a bit harder. This question is tough, and, more than likely, one you've grappled with yourself. Most people deal with these types of questions by turning to their religious or spiritual tradition, so you may want to rely on those roots. And you can always use compassion. Yes, your child's illness is breaking your heart, but hugging him close and telling him you love him goes really, really far. Let him know that, despite having to deal with CFS, he has the right to "life, liberty, and the pursuit of happiness" — just like everybody else.

Managing CFS effectively at and after school

When your child has a chronic illness, feeling alone in your school community may be difficult for you and your child. Other kids can be sent off to school with just a kiss and lunch money. Your CFS child has to be reminded to rest when she's tired, and may even have to take special foods for lunch. She may often feel isolated and different. Your child may also need to go to the doctor more often, or have more tests done — further setting him apart from his peers.

Contact your child's teacher, the principal, the school nurse, and her guidance counselor. Let them know about your child's diagnosis and the routines you and your doctor have created for managing the illness. He may have to be tutored at home, or home schooled, because he is too ill to attend school.

At home, stick to the daily routine you and your child devised. Help her to eat on time, finish homework on time, and get to bed on time — so that she can wake up the next day feeling refreshed.

Contacting your child's school

Ah . . . to tell or not to tell? You may hesitate to let school officials know that your child has CFS. After all, you don't want your child to be singled out or to feel more different than he already does! On the other hand, you want your child's teacher to be aware of his condition, so she can be alert to symptoms and watch out for your child. So what do you do?

In all likelihood, your child's teacher may have been the first to notice that something was wrong — your child may have seemed sleepy in class or slightly under the weather — so she may already be aware that something is wrong. The teacher's observations may have led you down the path to a CFS diagnosis to begin with. But do you want school officials to actually know what is wrong with your child?

The decision whether or not to tell is entirely yours, but you want your child to be educated and supported as he needs to be. You don't want your child to be accused of being lazy or unambitious. You also don't want your child to feel ashamed of having a medical condition. Once again, including your child in this decision-making process is helpful. Let him know you want to contact his school and his teachers — and why to give him some control over his CFS and doesn't leave him wondering what's wrong with him.

When you visit your child's school for the first time, consider some of the following suggestions:

- **Start by explaining what CFS is — don't assume they know!** If they're unaware of the nuances of CFS, offer to provide them with educational materials designed for health care professionals. Self-study courses and fact sheets are available through the CDC Web site at `www.cfids.org/treatcfs`.

- **Outline the symptoms your child is likely to display.** If any of them show up in class, make sure your teacher lets you know. You might have to keep your child at home for a while.

- **Clearly and carefully, make it clear that you aren't trying to get your child out of doing schoolwork.** After all, you want your child to succeed! If necessary, bring a letter from your doctor.

- **Depending on your child's workload, you may want to ask for extra time to complete some assignments.** You may also need to make special arrangements for taking tests, where more break times are allowed, because his CFS can affect his cognitive functioning.

- **Let the school know that while you want your child's CFS to be taken into account, you also don't want your child to be treated too differently.** Make sure the teacher knows that you still expect your child to be responsible for his actions and to participate in class. Sometimes teachers, although meaning well, may want to make the workload easier (or if they're really mean, harder) on the "sick" kid.

Don't be surprised if you meet with some resistance. Many people still don't believe that CFS is a real illness, and school officials may feel that you're making excuses or trying to get special considerations for your child. If you meet this resistance, have your doctor write a letter that you can give to the principal, teachers, and guidance counselors. You may have to educate them on CFS, so bring in the brochures and Web site links.

Pushing for an Individualized Education Plan (IEP)

Children with CFS often miss a lot of school. Your child may need to have a shorter school day, more time to complete assignments, a school day that includes a period of rest or a nap, or if severely affected, to be tutored at home. No matter what your child's needs are, she has the right to an education, and you have the right to a school or a setting that can meet your child's needs.

With the passage of the Individuals with Disabilities Education Act, parents of children with special needs gained the right to set up Individualized Education Plans (IEP) for their children. An IEP is an individualized program for your child made via a consensus between his teachers, his principal, and you.

Don't let the words *special needs* put you off. Special needs don't apply only to children who are developmentally delayed, but also to any need that puts your child outside the norm. On a positive note, an IEP can also mean that your child is ahead of her peers academically and needs advanced placement. Your child could have CFS *and* be a genius! The fact is, whatever her status, your child deserves to be educated in a way that best serves her needs.

Working with your child's teacher, principal, guidance counselor, and others, you can devise a program that can help your child succeed. However, bear in mind that you may encounter the same resistance in the school system as adults do in the work environment — where employers may not regard CFS as a real illness. You may need to present medical evidence to prove that your child is indeed ill and needs special consideration.

The school may also want to do an evaluation of its own. The evaluation team usually consists of a multi-disciplinary group of professionals chosen because of your child's particular needs. After the evaluation, set up a meeting with the team of professionals and your child's teacher to discuss a plan. Here are some things to keep in mind for these meetings:

✔ **Come prepared to all meetings.** Learn the CFS jargon (you can do research on the Internet), take notes, and ask questions. You and the team decide what goes into the IEP. If you feel your child needs additional support services, be sure to bring this concern up. If you need to consult with other professionals, bring their recommendations to the meeting as well.

> ✔ **Don't forget to speak up.** You have the right to disagree with any part of the plan that you feel will not be good for your child. If you need an advocate, you can get information about attorneys who specialize in education matters, and who can offer their services for free or at low cost.

The IEP is reviewed annually to ensure that its goals are being met and the level of services remains adequate to your child's needs. If you think that your child's needs have changed, be sure to bring this up at that time.

All public schools have specific laws and regulations regarding services they must provide for children with special needs. The rules vary from state to state, although all schools must adhere to a certain federal standard. Check with your school district or your state's Department of Education for more information.

Garnering peer support for your child

A cliché about children that adults often have ready is that "children can be cruel." While this saying can be true because *some* children can be mean to other children, especially if a child appears weak or different, children can also be extraordinarily kind and understanding. Most often, the cruelty that children exhibit is simply a defense mechanism. They fear what they don't understand, and their reaction is to make fun, be angry, or belittle in an attempt to not be affected or made fun of themselves.

One of the best ways to deflect bad behavior and to elicit support is to be upfront and forthright. Talk to your child to find out who his true friends are. Encourage him to come clean with them, letting them in on his condition and why he has special needs.

If your child is particularly confident and willing to take on the whole class, you can even arrange — with the school's permission, of course — for your child to address the entire class. This direct approach can be an excellent opportunity for her to educate her classmates about CFS and its symptoms. Addressing the class also goes far in having the other children believe that your child isn't faking it and gives them an opportunity to pitch in and help.

Dealing decisively with bullies

Bullies are the bane of childhood existence, and they can make life miserable for your CFS child. Other children who bully may feel jealous that your child gets special considerations, such as more time for class work or time out for rest, and as a result, they feel the need to act out.

If your child is being teased or bullied, give him a range of strategies he can use to counter the attacks. Talk to your child. Let him tell you how he is being bullied. Different tactics may be needed to deal with various situations, and, rather than you telling him what to do, let *him* come up with some of the strategies himself. After all, he is the one who has to face the bully on a daily basis!

Here are some tips you can tell your child to try when next faced with a problem schoolmate:

- **Act brave and ignore the bully.** Bullies thrive on intimidation and fear. If your child can ignore the bully and pretend that he isn't bothered, it often takes the fun out of it — for the bully. And tell your child not to try bullying back, which only makes things worse. Bullies have a lot of tricks up their sleeves and reacting could escalate the situation.

- **Defend yourself verbally.** Bullies like to feel powerful, but often they're just scared kids themselves. If ignoring a bully doesn't work, talk back. Tell the tyrant to stop, and then walk away.

- **Tell an adult.** No kid likes a snitch, but all kids dislike bullies. Tell your child to let the teacher, coach, or other adult that she trusts in the school know that she's being bullied.

- **Get a buddy.** If your child has a best friend, or a group of friends, then they can stick together and stand up to the bully together.

Make sure your child feels comfortable enough to let you know if these tactics aren't working. You may need to talk to your child's teacher or principal about the bullying situation. Yes, your child will hate it, but you need to know that the school environment is safe. Dealing with CFS is a bad enough stress without having to add worrying about bullies.

Nurturing Your Child's Understanding of Your CFS

Talking to a child about illness is never easy or pleasant. Getting her to understand that you have CFS is hard, especially if your child is very young.

Making sure your child understands that you aren't mad at her, that she hasn't done anything wrong, is important. You also don't want your child to worry about you. She needs reassurance. This task may sound impossible, but you can do several things to help put your child's mind at ease when it comes to your CFS. This section gives you some ideas to help your child — and you — cope with your CFS.

Describing your CFS in plain English

Keep it simple. When you sit down with your child to explain your illness, use terms that children can easily grasp and take it step by step. You'd be surprised how much your child can pick up, especially if you speak clearly and lovingly. Consider some of the following suggestions:

- **Tell him only what he needs to know.** You've probably heard the joke where a 4-year-old asks his dad the dreaded question, "Where do babies come from?" The father, long prepared for this question and determined to be more honest than his own parents were, launches into a detailed explanation, complete with diagrams and terminology. After he's done, the child looks up at him and replies, "No, they don't. Babies come from the hospital."

  The moral of the story is: Don't overdo it. Keep your explanations to the level of your child's ability to comprehend.

- **Use the right terms.** After you name things, they tend to be less scary. Most children can grasp the meaning of the words *chronic fatigue syndrome,* so tell them the name as well as the acronym for your illness.

- **Explain why mommy needs to have so many medical tests and take medicine.** Watching you leave the house for hospital visits and tests or watching you take a whole slew of medicines can be scary for most children. Explaining what the procedures are and why they need to be done can help your child to understand why you're doing what you're doing. Offering an explanation can go a long way in alleviating your child's fears.

- **Be honest.** Answer your child's questions as honestly as you can. If you don't know the answer, say so, but that you'll find out. Then find out the answer and get back to your child with it. Let him be part of your team.

- **Don't minimize, but don't exaggerate.** Of course you don't want your child to worry, but you also want him to be realistic about your condition. The worst thing you can do is give him false hope. He may never believe anything again! Stick with the facts. Talk about new research and possibilities. Talk about him — his dreams, his goals, the colleges he wants to visit. Let your child know that even though you may be ill, you're still his parent, and you love him very much.

- **Respect her emotions.** Your child will feel the same rage, fear, and grief that adults do — she just may not show it in the same way. She may feel that your getting sick is all her fault. She may start acting out at home, picking a fight with her sister, or crying. She may start acting out in school as well. Let your child know that she has a right to whatever emotions she feels, that the feelings are normal, and then help her find suitable ways to get her mind off your CFS, such as more exercise, a new hobby, or a trip. If necessary, make an appointment with a child psychologist.

✔ **Provide an outlet.** Your child may benefit from keeping a diary where he can record his thoughts and feelings about your CFS. You may also want to encourage him to draw or write poems about how he feels. These forms of expression can not only provide him with an outlet for his emotions, but also give you insight into how he's feeling.

✔ **Get outside help.** All sorts of support are out there. Look for books, videos, or Web sites that can help you talk to your child about your illness (like this book). You may also get some good advice from a therapist or your support group.

✔ **Be truthful.** Just like any other person with CFS, you have good days and bad days. Let your child know about this in advance, so she can be prepared and not be worried.

Listing and meeting your child's needs

All children need a healthy diet, the appropriate amounts of exercise and rest, and time for play. Those needs shouldn't change just because you have CFS. Making a list of your child's basic needs and then adding strategies for how you can meet them despite your illness can help take the edge off your child's fears — and yours.

In this section, I go over the ways to ensure your child's health physically, mentally, and emotionally.

Keeping your child healthy

If you can keep your child healthy, you have one less thing to worry about. Getting help from your support network, your spouse, a babysitter, or family friend can ensure your child gets what she needs. Make sure your child has the following:

✔ **Regular exercise:** Arrange for your child to continue any team or individual sports. That's why they invented carpools.

✔ **A healthy diet:** The good news is that even fast-food chains are getting into the health game. On the days where you just can't cook, take your child to a diner or restaurant and make sure he doesn't just get French fries or a dessert. Or, if you are too ill to go out to dinner, it's time to call for a pizza delivery — or have a bowl of soup.

✔ **Proper dress:** Make sure your child is dressed appropriately for the weather. It's easy enough for your spouse to handle coat buttons and mittens when the weather's cold.

You can also make sure that you have specific hooks by the door where your child can put her coat, boots, hat, and scarf. This way, you don't have to spend precious energy looking for that lone boot.

Attending to your child's emotional needs

Your child's psychological development will be impacted by your CFS. But that impact doesn't have to pack a wallop. Take time every day to spend with your child. You don't have to do something that requires a lot of energy, like throwing a ball or jumping rope. You can do a jigsaw puzzle together or help with homework. And you don't even have to get out of bed!

Your child needs time to adjust to your diagnosis and come to terms with it. Letting him know that his emotions are normal, no matter how dark and unpleasant, goes far in helping him cope. If you feel that your child isn't adjusting well, consider consulting with a professional who specializes in counseling families and children with chronic, long-term illnesses. (See Chapter 8 for more on finding a therapist.)

Fostering supportive friendships

Having friends is important to the normal psychosocial development of all children. Don't let your CFS limit your child's social circle. Let her friends' parents know that you have a chronic illness and you will have times when you won't be able to do the carpooling or make the cake for the party. You can also suggest that her friends come to your house.

Meeting your child's need to be needed

As long as your child knows she's loved, she will grow up strong and confident. But love is a two-way street. Let your child show you love as well. If she wants to make you breakfast one Sunday, let her! If he draws a picture for you, hang it on your bed frame. If she wants to go with you to the doctor's office, let her. Going with you can be a way to ease her fears (the doctor's office isn't filled with scary aliens), and the fact that she shows an interest should be encouraging to you. Depending on the age of your child, just make sure you bring plenty of games and books to keep her occupied. If possible, bring along another adult to stay in the waiting room and watch your kiddo when you're inside.

Chapter 16

Peering into the Future of CFS

In This Chapter

▶ Analyzing the newest scientific research

▶ Locating new CFS information

▶ Being a part of clinical trials for CFS

*Y*ou can't find established, by-the-book treatments for CFS. And, despite nearly 20 years of investigation by researchers in the United States and abroad, the cause of CFS remains unknown. But no one lives in a vacuum — nor does your illness. Researchers and clinicians are constantly on the lookout for the root cause of CFS. They're always seeking possible cures, potentially effective new treatments and therapies, and the elusive "magic pill" that can quickly eliminate CFS symptoms, or the illness itself. Inroads have been made into the mystery called chronic fatigue syndrome. We researchers are continuing to learn more and more about CFS.

You and your doctor may not be aware of the latest discoveries and breakthroughs. By keeping yourself posted and well informed, you can work with your doctor to identify innovative tests and treatments and perhaps even test them out before they go to market. In this chapter, I cue you in on some research in the works and give you some ideas of where you can look for the latest information on CFS, to keep yourself as up-to-date on the illness as possible. I even tell you how you yourself can participate in the research to bring about new treatments and cures for CFS!

Checking Out What's in the Works

It's important to stay current on the latest research, medications, and treatments so that you can take advantage of any new discoveries that come down the pike. It there is something that will help your CFS, then you need to know about it!

Diving into CFS studies

I've included studies here on inflammation and CFS, genetic research and CFS, and the newest medications on the fight against CFS. Although the conclusions of the studies presented here sound exciting, you have to remember that they are still in the development stage — and things can change. I suggest you keep tabs on them, checking them out on the Internet and in the news, to see if any have been completed and what the final results were.

Recent studies have indicated that CFS may be caused the body's response to inflammation in the pathways of the nervous system. This response has nothing to do with fire — except that it is your body's way to "put out fires." When you get a virus, infection, or injury, your body's response is inflammation, which destroys germs and intruders. But sometimes inflammation hangs around after the crisis is over. This chronic inflammation causes your immune system to break down, which may result in CFS.

Genes are another hot topic in the field of CFS studies. In April 2006, the Centers for Disease Control and Prevention (CDC) announced that scientists have identified clusters of genes that seem to be involved in the development of CFS. The CDC team of specialists included experts in such varied fields as molecular biology, epidemiology, physics, and the emerging field of genomics. They studied 227 controls and 227 CFS patients, analyzing such factors as sleep physiology, cognitive function, and *autonomic nervous system function* (the involuntary controls for breathing, reflexes, and body temperature). The team ultimately evaluated the activity of 20,000 genes and concluded that people with CFS are less able to adapt to life's major stresses,including physical illness, injury or major life events (such as a death in the family. . But these findings are not written in stone. More research is still needed, however, to determine just how much genes and CFS are linked.

Dubbed the *C3* (the CFS Computational Challenge), the research in this multidisciplinary team are an example of the new approach to studying chronic illness. Instead of isolating a specific gene, the C3 brought experts together to analyze similarities among the people studied and their genetic structures that may be different than the general population. With the C3 approach, more information is gathered — and researchers have a better chance of understanding CFS and how to successfully treat it in the future. This multidisciplinary, computational approach is also being used for Lupus and other chronic disease studies.

Discovering the latest, most-promising drugs

Science marches on — and hopefully towards a cure for all human illnesses. With the mapping of the human genome, scientists hope to develop new CFS medications based on gene therapy, clinical trials, and long-term studies.

Some of the newest medicines out there include:

- **Ampligen:** This experimental drug is actually a synthetic piece of a gene (nucleic acid) made in the laboratory. It works synergistically with *interferons* (viral-fighting, immune-system chemicals in the body), and is a potent immune system stimulant. With more interferons in the bloodstream, the theory goes, the more the body can fend off illness, including CFS.

  Ampligen is showing promise in both cognition and performance capability, but it isn't yet approved by the Food and Drug Administration (FDA) for widespread use. It's also extremely expensive and most insurance companies don't pay for it. Some negative reactions have also been reported, including liver damage. Amligen is manufactured by Hemisphere Biopharma, Inc.

- **Gamma globulin:** This is one of the bloodstream's antibody molecules and one of the body's prime defenses against infection. Gamma globulin may be injected intravenously into patients whose immune systems have been compromised and need a boost. Studies so far haven't shown any effectiveness in CFS, but the jury is still out. Adverse reactions are rare and include anaphylactic shock (a dangerous allergic reaction). It is also very expensive.

- **Corticosteroids:** In some people with CFS, their symptoms may mimic the symptoms of *Addison's disease,* an illness in which the body doesn't produce enough of the hormone cortisol. The result is a compromised immune system. Although a few studies have shown that corticosteroids can counteract these symptoms in people with CFS, nothing is definitive. Any observed benefit from corticosteroids has disappeared within one month — so far.

Doing a background check on cytokine

One of the suspected culprits in CFS is cytokines. So what are these pesky critters — and what role do they play in making you feel lousy?

Cytokines are proteins secreted by the immune system. They act as chemical messengers, carrying information to and from the body's cells. The Centers for Disease Control and Prevention (CDC) cites a study conducted in collaboration with Australian researchers that found that cytokines may play a role in CFS. How? When someone gets an infection, cytokines are stimulated. The patient begins to show what the CDC describes as an acute sickness with behavioral symptoms, such as fatigue, listlessness, and sleep dysfunction, with cognitive symptoms such as poor memory and an inability to focus, along with a fever. Sounds like CFS doesn't it?

Some researchers have long hypothesized that cytokines play a role in CFS. The CDC-Australian study found that 10 percent of two groups of patients, those who had infectious mononucleosis and others who had a mosquito-transmitted disease called Ross River virus (RRV), went on to develop an illness similar to CFS. Two cytokines, IL-1b and IL-6, were consistently implicated in the patients who reported the CFS-like symptoms. The study, though small, indicates that cytokines may be biological markers for an acute physical, behavioral and cognitive sickness, and by extension, CFS. Further work is needed to confirm or refute this hypothesis.

Keeping Your Eyes Peeled for New Findings and Treatments

The good news is that information is everywhere, including the latest, greatest findings on CFS. But that information won't just weasel its way into your brain on its own. In most cases, you need to search for it.

One of the best ways to find out the current — and legitimate — research being done on CFS is via a doctor or therapist you trust. If she specializes in CFS, she should be completely up-to-date. She should also be able to steer you toward sources so you can do your own research.

To make your search more efficient and more informative, in this section I've outlined some places to go for the best in CFS.

Surfing the Web for innovations

You have a wealth of information available to you on the Internet, sometimes *too* much, and not all of it good. How can you determine which advice is good or harmful or just plain useless?

If you typed the phrase *new treatment options for CFS* into the Google.com search engine, you would get over 600,000 hits (and in 0.22 seconds nonetheless)! And, by the time you're done reading this paragraph, that number will have most likely increased — perhaps dramatically. With numbers like this, reading everything is clearly impossible. Nor can you always trust the order in which the information is presented. Being the first Web site listed on the search engine's results list is no indication of accuracy. It can be the result of advertising, strategic word placement, and key word topics. In other words, don't limit your search to just the first few pages of the search engine results.

So how do you make sense of all that information? Consider some of the following tips to finding reputable CFS information on the Internet:

- ✔ **Don't get overwhelmed.** Set a time limit of, say, half-hour intervals and take frequent breaks. Print out information that you can read later. Remember, you're not going to get all the information you need in one day!

- ✔ **Check the source.** Can you trust where the information is coming from? Just because something is on the Web doesn't make it true. If the Web site ends in .gov (like www.CDC.gov), chances are that you're getting an accurate report.

    Finding an Internet address with .org used to mean that you were getting the real deal. Because *org* stands for an organization or nonprofit, you would assume that the information was there for the common good. But almost *anybody* can get an .org Web address if they request it. Make sure the .org is an association or organization that is extremely reputable, such as the American Heart Association or the Chronic Fatigue and Immune Dysfunction Association of America; chances are, the information you're receiving is valid.

    Any Web source you're unsure of is fair game and needs to be checked out. Make sure you investigate the *About Us* section and closely examine the small print. (And if they don't have a section like this, run away!)

One good thing about the Internet is that it is truly worldwide. A lot of people in other countries are conducting research, and, as you conduct your Web search, you can find information from Europe, the United Kingdom, and Australia, among other places. Research into innovative treatments even seems to be further ahead in these countries than in the United States.

But as you begin to expand your research to international waters, a word of caution: Many people tend to think that the pharmaceutical grass is greener on the other side of the pond. Not true. Apply the same level of skepticism you would for treatments you find on foreign Web sites as you would if the same treatments were being offered by your local doctor.

However, the following international Web sites about CFS treatment innovations are worth your while:

- The M.E./Chronic Fatigue Syndrome Society of Victoria is a nonprofit charitable organization serving people affected by CFS in Victoria, Australia, and Tasmania. Run entirely by volunteers, the society publishes a quarterly magazine, *Emerge,* that includes the latest in research, as well as articles from readers and other CFS information. The Society also has an E-mail Pen Friends section on the site where you can connect with other CFS patients. To visit this organization's Web site, head to `http://home.vicnet.net.au/~mecfs/`.

- The International Association for CFS (IACFS) has a Web site offering a lot of information on CFS, including current research being done across the globe. You can find the IACFS at `www.iacfs.net`.

For more online CFS resources, check out the appendix of this book.

As always, be sure to check with your doctor before acting on any medical advice you find on the Internet, even if the source seems reputable.

Listening to fellow CFS sufferers in support groups

If you aren't a part of a support group, get plugged into one (for more info on finding a support group, see Chapter 15). Once you're a part of a CFS support group, you need to keep your ears peeled! You never know when another member or the leader of your group has discovered something revolutionary about CFS treatments or the illness itself.

Make sure you trust the source. Just because Betty has CFS doesn't mean she's cured her tendency to exaggerate or even tell a fib here or there. Also, make sure you're a part of a credible support group, so you know the new information you hear from a buddy is reliable. (You still need to check with your health care professional just to make sure any new treatment or suggestion is right for you.)

To put your mind at ease about whether you can trust your current support group to provide valid information on CFS (or if you're beginning your search for a credible group to join), you can use the following tips (and if the support group doesn't make the cut, move on):

- ✔ **Find out who sponsors the group.** Many groups are run out of a hospital or house of worship. There are also many established local and national organizations you can choose from. Usually these groups have a track record, so you can check their effectiveness. The actual group may just use the facilities and have no actual ties to a hospital or church.

- ✔ **Check out the group's leader.** The *facilitator* (the leader of a support group) is an important factor in a support group's success. Although the facilitator doesn't need to be a professional counselor or therapist, you may want to find out more about the leader's background and training. The facilitator should be familiar with CFS, either because she suffers from the condition, or she is the caregiver of a person who has it. She needs to speak from experience.

  If you aren't already part of the group, try to talk to the facilitator before committing to the group, so you can get a feel for the person's abilities and how comfortable you feel with her.

- ✔ **Read over the support group's goals.** Some support groups focus more on the medical side of CFS. Others may focus on the psychological and social effects of the condition. Still others may be all about caregiving. Finding a group that focuses solely on CFS and not on other chronic diseases can help you get information specifically on CFS. Some smaller communities may have fewer options, and you might have to go to a group that covers broader topics. Just remember that the goals of the group should coincide with your own goals.

Locating and reading CFS studies hot off the press

You can stay up-to-date on CFS news by having CFS publications sent right to your door, chock-full of the most recent findings, treatments, and news. There are publications printed at various, established CFS organizations, including brochures, newsletters, and magazines. Some are even published through Internet news sites. I go over a few of these in this section.

- ✔ **The CFIDS Association of America** has published a 65-page special issue of its magazine, *Chronicle,* covering, as they put it, the latest "CFS research findings, profiles of key investigators, input from international researchers, a review of current best treatment practices, and stories about patients and families coping with the illness. Priced at $12.00, it can be ordered from the CFIDS Web site at `www.cfids.org/sparkcfs/magazine.asp`.

- ✔ **eMedicine,** an adjunct to the hugely successful WebMd, is a Web site that offers abstracts on the newest published articles on all conditions, including CFS. Go to `www.emedicine.com` for the latest news.

> ✔ **Medline** has long been used by health care professionals to find out the latest information on disease states, psychosocial theories, and clinical trials. Although you may have to pay to get an article in its entirety, you can find out the name of the most prominent researchers on CFS, as well as the journals that publish them. You'll also see some of the highlights of the study as well. Go to www.medline.com.

Keeping an eye on the Centers for Disease Control and Prevention (CDC)

The Centers for Disease Control and Prevention (CDC), based in Atlanta, Georgia, operates under the auspices of the United States Department of Health and Human Services. Founded in 1946, the CDC is the nation's primary vanguard to, as written on their Web site, "prevent and control infectious and chronic diseases, injuries, workplace hazards, disabilities, and environmental health threats."

So if the CDC has something new to say about CFS, you better be listening. The best way to stay current with the CDC's findings on CFS is to check out the CDC's Web site that has a page specifically for CFS. You can access this page at www.cdc.gov/cfs.

By visiting the CDC's CFS page, you have access to the latest research information, as well as basic information of CFS, fact sheets, free downloadable brochures, listings of support groups, helpful tips on such topics as how to talk to your doctor, and a glossary of medical terms.

Checking in with the National Institutes of Health (NIH)

The National Institutes of Health (NIH), a part of the United States Department of Health and Human Services, is a large organization comprised of 27 separate institutes and centers and is the nation's main vehicle for conducting clinical trials and supporting a great deal of medical research via grants.

The Office of Research on Women's Health is the division of NIH that addresses CFS. On its Web site, you can find the latest research information, news releases, and links to other resources. Go to http://orwh.od.nih.gov/cfs.html.

Helping Yourself and Other CFS Sufferers with Clinical Drug Trials

You don't want to be a guinea pig, but participating in a clinical trial is one way that you can contribute to science — and yourself. Clinical trials are one way scientists test to see whether a drug is useful or not. (I go into more detail about this process in a following section.)

Scientists need human subjects to test the efficacy and possible side effects (positive or negative) of the drugs they develop, and you, as a volunteer, can gain a sense of control — or at least a measure of satisfaction — that you are doing your part to help further medical research and the development of new treatments for CFS.

Other benefits to participating in a clinical trial include the following:

- ✔ You receive medical care from the doctors who are experts in the field. This care is at no cost to you.

- ✔ You are among the first to find out about new therapies.

- ✔ You have the opportunity to meet other people with your condition who are also participating in the study, thus giving yourself another source of emotional support.

Knowing the drug-approval process is important for keeping abreast of the newer information. So, what clinical trials are out there? You may want to look for some to participate in. In the following sections, I take you through the maze of drug testing and clinical testing, so you can keep informed and even get involved if you want to.

Familiarizing yourself with the drug-testing process

The approval process for new drugs in the United States is quite rigorous, probably the most rigorous in the world. Although recent movements to fast-track certain promising drugs and reduce the drug-approval process overall have surfaced, a report by the Congressional Office of Technology Assessment stated that it can take a pharmaceutical company upwards of $359 million, and 12 years to successfully bring a drug to market — and that was in 1993. Getting a drug approved costs even more in time and money today.

Further, only five out of 5,000 drugs make it to human testing, and of those five, only one is typically approved.

The Food and Drug Administration (FDA) is the regulatory body that governs the approval process. Clinical trials, conducted at hospitals or research centers, go through a rigorous multiphase process, as follows:

- Preclinical studies, lasting one to three years, are conducted in the lab or on animals to test a drug's potential.

- Phase I, lasting about a year or slightly more, is conducted on a small sample, between 20 and 80 volunteers, to determine proper dosing, how the drug is metabolized, and any side effects.

- Phase II lasts about two years and involves a larger group of volunteers — 100 to 300. The aim of this phase is to further study the drug's effectiveness and safety.

- Phase III lasts about three years. A much larger sample, 1,000 to 3,000 people, is usually involved. This phase further tests the drug's efficacy, and researchers look closely for any side effects. Because of the larger sample, the revelation of any negative side effects is more likely.

If obvious problems (such as severe side effects) arise at any stage in the testing process, the study is terminated. Conversely, if a drug is shown to have dramatic, life-saving effects, it can be fast-tracked to move through the process more quickly.

Placebo or nocebo?

Every physician probably has at least one patient who experienced a cure or remission in symptoms from a placebo. This phenomenon where patients report feeling better or having actual physical maladies clear up after being given an inert substance or a sugar pill is so well known that it has a name, the *placebo effect.*

There is power in expectation. Physicians and researchers have found that up to a third of patients report improvements in their condition after taking a placebo. This effect is often attributed to the patient's *belief* that they have been given a drug that will alleviate their symptoms,

but the actual psychological and physiological interplay that contributes to the placebo effect is still not fully understood. What is clear, though, is that for some patients, the placebo works.

The opposite phenomenon, called the *nocebo effect,* is where patients feel that their symptoms have worsened, even though they have been given an inert substance. Perhaps the placebo and nocebo effects serve to show that the mind plays an important part in the efficacy of any drug, separate from its measurable pharmacological results.

Some drugs may also be tested in a Phase IV trial after the drug has been pre-scribed for a number of years. Phase IV trials test for long-term side effects, and the use of the drug on other populations, who weren't included in the ini-tial testing.

In Phase I and Phase II trials, a control group generally receives a placebo or an inactive substance to compare to the test drug (for more on placebos, see the nearby sidebar). To remove bias from testing (after all, a researcher wants his theory to work), clinical trials are often *double-blinded,* which means that neither the researcher nor the participant knows who has received the drug or the placebo. In a *single-blinded study,* the researcher knows who has received the drug, but the participant doesn't.

Before you participate in a clinical trial, you are asked to give your informed consent. Risks are inherent in a clinical trial — you are, after all, allowing your body to be a living laboratory! Researchers don't take this responsibility lightly. In fact, the Investigational Review Board (IRB) is not a government body but rather an institution-specific group. Each hospital that has ongoing research has one of these groups of health care professionals review and approve clinical studies before they begin. The IRB protects your rights as a study participant, and it is their responsibility to make sure a proposed trial follows the strict guidelines of the FDA. So while a risk is still involved, remem-ber that if you choose to be a part of a clinical trail, you're in capable hands.

Finding out about available trials

At any given time, thousands of clinical trials are being conducted in the United States and abroad, on thousands of different illnesses and medical conditions.

In the U.S., a listing of all clinical trials can be obtained at `www.clinical trials.gov`, a Web site of the National Institute of Health (NIH). This site lists all the studies being conducted nationally, organizing them by condition, by the sponsoring organization, or by status (which means whether or not participants are being actively recruited).

You can also check out the following Web sites that list trials specifically for CFS:

- `www.cfids.org/about-cfids/clinical-trials.asp`
- `www.immunesupport.com/community/clinical-trials.cfm`

Part IV
The Part of Tens

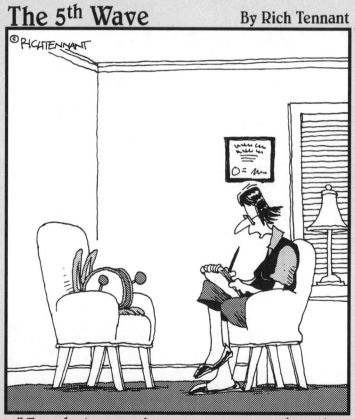

The 5th Wave
By Rich Tennant

"In what way do you see your Chronic Fatigue Syndrome affecting your job?"

In this part . . .

Many *For Dummies* book fans look forward to the Part of Tens chapters that appear at the end of every *For Dummies* book. This part features a rat-a-tat-tat of strategies, tips, facts, figures, and other fun stuff designed specifically to entertain and inform you without demanding that you do a whole lot of reading.

In this part, I reveal ten strategies to help you enhance your life, introduce you to ten famous people who have CFS, offer you ten drug-free ways to battle fatigue, and steer you clear of the ten most commonly suspected CFS symptom aggravators. I also bust ten common myths you may have heard about CFS.

Chapter 17

Ten Famous People with CFS

In This Chapter

▶ Finding inspiration in the ways famous people have coped with CFS

▶ Discovering that CFS can strike anyone, anytime

*F*lip through any issue of *Us* or *People* magazine, and you may begin to think that celebrities never get sick. Behind the jewels, designer fashions, and glamorous makeup jobs, famous people put their pants on one leg at a time just like you and aren't immune to disease. In this chapter, you discover ten celebrities who have had CFS. You witness first-hand how they've coped and, most importantly, how they've never given up.

Please note that this list isn't "for women only." There are many men who fall victim to CFS, too!

Michelle Akers

You may remember her as a 1996 Olympic gold medalist in soccer, but did you know that after the final game of the 1999 World Cup, Michelle Akers had to hobble to a team of doctors off-field who immediately attached her to not one, but two IV lines, an oxygen mask, and an EKG heart monitor machine? It's true. Ms. Akers suffers from chronic fatigue syndrome. Despite this, she continues to be a soccer legend — even in retirement. She scored a record 39 goals in 26 games in 1991's World Cup in China, and she didn't leave the sport until 2000 (when her CFS forced her to retire from soccer as a profession) — as one of only four women who scored over 100 career goals. Michelle was also inducted into the National Soccer Hall of Fame in 2004.

Of course, not every day is a good day. There are times when Michelle can't do anything, despite her untiring spirit. During the "bad times," she has terrible migraine headaches and has trouble getting through the day. What does she hate most about having CFS? She likes to play soccer for the full 90 minutes, and the illness makes this difficult! In 1997, Michelle wrote a book about her experiences with CFS called *Standing Fast: Battles of a Champion* (JTC Sports, Inc.).

Susan Blackmore

The author of over 60 academic articles and 40 books, either as author or literary contributor, Dr. Susan Blackmore is very well known in England, where she received degrees in psychology and physiology from Oxford University, and a PhD in parapsychology from the University of Surrey. She is also a contributor to the *Guardian* newspaper and is a frequent guest on British television and radio. Although she spent 30 years determined to prove her Oxford University colleagues wrong (that the paranormal does exist), she ultimately changed her beliefs. It was a devastating blow for her, turning her whole identity upside-down.

What saved her? Three things: science, Zen practices . . . and CFS. In 1995, after working too many long hours on too many different projects, she came down with CFS. She couldn't walk; she slept restlessly for 12 hours or more a day; she couldn't read or concentrate except in short bursts. Ironically, Dr. Blackmore's condition brought her to a whole new branch of science: cultural evolution, or memes, in which humankind stores ideas, art, stories, technologies, and science and passes them on to other generations just like genetic structure. If she hadn't come down with CFS, Dr. Blackmore wouldn't have had the time to speculate or think about the cultural evolution. She might possibly have never known about memes. Her disease gave her a new outlook on life.

Howard Bloom

What hasn't Howard Bloom done? In the 1970s and early '80s, he carved a legendary career in the entertainment business. As a music publicist, he developed the *raison de etre* of music publicity today: creating and maintaining a superstar profile. He worked with such rock greats as Prince, Michael Jackson, Bob Marley, Bette Midler, AC/DC, Talking Heads, and Simon & Garfunkel. During this time, he also worked with some of the biggest movie studios in the world — Paramount Pictures, Warner Brothers, and Disney. In addition, he helped build Amnesty International's and Farm Aid's music fundraisers.

In 1988, Howard contracted CFS and was forced to leave the entertainment industry. Did he fade away into oblivion? Did he take to his bed and stay there? No. Instead, he literally re-invented himself and journeyed to the far side of the spectrum — he became a prominent scientist, engineer, and cultural analyst. He's also become a prolific writer, authoring three books and publishing many articles in such publications as *Wired, The Washington Post,* and *The Village Voice.* CFS literally uprooted his career, forcing him to follow a new calling.

Cher

Not many people haven't heard of Cher. She's one of the world's most celebrated stars. Between her platinum albums, her sold-out concerts, her award-winning movies — even her famed television shows — she is the quintessential entertainer. She's done it all, and she's done it well.

But did you know that for three years Cher had CFS and that she had chronic bronchitis and pneumonia because of it? She had to drag herself to concerts and, in fact, cancel shows. Cher's battle with CFS happened in the late 1990s, and, as she told Larry King in 1999 after she'd recovered, no one believed her for two years. She found not one sympathetic doctor. Eventually, she found a sympathetic homeopathic doctor and she was on the road to recovery.

Blake Edwards

Yes, he received a lifetime honorary achievement award during the Academy Award ceremonies in 2004. Yes, he's the mastermind director of the *Pink Panther* movies starring Peter Sellers. Yes, he directed or collaborated on more than 50 movies, including *What Did You Do in the War, Daddy?, Victor/Victoria, Days of Wine and Roses, Breakfast at Tiffany's,* and *10.* But did you know that he's been suffering from CFS for years? Obviously, he has found ways to continue his career in spite of CFS.

Laura Hillenbrand

Laura remembers the exact day she was hit with CFS: Sunday, March 28, 1987. It was evening, and she and her friend Linc were returning to Kenyon College after spring break. Suddenly, out of nowhere, a deer ran into the road. They swerved and missed it. But Ms. Hillenbrand felt a warmth run through her. She felt nauseated and tired. It was that moment in time that she started a lifelong relationship with CFS, movingly chronicled in a 2003 *New Yorker* article, *A Sudden Illness — How My Life Changed.* She was 19.

You may find it difficult to imagine this bestselling author of *Seabiscuit: An American Legend* painstakingly writing her book and writing racing articles to earn money, while in the throes of CFS. Her symptoms were so bad, she literally couldn't get out of bed; her hand shook when she tried to write; she spent hours in delirium. She had to figure out how to pace herself. When she felt better, the slightest amount of work could send her back into CFS hell. It would come and go.

But necessity is the mother of invention. Helpless and in bed, Laura came across information about Seabiscuit the racehorse and began to write. The rest is history.

Andy Hunt

A famous English soccer player, or *footballer* as people in Great Britain call it, Andy Hunt scored 135 goals, appeared in 361 games, and was declared a top scorer in Charlton Division One Championship during the 1999–2000 season. Unfortunately, right after becoming a champion, he had to withdraw from soccer because of CFS. He quit and now owns an adventure travel agency. Two careers. Two lives. Would he have had the opportunity to travel to exotic places if he hadn't come down with CFS and had remained a soccer star? Who knows.

Keith Jarrett

In 1996, this renowned jazz pianist and composer had to curtail his performances: He had developed CFS. The illness, at first, was devastating. He'd been playing piano since he was a little boy of three, and, suddenly, whenever he sat down at the piano, he felt too sick to play! Worse, the connection between his brain and his hands disappeared; he *couldn't* play. As a composer quickly climbing to the peak of his career, this dysfunction was disastrous. He didn't know whether he would ever be able to play the piano again — he couldn't even bear to hear music because it gave him an awful headache. This particular CFS symptom lasted for two years.

By 2000, Keith had improved and was able to play some music. He slowly set up microphones and sound equipment around his piano whenever he had a burst of energy — even if it was only for a few minutes. He had gone over the music in his head the whole time he was incapacitated.

Today, Mr. Jarrett is much more economical in his composing. He told Terry Gross on National Public Radio that he had to get to the heart of the piece quickly because time is so precious.

At the time of this book's publication, Keith has made one public appearance since becoming ill with CFS.

Henry Percy, 11th Duke of Northumberland

CFS is indeed a great equalizer. Even English royalty can get it. Henry Percy, the 11th Duke of Northumberland and the godchild of Queen Elizabeth II, supposedly had CFS in his lifetime.

An active royal, the duke planted many trees at his ancestral home, Syon Park. He was also involved in politics. He died in 1995 at the age of 42 — supposedly the result of an amphetamine addiction. Could he have started taking the amphetamine to regain the energy he lost from CFS? No one will ever know for sure.

Ali Smith

Ali Smith, bestselling author of *The Accidental* (Pantheon) and *Hotel World* (Anchor Books), was born in 1962 in Inverness, Scotland. She studied in Aberdeen and then enrolled in Cambridge to work on her PhD. Before she completed her work at Cambridge, she became ill with CFS and spent an entire year struggling with the symptoms. Too exhausted to teach, she left her job as a lecturer and decided to do what she always had wanted to do — write.

Ali's writing conveys a unique blend of sensitivity, grandiosity, and humor, making one wonder whether her writing style and vision weren't somehow influenced by her bout of CFS. In any event, if Ali had never been stricken with CFS, perhaps she would have gone on for her PhD and kept teaching rather than doing what she really loved.

Chapter 18

Ten Drug-Free Ways to Fight Fatigue

*W*hen you find yourself too tired to go about your day, it doesn't always mean you have to stay in bed or on the couch. Many people have discovered strategies that are often successful in fighting fatigue. Look through this chapter for some re-energizers, and start breathing, stretching, and relaxing your way to a better day.

Boogie-ing to Your Favorite Tunes

Okay, I'm not talking Fred Astaire and Ginger Rogers here. That type of strenuous exercise would leave most people begging for mercy. A slow-paced cha-cha or salsa can get you moving (literally) and have you snapping your fingers, bobbing your head, and getting lost in the music. Because of your illness, it's best to start out slowly, simply listening to the music while lying or sitting, and gently moving your arms and legs. You can then gradually progress to actual dancing, and gently dance for a short period.

In other words: The right kind of dance exercise can actually make you forget you have CFS for a moment — and it also fights fatigue.

Here are some tips to help you dance away the fatigue:

- Don't think dance floor. Instead, think of a living room area rug. You aren't going to fly or swirl; you're just going to gently move your "booty."

- Try slower-paced music. Have you ever swayed to the sounds of the Big Band era? Or bobbed to a folk song? And what about Tony Bennett? Anything he does is perfect for a slow, safe — but completely enjoyable — workout!

- Don't forget the classics. I'm not talking early Beatles or Dylan here. I literally mean the true classics: Mozart, Beethoven, Bach. You can even sit one out and sink into the couch, your eyes closed, moving your head and arms.

- No obstacle courses, please! Make sure you move the end tables, loose cords, and slippery rugs out of the way (or recruit someone to do the work if the load is heavy). You want to concentrate on the music — not on falling.

- Make your dancing place private. In order to really get into the music and transport yourself, you need to feel uninhibited. You don't want the Smiths next door watching you dance. Nor do you need to worry about someone passing by. The best solution? Close the shades. Close the doors. Let everyone know this is your alone time.

Setting Sensible, Doable Goals

Something about goals can make people reach for the impossible. While having a dream is admirable, you need to have realistic goals in order to stick with it. And, like baby steps, they can lead the way to your dream.

You can use the following suggestions to help you set realistic goals:

- Don't get ahead of yourself. Until you know your limitations and strengths, you can't make realistic goals. Try planning your goals for just one day and see how you do.

- If you reach your daily goal, congratulations! But don't take that as permission to go further. Stay with that goal and if you continue to reach it for several days, then (and only then) add on.

- Accept that goals can't be written in stone. You have a medical condition and symptoms may flare up when you least expect them. You may have set a goal of completing two projects at work that day, but, wham — you wake up exhausted and can't move. In that case, change your goals! Instead of the impossible, go for the realistic. Change your goal to doing your personal grooming or even making a list for the next day.

✔ Take a tip from dieters. If someone has to lose 50 pounds and all she thinks about is those 50 pounds and how hard it will be to lose them, she won't get past dessert the next day. But if she thinks about losing one pound as a goal for the week, she just might make it. And the numbers add up: one pound a week for 52 weeks and, hey, that's a loss of over 50 pounds! Plan, say, for a ten-minute period of exercise one day per week, then two days per week, and so on. Or one night of yoga. Or getting to the halfway point on a project from work.

✔ Baby steps, baby steps. Yes, you have CFS and, yes, it does limit your abilities on occasion. Don't get mad at the disease. Don't get mad at yourself. Know that each goal you make is one step closer to learning to cope with CFS and having a better quality of life.

Breathing Deeper Than Normal

A deep breath can be like a time out. When you're feeling stressed, taking a breath to the count of eight and exhaling for a count of eight can help ease your anxiety. (See Chapters 8 and 9 for strategies to deal with stress.) Those same deep breaths can provide more oxygen to your body and help you feel less tired, too. Take a three-minute break (or write the planned break in your goals), and do the following:

1. **Sit in a chair with your feet on the floor, your hands in your lap, your head up, and your eyes closed.**

2. **Breathe in for a count of eight, hold your breath for a count of eight, and then gently exhale for a count of eight.**

3. **Do this breathing exercise three or four times, and then simply sit there for the remaining three minutes.**

If you start to feel restless, do the breathing exercise one more time. You will be more energized and ready to face the rest of your day!

Stretching Out

Have you ever seen a cat or dog stretch after a nap? They push out their legs, curl their back, and gently move forward and backward. They do this instinctively — we need to be reminded. When you're feeling fatigued, you can do the following stretches, either sitting in a chair or lying down:

✔ Try lifting your arms above your head (or out in front of you if your symptoms are too severe), spread your fingers, stretch, then gently bring your arms down.

✓ Lift one leg, point then flex your toes, then bring it back. You can do this sitting, standing, or holding on to a wall for support.

✓ Try some gentle yoga positions, such as Cat-Dog Pose or Child's Pose. (See Chapter 9 for diagrams and instructions.)

A few minutes of stretching and you may feel less tired!

Spending Time with a Positive Friend

Nothing can replace a good friend to help you through the day. Most people know someone who just exudes positive energy and encouragement. Allow this type of person into your life. And if you don't have a positive friend or an inspiring loved one? Seek out a CFS support group, or ask your therapist for help. He may help get that positive energy moving, too!

Kicking Back in Your Easy Chair

Knowing when to take a break is crucial for people with CFS. Too much exercise, stress, or exertion can bring back symptoms or worsen ones that never went away.

Relaxing is a good thing. Plan time in your daily goal schedule to relax. In fact, planning several breaks throughout the day is even better! To make the easy chair more enticing:

✓ Schedule breaks around your Tivo or favorite show.

✓ Keep a good book on the end table, your place clearly marked.

✓ Listen to a track of a book on tape.

✓ Close your eyes and listen to some relaxing music.

Celebrating Your Successes

No success is too small. Success is . . . success, and it needs to be acknowledged, especially when you have a chronic condition and can't do something that people without CFS take for granted — such as making dinner, staying at work until lunch, getting a good night's sleep, having a good yoga class, doing an errand, making a goal, or doing deep breathing after a particularly stressful incident.

Let your loved ones know when you've achieved something you've been working towards. Let them congratulate you — they want to feel good, too! And don't forget to tell your CFS support group. They will really understand what you've done.

When you feel good about yourself, you may feel less fatigued (or the fatigue may seem less noticeable). Less fatigue translates into a better quality of life.

Sleeping More . . . Or Less

Sleep is the foremost way to get your life regulated and fight fatigue. However, part of the problem with CFS fatigue is that sleep may not help. Normally, when you're tired, a good night's sleep is all you need. Not so if you have CFS. You can sleep 12 to 14 hours and still wake up fatigued!

Getting any amount of good sleep is the important issue here. It's a good idea to see a sleep specialist. A sleep specialist may be able to help you get refreshing sleep by looking for and treating a specific sleep disorder you may have.

Find out more about sleep and schedules in Chapter 11.

One of the very best stress reducers and sleep inducers is laughter. Watch a funny movie, or read a humorous book. Avoid depressing, violent, or action movies or TV shows just before bed.

Making Your Living Space Livable

People with CFS are more sensitive than other folks, not only when it comes to food or chemicals, but to the environment as well. Maybe your house or apartment warrants a top-to-bottom cleaning, getting rid of any dust and other potential allergens. If you're unable to clean it yourself, you can locate cleaning service franchises that are licensed and bonded and have them come in and clean your house in one day flat. If you can't afford the extra help, you can clean small areas at a time, pacing yourself so you don't overdo it.

The chemicals in many typical household cleaning products can provoke symptoms or trigger a relapse for some people with CFS. Choose one that is environmentally friendly and has a mild or no odor.

If your environment is causing you undue fatigue or added stress, the time has come to make some changes to your environment. Perhaps you need to call a strong loved one or your super to help rearrange your furniture. If rearranging isn't enough, here are a few solutions for problems you may face:

- ✔ **The glare from your windows is too much to handle:** You can order blackout shades to help fix the glare. People come in, measure, and put them up within a week. A much cheaper method of blocking out glare: eye masks! You can find them just about anywhere, from large discount stores to cosmetic boutiques.

- ✔ **You can hear your neighbors a little *too* well:** If the sound of your neighbor's TV or their lively children are too much for you, earplugs work pretty well. You can also listen to soothing music on your MP3 or CD player.

- ✔ **Your sleep area is messy or cluttered.** Being organized does more than ease your mind: It can also help you sleep. An uncluttered, quiet place for rest periods can help you get better quality rest.

Meditating Your Way to Feeling Refreshed

Meditation does more than calm you. It is a great way to feel energized — which is why many people meditate when they first wake up.

You can find morning meditations specifically designed to get you going, not put you to sleep. Dr. Wayne Dyer, a motivational speaker and author who is an expert on educational counseling, has a morning meditation that you can use for yourself. Go to www.drwaynedyer.com for more information.

Chapter 19

Ten Common Myths about CFS

*Y*ou can find all kinds of myths out there. Urban myths are supposed to take place on dark city streets. Greek myths are ancient stories about a group of strong-willed gods who lived on a mountain. And CFS myths? Well, you have them as well — faulty beliefs that continue to live on in your families, your colleagues, and even in yourself. The time has come to put these myths to rest and discover the real facts, so here you can debunk the top ten myths about CFS.

Only Young, White Females Get CFS

For a long time, people considered CFS a "yuppie disease," and one that Caucasian women fell victim to more often than anyone else. This misconception is just not true. Community studies show that CFS appears to be more prevalent in Hispanics and African-Americans and people in lower socioeconomic groups. The yuppie disease myth is shattered even further by the fact that, according to the Centers for Disease Control and Prevention (CDC), CFS is more prevalent in people in their 40s and 50s than in young professionals.

Yes, four times as many reported cases are in women than in men, but men aren't immune — nor are children. Kids as young as 5 years old have been diagnosed with CFS. Remember that *anyone* can get CFS.

CFS Symptoms Are Really Due to a Different Depressive Disorder

Part of the problem with CFS is its so-called invisibility. The diagnosis, for the most part, is based on symptoms described by the patient. These symptoms are usually initially attributed to a different depressive disorder or condition, such as in the following:

- **Fatigue and irritability?** These symptoms could be the result of clinical depression or generalized anxiety disorder.

- **Inability to concentrate?** Your doctor may tell you that your inability to concentrate may signal that you have attention deficit disorder or a symptom of bipolar disorder.

- **Body aches and pains?** These symptoms may bring your doctor back again to clinical depression.

- **Unrefreshing sleep?** Clinical depression, an anxiety disorder, a manic episode, attention deficit disorder — these illnesses are all possibilities your doctor may consider based upon your lack of fulfilling sleep.

Even more confusing is the fact that many people who get CFS *become* depressed. They may not have started out with any signs of depression other than fatigue, but, after several months, feelings of hopelessness and helplessness may appear.

Further, thanks to extensive research, the official classification of CFS has become more specific. Fatigue alone isn't enough. Headaches, swollen lymph nodes, joint and muscle pain, a sore throat, and more — these physical symptoms, when combined, are all considered part of the CFS makeup. (See Chapter 2 for more details.)

Overachievers Get CFS More Than Anyone Else

Overachievers are considered Type A personalities, perfectionists who must be perfect in everything they do, whether it be a PowerPoint presentation or a sparkling clean floor. Being an overachiever may raise the bar on your stress level, but it's probably not enough to cause full-blown CFS. The only exception to this guideline is if you're a high-performance, Ironman-level athlete, because strenuous exercise may trigger "overtraining syndrome," which may mimic CFS.

However, if you *are* an overachiever, it likely makes a diagnosis of CFS that much harder to swallow. Many people find it very difficult to adjust to a brave, new world where perfectionism, on occasion, is getting out of bed without help.

CFS Is Due to Burnout

If you work too hard, if you push yourself too far, and if you've had too many days and nights of burning the candle at both ends, you'll get tired. You don't have to be a psychic to know that doing too much for too long is going to have consequences. But the idea of burning out and CFS are, in reality, polar opposites. Burning out may cause CFS-like symptoms, but only because you're exhausted. Burnout can often be easily reversed with rest, a vacation, or a reduced workload. CFS, on the other hand, can strike anyone, from the idle rich to the factory worker that works overtime, and it can't be fixed with a Caribbean vacation.

The only way burning out can even be considered in the same breath as CFS is when you're pushing yourself too hard and your immune system becomes very vulnerable. And a vulnerable immune system can make you susceptible to illness.

CFS Was Discovered in the 20th Century

Wrong again. Over the past 15 years, more attention has been given to CFS, and this awareness has made CFS seem as if it came about only a few decades ago. However, reports of CFS-like symptoms date back to the 1750s. Of course, doctors don't have specific statistics or clinical studies, nor can they go back in time to actually diagnose people, but it's possible that those people who "took to their beds," who had flu-like symptoms that didn't go away, who had brutal headaches and aches and pains, in actuality, had CFS.

Eventual Recovery Is a Given

If only it were true! Unfortunately, no cure exists for CFS — yet. Various medicines, cognitive therapies, physical programs, and support teams can help you cope much better and help symptoms and day-to-day functioning improve. But the fact that you had CFS once does mean that you're predisposed to the condition. But . . . learning to cope better means less stress, a better quality of life, and less chance of a relapse.

The ability to improve over time, however, has been related to the length of time you've had the disease. Unfortunately, people who have had CFS long-term have a worse prognosis of recovery than someone newly diagnosed.

Getting More Sleep Can Help

This one's tricky because getting more sleep may actually reduce some of your symptoms. *But* the amount of sleep isn't what's causing the problems. If you have CFS, you know that sleeping for even 10 to 12 hours a night isn't going to help. You wake up as exhausted as if you never slept at all. Whether or not you're sleeping isn't the problem; the *quality* of sleep is what counts. See Chapter 11 for better sleep strategies.

CFS Comes from AIDS

A few theories floating around out there claim that CFS comes from HIV-AIDS. There are no studies that show that CFS is caused by HIV-AIDS, so right now it appears highly unlikely that there is a connection between CFS and these conditions. And — and this is a very important "and" — getting CFS doesn't mean you will get AIDS!

Exercise Cures CFS

No. In fact, strenuous exercise only makes your CFS worse. Often, when people with CFS start to feel better, they feel they want to get back to their lives: going to the grocery store, shopping at the mall, cleaning the house, going on field trips with the children — all the regular things they haven't been able to do. They also may want to get back to the treadmill or exercise class they loved. And sometimes exercise *does* feel good — for about 24 to 48 hours. You may not turn into a pumpkin at that time, but studies have shown that many CFS sufferers have a relapse within 24 to 48 hours after strenuous exercise. A study done in 2005 found that with a 28 percent increase in exercise over a four-week period, people with CFS had more intense muscle pain, more fatigue, and became moodier.

However, saying that people with CFS can't benefit from exercise is just as big a myth. In reality, a monitored, structured exercise plan can help prevent deconditioning and tone and strengthen your muscles. See Chapter 10 for more on exercising and CFS.

CFS Is a Rare Disease

According to the CDC, CFS affects over 1 million Americans. And this statistic doesn't include those people who don't report their symptoms and try to push past them on their own. This number alone makes CFS one of the most common chronic conditions around.

Chapter 20

Ten Things to Avoid if You Have CFS

- -

In This Chapter

▶ Discovering how much exercise you really need

▶ Recognizing when you're overdoing it

▶ Figuring out how to balance your activities

- -

*J*ust because you have CFS doesn't mean that life has to stop. You can still do certain things — but some things you can't. Of course, if you're in the throes of a severe case of CFS, you aren't going to be up to doing much beyond taking your medication, staying calm, and getting the support and help you need, most likely from your bedside.

But when you do get a break (and I hope that it just gets better and better for you!), you should avoid doing some things at all costs. Otherwise, you may find yourself back in bed, your symptoms more severe.

In this chapter, I point out ten activities you should stay away from for your own good.

Exercising Beyond Your Capacity

There you are, riding a stationary bike in the gym, your MP3 player blasting in your ear. You're feeling good! The last thing on your mind is your CFS. In fact, you're feeling so good that you figure you've gotten past the problem. You're free from your illness. How exhilarating! You can go another 15 minutes, easy. Maybe put the treadmill in "Hill Mode." Why not? And after that, maybe you can pump some iron; 8 pounds or 10 pounds will do just fine.

And then, the next morning, it suddenly hits. You're in the supermarket reaching for a jar, and you can barely move your arm or walk. Your head's on the shopping cart handlebars. It takes all your energy to call a friend and tell her to pick you up — fast! The clerk stocking the shelves has already called 911. What did you do?

Exercising more than your capacity is dangerous. You'll feel like a ton of bricks hit you — and you'll have reversed all the good you've done. Your CFS symptoms will be back with a vengeance. I know that when you're feeling good you may find it very tempting to keep going. Who doesn't want a great workout? But beware and remember that you have CFS, a chronic condition. You shouldn't push yourself. Know your limits and stick to them. (For more exercising advice, see Chapter 10.)

Hanging Around "Negative Nancies"

Sometimes when you're depressed, hanging out with other folks who are also depressed may feel comfortable. It makes sense — who wants to hang out with perky, happy friends when you feel so awful?

But resist the temptation to be negative. Remember, negativity is catching. Hanging around with Negative Nancies, or people who always seem to look at things in a negative way, can make you feel worse — *more* depressed, *more* hopeless, *more* helpless.

 Similarly, positivity is catching, too! If you spend time with your good friends, the ones who encourage you, who try to make you laugh, who show you love and compassion, you can do yourself a world of good. You can feel better about your illness, and, as studies show, that positive thinking can have a positive affect on your immune system and your health.

Heaping on Huge Meal Portions

A long time ago, I saw a television ad about a guy who couldn't sleep. He sat, like a sad sack, on the edge of his bed, crying, "I can't believe I ate the whole thing." Most people have been there: Eating too much of that delicious birthday cake. Heaping your dish at the all-you-can-eat buffet. Mindlessly going through a bag of chips or a pint of ice cream while watching TV. And you can probably remember how that feels: delicious while your eating, but *bad* right afterwards!

If a healthy person gets indigestion, feels bloated and gassy, or feels nause-ated from overeating, he can pop an antacid and call it a day. But if you have CFS, that indigestion, that acid, and that nausea can make you even more fatigued, more depressed, and more sick. Avoid huge meals, you can to help avoid an energy drain and an increase in other symptoms. You'll feel better. An added plus: The number on your bathroom scale may also drop. (For more on sensible eating, head to Chapter 11.)

Partying Past Your Bedtime

The worst thing a person can do if she has CFS is to stay up past her bedtime. Routine is crucial for someone with CFS and regular sleeping hours are an important part of the treatment process. Blow off that routine, and your fatigue can come back to haunt you — as will the aches, pains, and low energy.

If you're having a great time at a party, that's wonderful! It means you feel well enough to go out. But, like Cinderella, you don't want to get caught at the ball past midnight. It's all about conserving energy and staying within your limits.

Medicating Yourself with Alcohol and Drugs

Too many people attempt to drown their sadness with booze and drugs — a downfall of many famous people, and infamous ones, too. But that vodka on the rocks can interfere with the good work your medication is doing. Studies show that alcohol can negate the benefits of antidepressants, for example. And who knows how a pill or some weed can affect the other medication you're on? Don't do it — as tempting as it may seem. When the effect has worn off and you're left with a horrible hangover, you'll be a lot worse off than before. I don't mean to sound trite, but, "Just say no!"

Volunteering for Overtime

You're back on the job, feeling great. You were out for two weeks with severe CFS symptoms, but you're fortunate to have such an understanding boss. And you're going through the pile of mail on your desk with zeal. In fact, wouldn't it be a great idea to impress the boss by volunteering to stay late and get that Jones report done? He'll see how dedicated you are. And, more importantly, he'll see how healthy you are now.

Don't do it. Avoid the temptation to push yourself at work. You have a chronic condition — I can't say this enough. Just like a diabetic needs to avoid that piece of cake, you need to avoid overdoing it. You're feeling better — great! You have a good boss — great! But don't rock the boat.

Signing Up for a Split Shift

Splitting your workload with someone else may sound like a good idea in theory, giving you more free time and making your job less taxing. It sounds like the perfect solution for your CFS symptoms. Wrong! If you do a split shift, you are locked in to those hours, no matter what. What if you wake up one morning when you're due at the office and feel horrible? Too bad. You can ask your "split shifter" to make up the time, and the first two or three times, I'm sure she may be glad to help. But by the seventh or eighth time? I don't think so. You'll find out your life has just become more complicated — instead of easier.

The best work situation for someone with CFS is flexibility. You need to be flexible so that if a CFS episode strikes, you can take the time off and not inconvenience the world.

Overtaxing Your Brain

Doing a crossword puzzle is a great way to keep the brain sharp. So are word scrambles and Sudoku. Sounds like fun! It is — and keeping yourself open to new ideas, to learn and stay smart, is important. But with CFS, some people have problems concentrating or remembering simple things (like finding words or adding simple numbers), so these types of brain exercises may not be doable – and may highlight a person's disability, making them feel helpless and stupid. Even if you can participate in these activities, you have an added element: Too much of a good thing is, well, too much. If you have "brain strain" or feel burned out, overtaxing your mind, just like overtaxing your body, just fuels your feeling of fatigue and depletes your energy. So be sure to pace yourself when you're doing your brain exercises.

Picking Fights with Loved Ones

It's true. People fight with those they love. One reason for this is that you feel safe with someone you love — and you can take out your frustrations, anger, and fear on him. You can't do that with your boss — you'll just get fired. You can't unleash your emotions on a friend — you can lose the friendship. But your spouse? Your parent? They are with you for the long haul; they are there for you in times of stress.

However, fighting is going to bring on *more* stress, whether it be with someone you love or even someone you hate. Remember how you feel when you get angry? That extra adrenaline pumping, the heart racing? These physiological reactions are probably not good for your CFS. You must also consider the underlying hurt you may be causing. There you are, yelling at the top of your lungs, with your mom looking like you just hit her. You don't want to hurt the ones you love; they're the ones who care the most. And even loved ones have a limit. Too many arguments and your loved one may just go through that door marked "Exit." (For more on maintaining relationships when you have CFS, you can check out Chapter 13.)

Under- or Overestimating Your Abilities

Which is worse — doing too much or doing too little? That question is a hard one for someone with CFS. Both can be detrimental to your CFS. But when do you know when you're underestimating your abilities, or when you're over the top?

Volunteering to do something is a kind gesture — a way to learn, socialize, help someone, or stay in good graces with the outside world. But if you volunteer to do the books and you failed math in college, you aren't going to do anyone any favors! You won't be able to do it, and stress, that archenemy of CFS, will rear its ugly head.

On the other hand, if you can do complicated equations in your head and you *don't* volunteer to do the books, you're shortchanging yourself and may become bored with your lack of activity.

So how do you know when you're doing too much or not enough? Sometimes it takes a little trial and error. The best way to judge what you can and can't do is to be realistic about your skills and talents, and, as the Greeks said a gazillion years ago, "Moderation in all things." Follow that motto and you can't go wrong.

Chapter 21

Ten Strategies to Enhance Your Life

. . . .

In This Chapter

▶ Learning how to ask for help — and when

▶ Getting rid of stress and discovering the joy of being pampered

▶ Figuring out a newer, better daily routine

. . . .

*W*hen you have CFS, your quality of life may take a nose dive. The exhaustion you feel is often compounded by the fact that you may be keeping your condition secret from the very people who can help make things better. By disclosing your condition to trusted confidants, you can often reduce the burden of keeping a secret and may discover that you have a strong support network willing to lend a hand.

You can also employ several strategies to make your daily life less complicated. I've gone over some of these important life changes throughout the book, particularly in Part III, illuminating them as treatment "prescriptions" to make you feel better. In this chapter, you get a fast refresher course in quality of life with ten savvy tips to help you pull out of a (very exhausting) tailspin. Refer to this chapter often for a quick reminder of how to help your life stay on track.

Coming Clean about Your Condition

Honesty is the best policy — or so they say. But the truth is that sometimes honesty can push an issue a little too far. Some people won't care that you have CFS, some may dismiss it as something that's all in your head, and some people may even hold it against you, as though you've done something to deserve it or you're using it as an excuse to be lazy.

The truth can set you free only if the people who hear it are sensitive to your situation and are willing to offer understanding and guidance. So, depending on the situation and the people involved, you basically have three options:

✔ Keep mum.

✔ Provide details only on an as-needed basis.

✔ Come clean with a full disclosure.

The following suggestions offer guidance on just how honest to be:

✔ If your CFS is affecting your work, you need to speak either to your superior or the head of human resources so that colleagues don't think you're slacking on the job. In addition, if you require any workplace modifications, you must provide them in writing, before your employer is legally obligated to provide those modifications.

✔ If you work in a virtual office, or if you can work at home some days, hiding your symptoms is much easier. In this case, as long as you can keep up with the work, you really can't find a good reason why anyone associated with your job has to know your personal business.

✔ If you're on a business trip and you've just finished an exhaustive presentation, you can tell your co-workers that you're too tired to go out to dinner. They don't have to know the specifics.

✔ Your friends and loved ones are a whole other matter. They are there for you; they can provide the support you need to get through the day. By all means, come clean to the people you love. To quote a cliché — that's what friends are for.

✔ Your doctor is your confessor. You must tell him how you're feeling, what your symptoms are, and whether they're getting worse or better. He can only help you if you're honest. And, if he is skeptical of your condition, then consider it time to seek out a new doc.

Outsourcing Exhausting Tasks

If you were a do-it-all before CFS, CFS can change all that in a hurry. Perhaps you were supermom before symptoms set in. You worked at least part time during the day, picked up your kids after work, cooked dinner, cleaned the house, tucked in the kiddies, and spent some time with your husband so that he knows he's important in your busy world. When CFS strikes, you may have to offload some of that work.

A lot of people are reluctant to ask others for help. First of all, they feel embarrassed that they can't do it themselves. Forget it — the smartest and most successful folks today have figured out how to delegate.

Friends and family are the first resources to check for affordable (free) help. When CFS saps your strength, rally the troops and let them know that the time has come for them to help you. Delegate the cooking, cleaning, and other chores that you find most exhausting. In most cases, friends and family members really want to help, but they don't know exactly what to do. Tell them what you need done.

If assistance from family and friends isn't forthcoming, consider hiring professional help such as housekeepers, personal shoppers, babysitters, and meal-delivery services that can to make your life easier, especially when CFS steals your strength. These specialists can often do the job better and more efficiently than you — especially when you're sick. If you can afford to hire some help, especially to take care of the daily chores so you can function better at work, consider hiring a professional.

If the cost of professional help is an obstacle, reconsider. You may be surprised at how inexpensive it can be. In many cases, you can have a cleaning service come in once a month to give your home or apartment a thorough cleaning for almost the same price as the cost of monthly cleaning supplies. From online grocery stores, such as Peapod (www.peapod.com), to music and movie downloads, the world can literally be at your fingertips.

If hiring help is unquestionably not affordable, as is the case with a great many people with CFS, consider contacting local support and social service agencies to inquire what type of help is available free of charge or for a small fee. These agencies include the United Way, churches, and government agencies, such as the Department of Health and Human Services.

Check with your health insurance company — many companies pay for allied health care, day nurses, and physical therapists, all of whom can assist you in getting through the day. However, don't be greedy! Some individuals easily lose sight of realistic expectations placed on other people when the whole world has become centered around their illness, so keep in mind those things that you can do for yourself and what things that require help you can reasonably expect from others. Remember to keep expectations of others (*and* yourself) both reasonable and realistic Also, be aware and take care not to outsource *everything* — it makes people feel replaceable, including you!

Identifying and Removing the Worst Stressors

De-stressing your life sounds easier than it really is. Maybe one of your biggest stressors is the evening news. You don't even think about it (it's just the news!), but the pervasive global trouble could be creating havoc in your head. Or maybe one of the stressors is too easy to identify — perhaps that child of yours who needs *a long time-out*. But the basic rule is this: You can't get rid of stress — it's a fact of life. But you can acquire skills to cope with it more effectively.

Here are some tips to get you thinking in the right (unstressed) direction:

- **Think aummmm (Om. . .).** Meditation is a great way to dissolve the pressures of the day. Plenty of CDs and DVDs can put you on the right path — from proper sitting to keeping your mind focused.

- **Ignorance is bliss.** No one wants to be ignorant, and everyone needs to know what's going on in the world. But sometimes choosing to not read the paper, listen to the news, or debate world affairs is okay. Besides, do news stories really change all that much from one day to the next?

  Some people recommend that the first hour of each day should start out without these external traumatizing stressors — no TV news, no newspaper, no radio news. There's plenty of time to inundate yourself with the negatives of the world — and you don't want to set the tone of your whole day on "down." Fill that first hour with something uplifting and positive, such as listening to music, meditating, eating breakfast, or reading a good book.

- **Go caffeine free.** Remembering not to drink coffee or tea is easy, but what about diet sodas, iced teas, or even juice drinks? Check the labels of your afternoon beverages and make sure *decaffeinated* is the word of the day, especially around bedtime.

- **Outsource! Outsource! Outsource!** As I say in a previous section, having help isn't being lazy, and it doesn't have to be expensive. In fact, getting someone to assist you with your rambunctious child is smart — it may even add more *quality* to your quality time together. Just be careful not to outsource too much!

Reducing the Clutter in Your Life

A messy home supposedly reflects a messy mind. As someone who finds that clutter magically appears all the time, I'd have to refute that. But I do know that when I put things away, organize my closets, and throw things out that I haven't looked at in three months or sell them on eBay, I feel much better. I feel peaceful.

If you have CFS, that sense of peace is critical for your health and to help alleviate symptoms. Dust and dirt can also aggravate any allergies, adding that to your problems. Use the one-year axiom: If you haven't used it, worn it, or noticed it for a whole year, out it goes.

Restructuring Your Day

Here's a fact of life: If you have CFS, you have to change your routine. You can't do as much as you did before, and trying harder only makes you feel worse.

The best way to restructure your life is with a pad and pencil. Write out your typical day, using an hourly measure. Then see where you can cut back. Maybe you can sleep or rest an extra hour. Maybe someone else can pick up the kids from school. Maybe you can bring lunch to work so you don't have to go out and deal with crowds and lines.

Budget your time as carefully as you budget your household expenses. Jot down a complete list of your time expenditures, and you can immediately begin to notice the biggest time wasters.

Training Yourself to Say No

Saying no has a lot in common with outsourcing (see the section "Outsourcing Exhausting Tasks"). Essentially, when you say no, you're making someone else do a task, because eventually everything needs to get done. By saying no, you're simply saying that you're not going to be the one doing what needs to be done. Don't worry. It'll get done. If you don't do it, someone else will, particularly if you can successfully delegate the duty.

Try saying no to yourself. It's easy. One syllable. The next time someone asks you to do something, even if the request is hedged in a compliment (such as "You're the perfect person to organize the neighborhood block party!"), just say no. After you do it once, you begin to feel liberated. The world didn't end, and no one stopped talking to you. And, if need be, remember that saying no may even help ease your CFS symptoms. That alone is motivation.

Pampering Yourself: You Deserve It!

Many people haven't learned the "art of me"; they put everyone — from spouses to kids to friends to the family pet — ahead of themselves. But until you take care of yourself, you can't have the energy to take care of anyone else, which is especially true with CFS. Energy is at a premium, and the more self-care you do, the better you feel. Following are some suggestions for taking a little time for yourself:

✔ Try a relaxing bath, using lavender essential oils. The lavender helps relax you, the oil helps smooth your skin, and the bath itself eases some of your pain. If you're sensitive to strong scents, you may want to go with a milder scent, such as vanilla. You may even want to choose a gentle baby oil or unscented bubble bath.

✔ Even if your symptoms are too intense for you to go to the mall and buy something for yourself, you can always shop the Web. Check out the department stores online, eBay, and Overstock.com, and, of course, the old standby, Amazon.com. Even if you end up not buying anything, you can easily have a few hours of enjoyable distraction.

✔ Treat yourself to a treat. Watching your diet is vital for a healthy lifestyle, and sound nutrition is one of the ways to help relieve CFS symptoms, but a once-in-a-while treat isn't going to move you backward. If anything, that hot fudge sundae, chocolate-chip cookie, or fresh-baked croissant will make you smile.

Regulating Your Social Time

If you've ever needed support, now is the time. Make a list of your friends and loved ones and contact them. A great way to get the help and support you need without feeling guilty that you're a burden is to schedule time with your friends and family — specify who's going to see you on what day and at what time.

A schedule ensures that people aren't showing up at all hours, that you're not having to entertain crowds of visitors, and that you have a steady flow of helpers who can share the workload.

Finding More Rewarding Work

In Chapter 12, I reveal tips and techniques to deal effectively with work issues related to CFS, but if your employer refuses to make the workplace modifications you need, and you decide not to take legal action, or you simply decide that you want to try your hand at a different line of work, you may be in the market for a new job.

When looking for a new job, avoid the natural impulse to snap up the first job that comes your way. Look for an employer that offers a CFS-friendly environment with the following criteria:

✔ **Low-stress setting.** A pressure-filled environment isn't the most conducive for those with CFS to remain productive.

✔ **Less physically demanding work.** When even some moderate exercise leaves you exhausted for several hours or days, a physically intensive job will quickly use up your precious energy.

✔ **Less mentally demanding work.** Most people want their jobs to be somewhat challenging, but if you have CFS, an intense mental workout can be just as exhausting as physical labor.

✔ **Flexible work hours.** With CFS, you may have good days and bad days. If your employer understands this, she may be willing to allow you to flex your schedule, so you can put in more time on the good days and less time on the bad days. Flexible work hours also enable you to keep doctor appointments during the day. Many companies offer virtual offices, where you can work from your house by telecommuting by phone and e-mail.

Letting Go of the Little Stuff

There's an old story about a dad driving in traffic, his heart racing because his son, sitting in the passenger seat, is late for school, and he has a meeting at the office. He's pounding the steering wheel, swearing under his breath, and checking his cell phone. His son taps him on the shoulder and says, "Relax, Dad. It's not worth it." Out of the mouth of babes!

But his advice is true. Traffic is nothing, especially when it comes to health. Stop fussing about your hair or your deadlines or why you weren't invited to a party. Life is too short. Besides, worrying about the little stuff is the antithesis of pampering yourself. Few things in life are more exhausting than rage. Yes, you have CFS, but you don't have to let it ruin your life!

Appendix

CFS Reference and Support Sources

∙ ∙

*O*f course this book is comprehensive and authoritative, but it can't possibly cover information that wasn't available at the time it was written, and it can't provide you with the immediate support and understanding of a compassionate human being. Nor can this book hold every single fact on CFS — it would have to be thousands of pages! So, in this appendix, I point you to the sources of information and support where you can find more research on CFS. Think of this book as CFS 101, and these sources as extra credit.

Top Five Recommended CFS Web Sites

These sites can give you the most comprehensive and up-to-date information *specifically* on CFS — including facts, statistics, clinical trials, newest research, and links to other helpful sites.

Centers for Disease Control and Prevention Online: www.cdc.gov/cfs

Consider the Centers for Disease Control and Prevention (CDC) as the command center. This government Web site has the most facts and figures on just about every disorder — it also points you in the direction of other research, organizations, and studies. You can find everything from PDF brochures to download (for both patients and health care professionals) to the newest clinical trial information (most of which involves only CDC research), from pertinent facts about CFS to details on a national campaign from the CDC, the Department of Health and Human Services (HHS), and the CFIDS Association of America to build public awareness of this debilitating illness.

If you have access to a computer, checking out the CDC's Web site is your best option (available both in English and in Spanish), but if you don't have a computer, you can also request information on CFS by contacting the following: Centers for Disease Control and Prevention, Public Inquiries/MASO, Mailstop E11, 1600 Clifton Road, Atlanta, GA 30333; phone 800-311-3435.

CFIDS Association of America: www.cfids.org

Think of the Chronic Fatigue and Immune Dysfunction Syndrome (CFIDS) Association of America as home. This entire organization is dedicated to CFS, from building public awareness to helping you determine whether you have CFS and making available books and brochures on the subject.

Some of the pertinent information you can find on the CFIDS Web site includes the following:

- Community resources and links for help in your area
- Guidance on starting and joining a support group in your community
- Information on children with CFS
- Tips on finding assistance for your caregivers so they can better help you
- The CFIDS periodical, *The CFIDS Chronicle,* both past and current issues, for subjects of particular interest to you
- A step-by-step online questionnaire to help you figure out whether you have CFS
- Information on participating in grassroots advocacy efforts to support CFS research and federal government attention to the illness

You can even subscribe to the CFIDS*Link,* a free e-newsletter with the latest news that comes directly to your e-mail address by clicking on the E-NEWSLETTER tab at the top of the home page and following the instructions.

You can also direct any inquiries you may have regarding CFS or this organization to: The CFIDS Association of America, P.O. Box 220398, Charlotte, NC 28222-0398; phone 704-365-2343, fax 704-365-9755.

International Association for Chronic Fatigue Syndrome: www.iacfs.net

The International Association for Chronic Fatigue Syndrome (IACFS) is geared toward health care professionals and research scientists. Originally the American Association for Chronic Fatigue Syndrome, the organization now has clinicians, researchers, and board members in Japan, Sweden, and Belgium. This nonprofit organization consists of scientists, physicians, and other health care professionals, as well as individuals and institutions interested in CFS. Its goal is to promote and coordinate research, patient care, and treatment modalities for both CFS and fibromyalgia.

In addition to both international and national conferences held every two years, IACFS also publishes an online newsletter. Although created for the professional, IACFS is now branching out to patients and patient support groups. You can find the latest clinical studies on its Web site, as well as material on myths and more.

If you can't find the answers to your questions on the IACFS Web site, you can send an e-mail to Admin@iacfs.net to contact the organization directly. To reach the IACFS without the use of a computer, use the following: The International Association for Chronic Fatigue Syndrome, 27 N. Wacker Drive Suite 416, Chicago, IL 60606; phone 847-258-7248, fax 847-579-0975.

Medline Plus: medlineplus.gov

Medline Plus is the place to go if you want information about medical research right at your fingertips (and the site is available in both English and Spanish). The brainchild of both the National Institutes of Health and the United States National Library of Medicine, this site offers health information on over 700 conditions, including CFS (of course!). You can also find articles and journals, as well as information on current clinical trials. You can also check out the following resources:

- A medical dictionary for correct terminology and spelling
- A reference tool on drugs and supplements
- A medical encyclopedia complete with diagrams and illustrations
- Current medical news

If you don't have access to a computer, you can reach Medline Plus via the following: The National Library of Medicine, Medline Plus, 8600 Rockville Pike, Bethesda, MD 20894; phone 888-346-3656 or 301-594-5983.

Sleepless in America: sleeplessinamerica.org

Designed to be user-friendly, Sleepless in America's Web site offers a Sleep Kit, a valuable tool that includes a sleep diary and a sleeplessness scale. Created by the Depression and Bipolar Support Alliance (DBSA), the site also gives answers to questions such as:

- ✔ What's keeping you up at night?
- ✔ Why is sleep so important?
- ✔ Are you moody and irritable?

Although not related to CFS per se, the site does address one of its most common symptoms: fatigue. The site is available in Spanish and English.

To contact Sleepless in America via conventional methods, you can use the following contact info: Depression and Bipolar Support Alliance (DBSA), 730 N. Franklin Street, Suite 501, Chicago, IL 60610-7224; phone 800-826-3632, fax 312-642-7243.

More CFS Help and Information

In addition to the top five Web sites from the preceding section, many other Web sites and organizations can help you figure out more about CFS. To help you navigate away from the quacks and false claims to the truly helpful sites and organizations, I have included a brief list of reputable resources.

Many of the Web sites I list, including the five above, have links to other Web sites — which makes surfing the Web a breeze. All you need is a computer, a mouse, and access to the Internet. (But just in case you don't have access to the computer, I also supply you with an address and phone number when I can, so that you aren't left in the dark.)

Many of the sites that I list in the following section are general medical sites or sites that deal specifically with a symptoms or condition related to CFS. To find information specifically about CFS or a specific symptom, simply type *CFS* or the type of symptom you want to know more about into the site's Search box and click Go. (**Note:** Because some sites deal only with related conditions or symptoms, such as the International Foundation for Functional Gastrointestinal Disorders, these sites may not have information that is geared specifically to patients with CFS. However, you can still find helpful information on the symptom or condition itself.)

CFS and related conditions and symptoms

Agency for Healthcare Research and Quality Office of Communications and Knowledge Transfer
540 Gaither Road, Suite 2000
Rockville, MD 20850
Phone 301-427-1364
Web site www.ahrq.gov

American Academy of Family Physicians
P.O. Box 11210
Shawnee Mission, KS 66207-1210
Phone 800-274-2237
Web site www.aafp.org

American Academy of Sleep Medicine
One Westbrook Corporate Center, Suite 920
Westchester, IL 60154
Phone 708-492-0930
Web site www.aasmnet.org

American College of Rheumatology
1800 Century Place, Suite 250
Atlanta, GA 30345-4300
Phone 404-633-3777
Web site www.rheumatology.org

Arthritis Foundation
P.O. Box 7669
Atlanta, GA 30357-0669
Phone 800-568-4045 or 404-872-7100
Web site www.arthritis.org

U.S. Department of Health and Human Services (DHHS) National Women's Health Information Center
8270 Willow Oaks Corporate Drive
Fairfax, VA 22031
Phone 800-994-9662, 888-220-5446 (TDD), or 202-690-7650
Web site www.womenshealth.gov

eMedicine Health (a division of WebMD)
Web site
www.emedicinehealth.com
Note: Address and phone number not available.

International Foundation for Functional Gastrointestinal Disorders
P.O. Box 170864
Milwaukee, WI 53217-8076
Phone 888-964-2001 or 414-964-1799
Fax 414-964-7176
Web site www.iffgd.org

The Mayo Clinic
Web site www.mayoclinic.com
Note: Address and phone number not available.

National Fibromyalgia Association
2200 N. Glassell St., Suite A
Orange, CA 92865
Phone 714-921-0150
Web site www.fmaware.org

National Digestive Diseases Information Clearinghouse
2 Information Way
Bethesda, MD 20892-3570
Phone 800-891-5389
Fax 703-738-4929
Web site
www.digestive.niddk.nih.gov/ddiseases/pubs/ibs

National Institute of Health National Center on Sleep Disorders Research
P.O. Box 30105
Bethesda, MD 20824-0105
Phone 301-592-8573
Fax 240-629-3246
Web site
www.nhlbi.nih.gov/about/ncsdr

Pro Health Immune Support
Phone 800-366-6056 or 805-564-3064
Web site www.immunesupport.com
Note: Address not available.

U.S. Department of Health and Human Services (DHHS) Chronic Fatigue Syndrome Advisory Committee (CFSAC)
200 Independence Avenue, S.W.
Washington, DC 20201
Phone 202-690-7694
Web site www.hhs.gov/advcomcfs

CFS in children and adolescents

National Dissemination Center for Children with Disabilities (NICHCY)
P.O. Box 1492
Washington, DC 20013
Phone 800-695-0285 or 202-884-8200
Fax 202-884-8441
Web site www.nichcy.org

The Pediatric Network
Web site www.pediatricnetwork.org

Note: Address and phone number not available.

Caregivers

Family Caregiver Alliance
180 Montgomery Street, Suite 1100
San Francisco, CA 94104
Phone 800-445-8106 or 415-434-3388
Web site www.caregiver.org

Medline Plus: Caregivers
Web site www.nlm.nih.gov/medlineplus/caregivers.html

Note: See previous section on Medline Plus for more contact info.

National Organization for Empowering Caregivers
425 West 23rd Street, Suite 9B
New York, NY 10011
Phone 212-807-1204
Fax 212-645-5143
Web site www.nofec.org

National Family Caregivers Association
10400 Connecticut Avenue, Suite 500
Kensington, MD 20895-3944
Phone 800-896-3650 or 301-942-6430
Fax 301-942-2302
Web site www.nfcacares.org

Disability benefits and queries

Job Accommodation Network
P.O. Box 6080
Morgantown, WV 26506-6080
Phone 800-526-7234 or 304-293-7186
Web site
www.jan.wvu.edu/media/cfs.
html

**National Organization of Social
Security Claimants' Representatives**
560 Sylvan Ave.
Englewood Cliffs, NJ 07632
Phone 800-431-2804
Web site www.nosscr.org
Note: This site is for lawyer referrals.

Social Security Administration
Office of Public Inquiries
Windsor Park Building
6401 Security Blvd.
Baltimore, MD 21235
Phone 800-772-1213 or your local
listing
Web site www.ssa.gov

Note: This site is listed so you can
figure out whether you're qualified to
receive any benefits because of your
condition.

U.S. Department of Labor
Frances Perkins Building
200 Constitution Ave., NW
Washington, DC 20210
Phone 866-487-2365
Web site www.dol.gov
Note: This site is listed so you can
see whether you qualify for
Workmen's Compensation.

Glossary

*I*t's expected that when investigating all you can about CFS, or any illness, you encounter a lot of words that probably aren't familiar to you, or that are familiar but you aren't quite sure of the precise definition. Here is a list of words that you're most likely to encounter. For any words that aren't included here, don't be afraid to ask your doctor for clarification. The more you know, the better you'll be able to get a handle on CFS.

acute: When symptoms appear quickly, and usually disappear quickly, too.

Addison's disease: A hormonal dysfunctional disease in which the adrenal glands aren't producing enough adrenal hormones, particularly cortisol.

allostatic load: The physical damage done by chronic stress, referring to the strain put on various organs like the adrenals and the autonomic nervous system.

analgesic: A type of over-the-counter medicine that combats pain.

anaphylactic shock: An acute (sometimes fatal) allergic reaction in which a person is unable to breathe and has a drop in blood pressure. An injection of epinephrine must be given immediately.

anemia: The most common blood disorder that results in fatigue and weakness and can usually be easily treated with supplements.

antidepressants: Medications used to treat depression by controlling the amount of chemicals in the brain that have been linked to the illness. These chemicals include serotonin and norepinephrine.

arthralgia: Pain in the joints.

autoimmune: Pertaining to one's own immune system. Used in *autoimmune disease,* meaning a disease in which your immune system gets confused and begins to attack itself, such as in AIDS.

autonomic nervous system: The more instinctive part of a person's nervous system that regulates temperature, as well as the heart, breathing, and even saliva amount.

axillary lymph nodes: These lymph nodes are located in the armpit and drain lymph channels from the breast.

CAT scan: CAT stands for *computed axial tomography,* an imaging device that provides a more detailed picture of the body than a regular X-ray. The machine itself looks like a huge doughnut.

cataplexy: A condition caused by narcolepsy in which a person's muscles, including facial muscles, become very week.

cerebrospinal fluid: A clear liquid found in the central nervous system, including the spinal cord and the brain (in which the fluid fills the cavities and protects them).

cervical lymph nodes: Lymph nodes located in the neck.

CFS Computational Challenge: Also called the C3; an intense comprehensive collaboration of 14 different studies lead by clinicians in several areas of medicine and biological sciences to help determine the factors that create or lead to chronic fatigue syndrome.

chemical sensitivity disorder: A syndrome in which a person becomes allergic to chemicals or airborne particles, resulting in CFS-like symptoms such as headaches and flu-like symptoms. Some people feel this disorder may be a cause of CFS, too.

chronic: A condition that is on-going or prolonged.

chronic fatigue syndrome (CFS): A syndrome affecting the central nervous system, immune, and many other systems and organs, resulting in chronic exhaustion and/or numerous other potentially debilitating symptoms.

cluster investigation: A research team pulls together to determine what causes an outbreak of a disease in a certain location and time period.

cognitive: An adjective used in describing mental functioning in the brain, such as thinking, organizing, and problem solving. It is the name of a type of short-term psychotherapy that has been found to work for people with CFS.

collagen: The tough protein that shapes your tendons and connective tissues. When the immune system becomes dysfunctional, these structures break down, creating collagen vascular disease.

comorbid: A situation when two medical conditions are present at the same time.

complementary medicine: Another term for alternative medicine, emphasizing its use alongside traditional medicine.

connective tissue: The tissue that connects and supports the body, such as tendons, cartilage, and ligaments.

control: A term used in clinical studies; it usually refers to a group of people without the condition being studied along side the group with the condition and the results can be compared.

corticotropin-releasing factor: A neuropeptide (a type of proteinlike molecule made in the brain) that plays an important role in how you deal with stress.

cortisol: A stress hormone produced in the adrenal glands.

cytokines: Proteins of the immune system that enable cells to communicate with each other.

cytomegalovirus (CMV): A type of human herpes virus (HHV-5) that can cause illness in people with immune disorder dysfunction.

enzymes: Proteins that act as catalysts to make chemical reactions in the body happen.

epidemiologists: Clinicians and researchers who study the incidence of disease in a particular population.

epidemiology: A type of medical study that looks at the prevalence and spread of an illness in a community.

Epstein-Barr virus (EBV): A virus that presents many of the same symptoms as CFS, so it is confused with it. But they are two separate entities.

fatigue: In CFS, fatigue is more than feeling sluggish after a bad night's sleep. Fatigue as a symptom is exhaustion not relieved by sleep and is present for six months or more.

fibromyalgia: A condition often confused with CFS, but very similar. The main difference is that the most crucial symptom with fibromyalgia is muscle aches and pains, and with CFS, the major symptom is fatigue. (For more info on fibromyalgia, check out *Fibromyalgia For Dummies* by Roland Staud, M.D., and Christine Adamec [Wiley].)

gallbladder: A ball-like organ near the liver that stores bile made by the liver and releases that bile to help the digestive system absorb fats.

HPA axis: The hypothalamus (in the brain), pituitary gland (pea-shaped gland below the hypothalamus), and adrenal gland (one on top of each kidney) "trilogy" that modulates reactions to stress and mood states, as well as controls such vital bodily functions as digestion and sexuality. They are part of the body's endocrine (hormone) system.

hypersomnia: Getting too much sleep, between 12 and 14 hours, (and in the case of CFS, still feeling tired).

interdisciplinary team: A group of health care professionals in different specialties who come together to research and diagnose and treat a condition.

interleukin: Important Immune system cells that perform many functions.

irritable bowel syndrome (IBS): A disorder of the gastrointestinal tract; symptoms include diarrhea or constipation, bloating, abdominal pain, and gas. Some people with CFS have developed this condition.

leukocytes: The white blood cells found in the blood that fight off disease.

Lupus: The clinical name is *systemic lupus erythematosus,* and this condition is an autoimmune disorder that is sometimes confused with CFS.

Lyme disease: A condition often confused with CFS; it is transmitted by a tick bite and can lead to fatigue, muscle aches, and memory problems. CFS can sometimes occur after a bout of Lyme disease.

lymph nodes: Organs of the immune system located throughout the body that filter and collect foreign invaders such as viruses. When inflammation invades the body, lymph nodes can become swollen and are responsible for activating cells to fight off the infection.

lymphocytes: Immune system Cells that enable the body to remember and recognize previous invading germs and viruses in case they come again. They serve as a major defense weapon in the immune system.

malaise: General physical discomfort.

mononucleosis: A condition also called the "kissing disease." Mononucleosis is linked to the Epstein-Barr virus and can be passed via kissing (saliva) as well as through mucus and sometimes tears. It has long been associated with CFS, but it doesn't have the same route. However, a long bout of mono may possibly cause CFS.

MRI: Magnetic Resonance Imaging (MRI) gives a 3-D picture of the brain by using magnetic particles and a computer screen.

myalgic encephalomyelitis: The term used for CFS in Great Britain and Canada.

narcolepsy: A neurological disorder in which a person has abnormal sleep-wake cycles. A person with narcolepsy sleeps in uncontrollable spurts throughout the day.

natural killer (NK) cells: These antibody cells are considered the first line of defense in fighting off foreign germs and viruses.

neurasthenia: Exhaustion usually accompanied with nervousness and weakness.

neuromyasthenia: Emotionally caused muscle weakness.

neuron: Also called a nerve cell. A neuron is the primary cell of the nervous system.

neuropeptide: Protein molecules found in the brain.

neurotransmitters: The chemicals that help transport messages from neuron to neuron in the brain.

orthostatic intolerance (OI): Two types of OI are associated with CFS, both of which can be diagnosed with a simple test: taking your blood pressure while lying down, and then taking it again while standing up. In people with CFS, the OI is delayed. It will be a few minutes before you feel faint or your heart begins to race. The two OIs are the following:

- ✔ **neurally mediated hypotension (NMH):** A sudden drop in blood pressure when you stand up. The drop usually causes an increase in CFS symptoms.

- ✔ **postural orthostatic tachycardia syndrome (POTS):** A sudden, rapid heart rate (read: pulse) within ten minutes of standing up. POTS is also called *chronic orthostatic intolerance,* or COI.

pacing and envelope theories: Pacing is An energy management strategy where a person paces his activity to avoid a crash via small chunks of activity and scheduled breaks. The envelope theory suggests that a person keep his available energy in an envelope as if it were a bank account. Too much energy used in one day means that person will have to put some energy back in the envelope the next day. The key is to find a balance, not overdrawing and not saving too much.

pathognomonic: Keeping within the pattern of a specific disease; having typical symptoms of the disease.

PET scan: PET stands for positron emission tomography. A PET scan takes imaging to an advanced level, in which cellular function can be seen in action.

phagocytes: Cells in the blood that literally chew up invaders.

postexertional malaise: The fatigue you experience *after* pushing yourself too much, either with physical or mental activity.

prostaglandin: A hormone-like substance that helps modulate muscle contraction, blood vessel constriction and dilation, blood pressure, and inflammation.

renal: Kidney-related.

rheumatologist: A doctor who specializes in treating rheumatoid arthritis, autoimmune deficiency diseases, fibromyalgia, and some CFS symptoms.

secondary condition: This condition (or conditions) is created by the primary condition. For example, depression can be the secondary result of having CFS, the primary condition.

sleep apnea: A condition in which breathing actually stops very briefly while sleeping. Often Accompanied by snoring.

SSRIs: Selective Serotonin Reuptake Inhibitors (SSRIs) are a class of antidepressants that make sure enough of the chemical serotonin is available in your brain; doctors have found a link between too little serotonin and depression.

subacute: A disease state between acute and chronic.

thrombocytopenia: A blood disorder that creates bruises.

tissue: A group or layer of similar cells that work together to perform one function.

tumor: An abnormal mass of tissue that can be either benign or cancerous.

Index

• B •

• E •

• Q •

• R •

BUSINESS, CAREERS & PERSONAL FINANCE

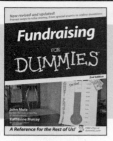

0-7645-9847-3

0-7645-2431-3

Also available:
- Business Plans Kit For Dummies
  0-7645-9794-9
- Economics For Dummies
  0-7645-5726-2
- Grant Writing For Dummies
  0-7645-8416-2
- Home Buying For Dummies
  0-7645-5331-3
- Managing For Dummies
  0-7645-1771-6
- Marketing For Dummies
  0-7645-5600-2
- Personal Finance For Dummies
  0-7645-2590-5*
- Resumes For Dummies
  0-7645-5471-9
- Selling For Dummies
  0-7645-5363-1
- Six Sigma For Dummies
  0-7645-6798-5
- Small Business Kit For Dummies
  0-7645-5984-2
- Starting an eBay Business For Dummies
  0-7645-6924-4
- Your Dream Career For Dummies
  0-7645-9795-7

HOME & BUSINESS COMPUTER BASICS

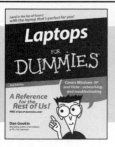

0-470-05432-8

0-471-75421-8

Also available:
- Cleaning Windows Vista For Dummies
  0-471-78293-9
- Excel 2007 For Dummies
  0-470-03737-7
- Mac OS X Tiger For Dummies
  0-7645-7675-5
- MacBook For Dummies
  0-470-04859-X
- Macs For Dummies
  0-470-04849-2
- Office 2007 For Dummies
  0-470-00923-3
- Outlook 2007 For Dummies
  0-470-03830-6
- PCs For Dummies
  0-7645-8958-X
- Salesforce.com For Dummies
  0-470-04893-X
- Upgrading & Fixing Laptops For Dummies
  0-7645-8959-8
- Word 2007 For Dummies
  0-470-03658-3
- Quicken 2007 For Dummies
  0-470-04600-7

FOOD, HOME, GARDEN, HOBBIES, MUSIC & PETS

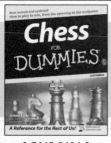

0-7645-8404-9

0-7645-9904-6

Also available:
- Candy Making For Dummies
  0-7645-9734-5
- Card Games For Dummies
  0-7645-9910-0
- Crocheting For Dummies
  0-7645-4151-X
- Dog Training For Dummies
  0-7645-8418-9
- Healthy Carb Cookbook For Dummies
  0-7645-8476-6
- Home Maintenance For Dummies
  0-7645-5215-5
- Horses For Dummies
  0-7645-9797-3
- Jewelry Making & Beading For Dummies
  0-7645-2571-9
- Orchids For Dummies
  0-7645-6759-4
- Puppies For Dummies
  0-7645-5255-4
- Rock Guitar For Dummies
  0-7645-5356-9
- Sewing For Dummies
  0-7645-6847-7
- Singing For Dummies
  0-7645-2475-5

INTERNET & DIGITAL MEDIA

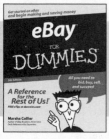
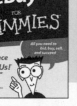
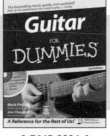

0-470-04529-9

0-470-04894-8

Also available:
- Blogging For Dummies
  0-471-77084-1
- Digital Photography For Dummies
  0-7645-9802-3
- Digital Photography All-in-One Desk Reference For Dummies
  0-470-03743-1
- Digital SLR Cameras and Photography For Dummies
  0-7645-9803-1
- eBay Business All-in-One Desk Reference For Dummies
  0-7645-8438-3
- HDTV For Dummies
  0-470-09673-X
- Home Entertainment PCs For Dummies
  0-470-05523-5
- MySpace For Dummies
  0-470-09529-6
- Search Engine Optimization For Dummies
  0-471-97998-8
- Skype For Dummies
  0-470-04891-3
- The Internet For Dummies
  0-7645-8996-2
- Wiring Your Digital Home For Dummies
  0-471-91830-X

* Separate Canadian edition also available
† Separate U.K. edition also available

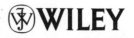

SPORTS, FITNESS, PARENTING, RELIGION & SPIRITUALITY

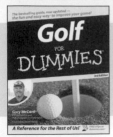

0-471-76871-5

0-7645-7841-3

Also available:
- Catholicism For Dummies
  0-7645-5391-7
- Exercise Balls For Dummies
  0-7645-5623-1
- Fitness For Dummies
  0-7645-7851-0
- Football For Dummies
  0-7645-3936-1
- Judaism For Dummies
  0-7645-5299-6
- Potty Training For Dummies
  0-7645-5417-4
- Buddhism For Dummies
  0-7645-5359-3

- Pregnancy For Dummies
  0-7645-4483-7 †
- Ten Minute Tone-Ups For Dummies
  0-7645-7207-5
- NASCAR For Dummies
  0-7645-7681-X
- Religion For Dummies
  0-7645-5264-3
- Soccer For Dummies
  0-7645-5229-5
- Women in the Bible For Dummies
  0-7645-8475-8

TRAVEL

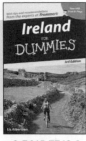
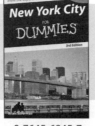

0-7645-7749-2

0-7645-6945-7

Also available:
- Alaska For Dummies
  0-7645-7746-8
- Cruise Vacations For Dummies
  0-7645-6941-4
- England For Dummies
  0-7645-4276-1
- Europe For Dummies
  0-7645-7529-5
- Germany For Dummies
  0-7645-7823-5
- Hawaii For Dummies
  0-7645-7402-7

- Italy For Dummies
  0-7645-7386-1
- Las Vegas For Dummies
  0-7645-7382-9
- London For Dummies
  0-7645-4277-X
- Paris For Dummies
  0-7645-7630-5
- RV Vacations For Dummies
  0-7645-4442-X
- Walt Disney World & Orlando
  For Dummies
  0-7645-9660-8

GRAPHICS, DESIGN & WEB DEVELOPMENT

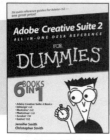
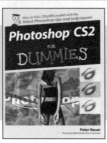

0-7645-8815-X

0-7645-9571-7

Also available:
- 3D Game Animation For Dummies
  0-7645-8789-7
- AutoCAD 2006 For Dummies
  0-7645-8925-3
- Building a Web Site For Dummies
  0-7645-7144-3
- Creating Web Pages For Dummies
  0-470-08030-2
- Creating Web Pages All-in-One Desk
  Reference For Dummies
  0-7645-4345-8
- Dreamweaver 8 For Dummies
  0-7645-9649-7

- InDesign CS2 For Dummies
  0-7645-9572-5
- Macromedia Flash 8 For Dummies
  0-7645-9691-8
- Photoshop CS2 and Digital
  Photography For Dummies
  0-7645-9580-6
- Photoshop Elements 4 For Dummies
  0-471-77483-9
- Syndicating Web Sites with RSS Feeds
  For Dummies
  0-7645-8848-6
- Yahoo! SiteBuilder For Dummies
  0-7645-9800-7

NETWORKING, SECURITY, PROGRAMMING & DATABASES

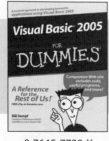
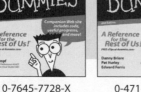

0-7645-7728-X

0-471-74940-0

Also available:
- Access 2007 For Dummies
  0-470-04612-0
- ASP.NET 2 For Dummies
  0-7645-7907-X
- C# 2005 For Dummies
  0-7645-9704-3
- Hacking For Dummies
  0-470-05235-X
- Hacking Wireless Networks
  For Dummies
  0-7645-9730-2
- Java For Dummies
  0-470-08716-1

- Microsoft SQL Server 2005 For Dummies
  0-7645-7755-7
- Networking All-in-One Desk Reference
  For Dummies
  0-7645-9939-9
- Preventing Identity Theft For Dummies
  0-7645-7336-5
- Telecom For Dummies
  0-471-77085-X
- Visual Studio 2005 All-in-One Desk
  Reference For Dummies
  0-7645-9775-2
- XML For Dummies
  0-7645-8845-1

HEALTH & SELF-HELP

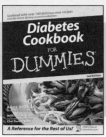

Diabetes Cookbook FOR DUMMIES
0-7645-8450-2

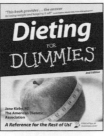

Dieting FOR DUMMIES
0-7645-4149-8

Also available:
- Bipolar Disorder For Dummies
  0-7645-8451-0
- Chemotherapy and Radiation For Dummies
  0-7645-7832-4
- Controlling Cholesterol For Dummies
  0-7645-5440-0
- Diabetes For Dummies
  0-7645-6820-5* †
- Divorce For Dummies
  0-7645-8417-0 †

- Fibromyalgia For Dummies
  0-7645-5441-7
- Low-Calorie Dieting For Dummies
  0-7645-9905-4
- Meditation For Dummies
  0-471-77774-9
- Osteoporosis For Dummies
  0-7645-7621-6
- Overcoming Anxiety For Dummies
  0-7645-5447-6
- Reiki For Dummies
  0-7645-9907-0
- Stress Management For Dummies
  0-7645-5144-2

EDUCATION, HISTORY, REFERENCE & TEST PREPARATION

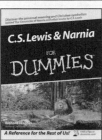

C.S. Lewis & Narnia FOR DUMMIES
0-7645-8381-6

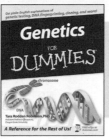

Genetics FOR DUMMIES
0-7645-9554-7

Also available:
- The ACT For Dummies
  0-7645-9652-7
- Algebra For Dummies
  0-7645-5325-9
- Algebra Workbook For Dummies
  0-7645-8467-7
- Astronomy For Dummies
  0-7645-8465-0
- Calculus For Dummies
  0-7645-2498-4
- Chemistry For Dummies
  0-7645-5430-1
- Forensics For Dummies
  0-7645-5580-4

- Freemasons For Dummies
  0-7645-9796-5
- French For Dummies
  0-7645-5193-0
- Geometry For Dummies
  0-7645-5324-0
- Organic Chemistry I For Dummies
  0-7645-6902-3
- The SAT I For Dummies
  0-7645-7193-1
- Spanish For Dummies
  0-7645-5194-9
- Statistics For Dummies
  0-7645-5423-9

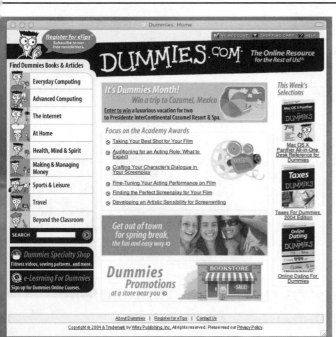

Get smart @ dummies.com®

- **Find a full list of Dummies titles**
- **Look into loads of FREE on-site articles**
- **Sign up for FREE eTips e-mailed to you weekly**
- **See what other products carry the Dummies name**
- **Shop directly from the Dummies bookstore**
- **Enter to win new prizes every month!**

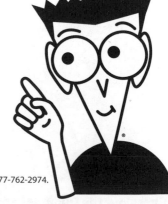

* **Separate Canadian edition also available**
† **Separate U.K. edition also available**

Available wherever books are sold. For more information or to order direct: U.S. customers visit www.dummies.com or call 1-877-762-2974.
U.K. customers visit www.wileyeurope.com or call 0800 243407. Canadian customers visit www.wiley.ca or call 1-800-567-4797.

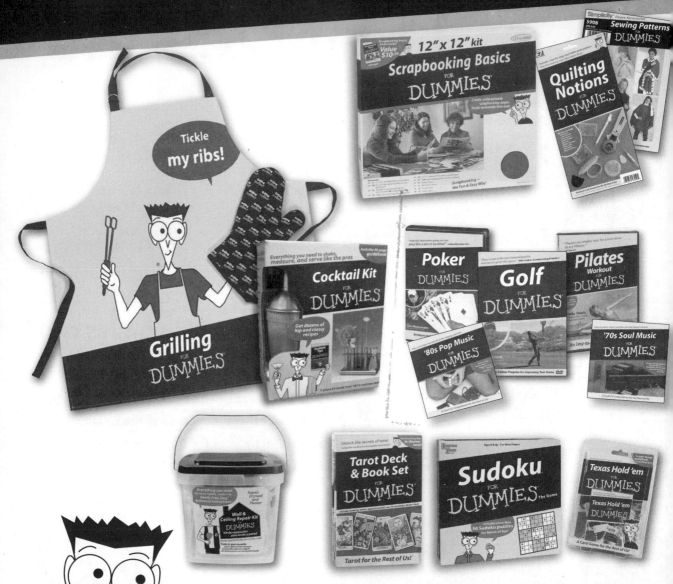
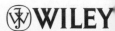